Image-Guided Neurosurgery

Clinical Applications of Surgical Navigation

Image-Guided Neurosurgery

Clinical Applications of Surgical Navigation

EDITED BY

Gene H. Barnett, M.D.

Vice Chairman, Department of Neurosurgery,
The Cleveland Clinic Foundation,
Cleveland, Ohio

David W. Roberts, M.D.

Professor of Surgery, Section of Neurosurgery,
Department of Surgery, Dartmouth Medical School,
Lebanon, New Hampshire

Robert J. Maciunas, M.D.

Professor of Neurological Surgery and Biomedical Engineering,
Department of Neurological Surgery, Vanderbilt University School of Medicine,
Nashville, Tennessee

QMP

Quality Medical Publishing, Inc.

ST. LOUIS, MISSOURI
1998

Printed in the United States of America.

This book presents current scientific information and opinion pertinent to medical professionals. It does not provide advice concerning specific diagnosis and treatment of individual cases and is not intended for use by the layperson. The authors, editors, and publisher will not be responsible or liable for actions taken as a result of the opinions expressed in this book.

PUBLISHER Karen Berger

EDITOR Beth Campbell

PROJECT MANAGER Katherine Spakowski

COPY EDITOR Carolita Deter

PRODUCTION Susan Trail and Judy Bamert

BOOK DESIGN Susan Trail

COVER DESIGN David Berger

Quality Medical Publishing, Inc.
11970 Borman Drive, Suite 222
St. Louis, Missouri 63146
Telephone: 1-800-348-7808
Web Site: http://qmp@qmp.com

LIBRARY OF CONGRESS CATALOGING-IN-PUBLICATION DATA

Image-guided neurosurgery : clinical applications of surgical navigation / edited by Gene H. Barnett, David W. Roberts, Robert J. Maciunas.
p. cm.
Includes bibliographical references and index.
ISBN 1-57626-083-6
1. Central nervous system—Surgery. 2. Central nervous system—Imaging. I. Barnett, Gene H. II. Roberts, David W., 1950- III. Maciunas, Robert J.
[DNLM: 1. Neurosurgical Procedures—methods. 2. Image Processing, Computer-Assisted. WL 368 I31 1998]
RD594.I43 1998
617.4'8—dc21
DNLM/DLC
for Library of Congress 98-13928
CIP

VT/WW/WW
5 4 3 2 1

To

My wife **Cathy**
and our children **Alex, Austin,** and **Addison**

– *G.H.B.* –

My wife **Kathryn**
and our children **Jane** and **Chris**

– *D.W.R.* –

My wife **Ann**
and our children **Nicholas** and **Joseph**

– *R.J.M.* –

Contributors

John R. Adler, Jr., M.D.
Associate Professor of Surgery, Department of Neurosurgery, Stanford University School of Medicine, Stanford, California

Eben Alexander III, M.D.
Associate Professor of Surgery and Assistant Professor of Radiation Oncology, Department of Neurosurgery, Harvard Medical School/Brigham & Women's Hospital, Boston, Massachusetts

Gene H. Barnett, M.D.
Vice Chairman, Department of Neurosurgery, The Cleveland Clinic Foundation, Cleveland, Ohio

William E. Bingaman, M.D.
Head, Section of Epilepsy Surgery, Department of Neurosurgery, The Cleveland Clinic Foundation, Cleveland, Ohio

Peter M. Black, M.D., Ph.D.
Franc D. Ingraham Professor of Neurosurgery and Neurosurgeon-in-Chief, Department of Neurosurgery, Harvard Medical School/Brigham & Women's Hospital/Children's Hospital, Boston, Massachusetts

Terrance M. Darcey, Ph.D.
Associate Professor of Medicine, Department of Neurology, Dartmouth-Hitchcock Medical Center, Lebanon, New Hampshire

Fernando Diaz, M.D., Ph.D.
Professor of Neurosurgery and Chairman, Department of Neurosurgery, Harper Hospital, Wayne State University, Detroit, Michigan

Barton L. Guthrie, M.D.
Associate Professor of Surgery, Division of Neurosurgery, Department of Surgery, University of Alabama School of Medicine, Birmingham, Alabama

Steven L. Hancock, M.D.
Professor of Radiation Oncology, Department of Radiation Oncology, Stanford University School of Medicine, Stanford, California

Zhaowei Jiang, Ph.D.
Assistant Professor of Neurosurgery and Chief, Computer Networks, Department of Neurosurgery, Harper Hospital, Wayne State University, Detroit, Michigan

Ferenc A. Jolesz, M.D.
Professor of Radiology and Director, Division of MRI and Image-Guided Therapy, Department of Radiology, Harvard Medical School/Brigham & Women's Hospital, Boston, Massachusetts

Wayel Kaakaji, M.D.
Chief Neurosurgical Resident, Department of Neurosurgery, The Cleveland Clinic Foundation, Cleveland, Ohio

A. Majeed Kadi, M.S.
Systems Development Engineer, Department of Neurosurgery, Harper Hospital, Wayne State University, Detroit, Michigan

Iain H. Kalfas, M.D.
Head, Section of Spinal Surgery, Department of Neurosurgery, The Cleveland Clinic Foundation, Cleveland, Ohio

Ron Kikinis, M.D.
Associate Professor of Radiology, Department of Radiology, Harvard Medical School/Brigham & Women's Hospital, Boston, Massachusetts

Miguel Lis-Planells, M.D.
Fellow, Department of Neurosurgery, Harper Hospital, Wayne State University, Detroit, Michigan

Mark G. Luciano, M.D., Ph.D.
Head, Section of Pediatric Neurosurgery, Department of Neurosurgery, The Cleveland Clinic Foundation, Cleveland, Ohio

Robert J. Maciunas, M.D.
Professor of Neurological Surgery and Biomedical Engineering, Department of Neurological Surgery, Vanderbilt University School of Medicine, Nashville, Tennessee

Michael W. McDermott, M.D., F.R.C.S.(C)
Assistant Professor of Surgery, Department of Neurosurgery, University of California School of Medicine, San Francisco, California

David W. Miller, M.D.
Staff Neurosurgeon and Head, Section of Pituitary Surgery, Department of Neurosurgery, The Cleveland Clinic Foundation, Cleveland, Ohio

Martin J. Murphy, Ph.D.
Radiation Oncologist, Department of Radiation Oncology, Stanford University School of Medicine, Stanford, California

Lutz Nolte, Ph.D.
Miller Institute of Biomechanics, University of Bern, Bern, Switzerland

Troy D. Payner, M.D.
Indianapolis Neurosurgical Group, Indianapolis, Indiana

R.L. Patrick Rhoten, M.D.
Department of Neurosurgery, Kaiser Permanente, Los Angeles Medical Center, Los Angeles, California

David W. Roberts, M.D.
Professor of Surgery, Section of Neurosurgery, Department of Surgery, Dartmouth Medical School, Lebanon, New Hampshire

Achim Schweikard, Ph.D.
Professor of Computer Science, Department of Computer Science, Institut für Informatik der Technischen Universität, Munich, Germany

Charles P. Steiner, B.S.
Department of Neurosurgery, The Cleveland Clinic Foundation, Cleveland, Ohio

James G. Walsh, R.N., B.S.N.
Nurse Clinician, Gamma Knife Center, The Cleveland Clinic Foundation, Cleveland, Ohio

Joseph P. Weisenberger, R.T.
Department of Neurosurgery, The Cleveland Clinic Foundation, Cleveland, Ohio

Lucia Zamorano, M.D., Ph.D.
Professor of Neurological Surgery and Radiation Oncology, Departments of Neurosurgery and Radiation Oncology, Harper Hospital, Wayne State University, Detroit, Michigan

Preface

The practice of neurosurgery has been fundamentally changed by the evolution of the electronic computer. Digital imaging techniques such as computer-assisted tomography (CT), magnetic resonance imaging (MRI), and digital angiography have revolutionized diagnostic neurosurgery, supplanting pneumoencephalography, myelography, and many other invasive procedures. Although they are powerful diagnostic tools, these technologies have not replaced the diagnostician; rather they complement and confirm thoughtful deductions based on a careful neurologic history and examination.

In the late 1970s several neurosurgical visionaries recognized that these computerized imaging systems were capable of more than just aiding diagnosis. These individuals devised equipment and techniques to harness the spatial information contained within these images for surgical guidance. Image-guided frame stereotaxy used a stereotactic reference frame and imaging modality–specific encoders to allow safe, accurate biopsy of imaged brain lesions. This technique was adapted to numerous neurosurgical procedures, including depth electrodes, functional neurosurgery, radiation implants, and craniotomy. Virtually any intracranial target could be accessed along predefined approaches or trajectories. Although the calculations to decode spatial information from neuroimaging could be done manually or with calculators, the availability of reasonably priced computers and workstations simplified the process for the surgeon.

As the ratio of computing power to cost increased, not only could points be defined stereotactically, but also volumes. Stereotactic radiosurgery and volumetric craniotomy benefited from these technological advances, but stereotactic craniotomy failed to be widely adopted in the neurosurgical community, perhaps because the benefit of guidance was not felt to outweigh the cumbersome logistics of the procedure.

In the early 1980s, three technologic advances occurred that allowed for the development of stereotactic systems that were not reliant on applied reference frames. First, neuroimaging progressed to the point where it was not only spatially accurate within a given image (i.e., a slice), but also accurate throughout the entire volume of data. Second, accurate, inexpensive three-dimensional digitizers became available. And finally, there was another incremental increase in low-cost computing power such that three-dimensional transformations and other calculations could be performed and displayed in near real time using image data sets several megabytes in size. Image-guided frameless stereotaxy could not only provide the guidance information of its frame counterpart, but provide truly interactive navigational information such as location and orientation during surgical procedures. These devices could provide instantaneous intraoperative answers to the questions "Where am I in this head?" and "What's on the other side of that structure?"

Experience with these surgical navigation systems is approaching a decade of use, most of which has been accumulated in academic research centers. Much has been written on how these devices function and the various benefits and disadvantages of one technology compared with another. Yet, as the first commercial systems come to market for neurosurgery at large, there is little information on how best to use them in clinical practice. Our focus, therefore, is not to dwell on the technologies behind surgical navigation systems (a brief review is provided for the uninitiated), but rather to demonstrate how to get the most from them, show how they are useful for selected clinical problems, and provide information on the clinical and economic results that may be expected when this technology is applied.

One final note. Just as computerized imaging has not replaced the diagnostician, these tools will not transform a bad surgeon into a great one, let alone replace the surgeon entirely. They remain an adjunct to the surgeon's experience, judgment, and technical skills—one more instrument at his or her disposal. We believe that this technology is the next computer-generated revolution in neurosurgery, and we hope that you find the information and experiences in this book to be a useful guide on the clinical application of interactive surgical navigation systems.

Gene H. Barnett, M.D.
David W. Roberts, M.D.
Robert J. Maciunas, M.D.

Contents

Image-Guided Neurosurgery
Clinical Applications of Surgical Navigation

PART I

Basic Principles

1

Fundamentals of Registration

David W. Roberts, M.D.

The ability to quantify and manipulate spatial information to relate one set of data to another is fundamental to surgical navigation. Numerous benefits are derived from establishing such spatial registration, including the identification of anatomic features from an atlas in an imaging study, the integration of multiple imaging modalities, and the tracking or delivery of a surgical instrument to a given location seen in an atlas or on a radiographic study.

This chapter will present an overview of stereotactic co-registration, including the basic mathematical principles of coordinate systems and their manipulation. Before the current, relatively inexpensive computing resources in the operating room became available, stereotaxy relied on frame-based instrumentation and registration strategies that could be readily implemented by the neurosurgeon in the operating room. These strategies necessarily constrained the registration problem and usually achieved their ends through simple arithmetic or graphic geometric steps. More recently, computer resources have altered this process as significantly as CT and MR scanning broadened the indications for stereotaxy and facilitated its application. Inexpensive computational power has provided more efficient algebraic solutions to many of the registration tasks required for stereotaxy frame systems. In addition, it has made possible sophisticated representation of a reformatted atlas and individualized neuroimaging and operative field information for two- and three-dimensional visual display during surgery.

Despite the increasingly intuitive interfaces of surgical navigation systems that facilitate their use without having to learn the underlying mathematics, an understanding of the fundamentals of this technology has obvious advantages for neurosurgeons. Foremost among these is that it serves as a safeguard during clinical application; errors that might arise may be better appreciated or prevented altogether. Equally compelling is the recognition that such understanding on the part of the surgeon can provide the impetus and direction for further developments.

COORDINATE SYSTEMS

In the early 17th century Pierre de Fermat and René Descartes independently recognized that a system comprised of two perpendicular lines could be used to identify any point within a plane.[1] The distances along each of these lines (what may be called x- and y-axes) from the origin (the intersection of the axes where each is usually assigned a value of 0) to a given point provide an ordered pair of numbers, or coordinates, unique to that point. Such a rectangular coordinate system is commonly called Cartesian, in honor of Descartes, and may be extended to three dimensions, with x-, y-, and z-axes. In such a manner each location in a given space may be uniquely and quantitatively defined.

There are other ways, of course, to describe a point's location in space as well. For example, the lines representing the coordinate system's axes need not be perpendicular to one another (although for each to provide independent information about each point they must be nonparallel). Alternatively, a point in a plane may be described by specifying its distance and direction from an origin, that is, a radius (r) and an angle (theta), using a polar coordinate system. This may be extended into three dimensions using a cylindric coordinate system by specification of a distance along an additional (z) axis perpendicular to that original plane, or a spherical coordinate system may be used to specify a radius and two angles (perpendicular with respect to each other) and describe the direction from the origin.

All of these systems are mathematically equivalent and achieve the same end in uniquely defining the location of a point in space. The coordinates of one system may be readily converted to those of another. It is an elementary exercise to show, for example, that the coordinates of a point (r and theta) in two-dimensional polar coordinate space may be converted to x- and y-coordinates in two-dimensional Cartesian coordinate space by the formulas x = r cos theta and y = r sin theta and that similar conversion from three-dimensional spherical coordinates is represented by the formulas x = r sin theta cos phi, y = r sin theta sin phi, and z = r cos theta.[2]

Various two- and three-dimensional coordinate spaces may be employed in a stereotactic procedure. As noted earlier, spatial information from imaging studies, atlases, stereotaxy frames, or other intraoperative digitizers may all be represented in such coordinate spaces. Considering imaging studies first, the coordinates inherent in a single CT slice are most intuitive. The computer graphic representation of such a slice is generated using coordinates inherent to the scanner, and these machine-specific or gantry coordinates are usually readily accessible at the scanner console. By convention, an x-coordinate is assigned along the right-left axis of the image and a y-coordinate along the posterior-anterior axis. Thus, on any given two-dimensional CT, MR, PET, or SPECT image, a given pixel's location may be specified in terms of an x- and y-coordinate; whether this is in gantry coordinate space or some other space based on part of a stereotaxy frame that may also be in the scan is immaterial at this point and will be revisited later in the discussion on transformations.

Neurosurgical procedures must account for the three-dimensional space of the intracranial volume, and imaging information must include this third dimension. The location of a slice with respect to a frame or to other slices in the study may be determined in several ways, the most common of which are monitoring the position of the scanner table relative to the gantry and using the geometry of frame components visible in the scanner that enable unique determination of the slice plane relative to the frame (i.e., the various N-shaped fiducial plates). A coordinate incorporating this third dimension may be added to the coordinates already derived in two dimensions to provide a three-dimensional address for any location within the imaging study. Aside from such traps as a gantry tilt that will introduce skew into the stack of slices (which can be accounted for), the Cartesian coordinate system of CT and MR imaging is intuitive, tractable, and convenient.

The projection geometry of conventional radiographs and biplanar angiography is not as simple—accounting in part for the esoteric mystique surrounding stereotaxy initially—but remains directly solvable as well. In this instance spatial information is obtained from two-dimensional images, and to derive three-dimensional information one must use data from at least two images obtained from different perspectives, identify the same object(s) in each image, and account for magnification and parallax. All of these issues have been well worked out mathematically in general and by multiple stereotactic systems in particular.[3] Geometric methods using plotting graphs or the spiral diagram provided nonalgebraic working solutions before computers were available. Analytic solutions for conventional angiography, however, have now been developed for multiple stereotaxy frame systems using fiducial-embedded plates attached to the frame.[4,5] Scalp-based fiducial markers in a frameless adaptation have also been described.[6]

Stereotactic atlases derive their utility from similar organization of their anatomic information into coordinate space. Nearly all stereotactic atlases are Cartesian, and from a mathematical perspective differ primarily in the selection of the coordinate system's origin, the orientation of its axes (i.e., what other natural reference points are used to align one or more axes), the methodology of scaling, the intervals of data sampling, and the occasional incorporation of statistical methodology. Independent of these issues, each atlas assigns a unique three-dimensional address (the stack of anatomic slices compiled into a three-dimensional volume in a manner entirely analogous to stacking CT slices) to each anatomic point of interest, enabling subsequent manipulation and incorporation of that information into a stereotactic procedure.

Multiple functions are made possible by stereotaxy frame systems: the definition of a coordinate space that includes the relevant portion of a particular patient's intracranial volume, the means by which co-registration of that coordinate space with information from imaging studies or anatomic atlases may be accomplished, and the delivery of an operative instrument to a selected coordinate address (stabilization of that instrument by the frame is an advantageous and convenient, but nonstereotactic additional benefit). The first of these tasks may be achieved using any type of coordinate system, and indeed the various stereotaxy frame systems use a variety of them. Leksell, Talairach, and Hitchcock frames, to cite a few, are all Cartesian based; target coordinates on these frames are specified as ordered triplets (x, y, z). Arc-centered systems (such as the Leksell system) have the attractive and convenient feature of enabling free adjustment of the angles of the arc and probe carrier (and thus the trajectory) with the target point always remaining centered. For applications of point targeting, these additional parameters need not be stereotactically defined. If a specific trajectory is to be stereotactically defined (e.g., one passing through more than one designated point), these angles, of course, must be specified; there are more than three parameters to such a localization, and information in addition to Cartesian coordinates of the target is necessary.

Non-Cartesian coordinate systems are employed by still other stereotaxy frame systems. The Reichert-Mundinger frame uses two angles on an arc, an additional two angles on the probe carrier, and a dimension of depth.[7] Determination of this combination of spherical coordinates was originally performed noncomputationally, by mechanically adjusting the trajectory probe until it reached the simulated target on a phantom. (The positioning of this phantom target would already have been set using radiographically determined rectangular coordinates, in turn derived through projection geometry from multiple two-dimensional image rectangular coordinates.) The inconvenience and potential contamination of this step by a phantom was eventually replaced by the mathematical calculation of the frame angles and length, exemplifying the integration of increasingly accessible computational power.

The coordinate space of the Brown-Roberts-Wells stereotactic system, in which targets and trajectories are defined by four angles and a length, is similarly non-Cartesian.[8,9] Its development at a time when computational resources were available—initially using the CT scanner's computer and later a programmable calculator—allowed computational conversion from Cartesian scanner coordinates to spherical coordinates, and its phantom base is used for mechanical confirmation only.

SURGICAL NAVIGATION SYSTEMS

The operative coordinate space is defined by the coordinate system of a particular stereotaxy frame. More recently developed stereotactic systems that do not use a mechanical frame nevertheless still require an operative coordinate space, and this requirement is fulfilled through the use of a three-dimensional digitizer within the operating room. Such a device can locate a point within its working volume, assigning it a coordinate address (usually within whatever kind of coordinate space is desired, the interconversion being straightforward as noted earlier). A variety of digitizing technologies may be employed to accomplish this localization task, including those based on ultrasound emitters and microphone arrays, articulated arms with potentiometers or optical encoders at the joints between links, light-emitting diodes (LEDs) and linear charge-coupled device camera arrays, stereo video or electronic cameras, and electromagnetic field transmitters and detecting coils.

The software running these various digitizers calculates the location of a selected point from the one or more sensors of the device, and this information is usually passed directly to further software determining co-registration, driving appropriate graphic displays, or interfacing with robotic instrumentation. The actual coordinate system and numeric coordinates for a selected point in operating room space in these implementations remain transparent to the procedure. A good illustration of how such a digitizer can define an operating room stereotactic space is found in the description of a sonic digitizer used to track an operating microscope by Friets et al.[10]

Registration Concepts

The establishment of the spatial relationship between the multiple coordinate spaces defined by imaging studies and by the intraoperative stereotactic system is the sine qua non of a stereotactic procedure. With the goal of minimizing calculation, particularly when computational aids were less available, most frame-based methodologies were developed using some degree of mechanical alignment of frame and imaging studies. The problem of determining the relationship between coordinate spaces is in this manner at least partially constrained and in turn made more tractable. Use of an orthogonal central beam a given distance from a frame's side is an example of working with projection geometry; placing a frame in a scanner perpendicular to the gantry and without rotation is another. In the latter example elimination of rotation along any of three coordinate axes reduces the transformation from Cartesian scanner space to Cartesian frame space to a calculation of only three translations (Fig. 1-1). Continuing the imposition of constraints to an extreme, if two coordinate spaces were concordant, with corresponding points in the imaging study and the intracranial working space having identical coordinates, co-registration would in effect already be accomplished and no further manipulation or computation would be required. This is the situation in the recent development of operating within an open-magnet MRI.

With increasingly fast and inexpensive computation, more and more of the task of determining the relationship between different coordinate spaces can be shifted from the mechanical to the software realm. An example of this is the registration process for the Brown-Roberts-Wells frame in which a full three-dimensional transformation is derived during the registration step; positioning of the frame within a CT scanner is thus less constrained at the expense of more elaborate, but still reasonably efficient calculation. Conceptually this shift toward computational derivation of necessary transformations has led to elimination of the stereotaxy frame altogether.

The correspondence between one Cartesian coordinate space and another at its most fundamental level consists of the definition of six parameters. These are three angles of rotation by which the x, y, and z coordinate axes can be made parallel to one another, respectively, and three distances (along each of these axes) by which the origins of the two coordinate systems can be superimposed. An additional parameter of scale must, of course, also be explicitly or implicitly accounted for as well. It is not difficult to intuitively appreciate these rotations, translations, and scaling (Fig. 1-2). In registering a patient's imaging study with the patient's head in the operating room, the most common method of registration involves determining a rigid-body transformation, with the assumption being made that the morphology of the brain is constant (i.e., without deformation) in both coordinate systems. In instances where this assumption cannot be made (e.g., registering a stereotactic atlas to an individual patient), an elastic transformation may be necessary, but such algorithms are not yet as well developed.

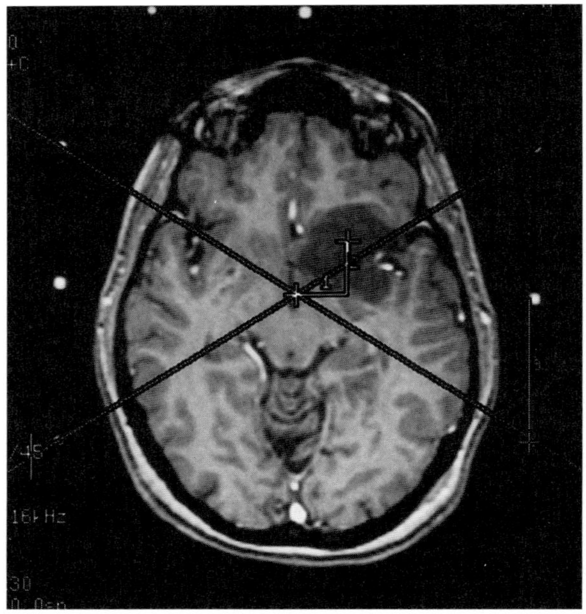

Figure 1-1. Calculation of stereotaxy frame coordinates at the CT or MRI console (in this instance using the Leksell stereotaxy frame and MRI for the biopsy of what proved to be an astrocytoma in a young woman) is facilitated by constraining the problem to one of straightforward translations. The left-right (x) and posterior-anterior (y) distances between the center of the frame (as determined by the intersection of diagonal lines passing through symmetric landmarks on the frame's imaged superstructure) and the target are measured using the scanner console's measure-distance function. The superior-inferior (z) coordinate is calculated from the distance between a vertical fiducial rod (posteriorly) and a diagonal fiducial rod whose geometric relationship to the frame's coordinate system is known.

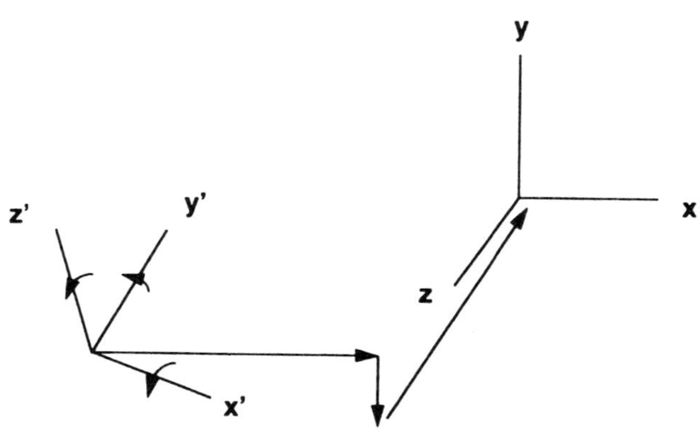

Figure 1-2. A rigid-body transformation from one coordinate space to another requires the designation of three angles of rotation and three translations.

Transformation Matrices

This process of moving between different coordinate spaces is often represented mathematically by transformation matrices.[3,11] Such a matrix for rotation about the x-axis has the form:

$$Rx(\theta) = \begin{bmatrix} 1 & 0 & 0 & 0 \\ 0 & \cos\theta & \sin\theta & 0 \\ 0 & -\sin\theta & \cos\theta & 0 \\ 0 & 0 & 0 & 1 \end{bmatrix}$$

and multiplication of the coordinates of a point by this matrix generates the new coordinates for that point:

$$\begin{aligned} P' &= P \cdot Rx(\theta) \\ &= [\, x\ y\ z\ 1\,] \cdot \begin{bmatrix} 1 & 0 & 0 & 0 \\ 0 & \cos\theta & \sin\theta & 0 \\ 0 & -\sin\theta & \cos\theta & 0 \\ 0 & 0 & 0 & 1 \end{bmatrix} \\ &= [\, x \quad y\cos\theta - z\sin\theta \quad y\sin\theta + z\cos\theta \quad 1\,] \end{aligned}$$

The new coordinates may be considered conceptually as either movement of the point to a new location within a single coordinate space or representation of an analogous point in a new coordinate system; the two are functionally equivalent.

A matrix may be derived for each of the other rotations, translations, and scaling as follows[11]:

Rotation about the y-axis:

$$Ry(\theta) = \begin{bmatrix} \cos\theta & 0 & -\sin\theta & 0 \\ 0 & 1 & 0 & 0 \\ \sin\theta & 0 & \cos\theta & 0 \\ 0 & 0 & 0 & 1 \end{bmatrix}$$

Rotation about the z-axis:

$$Rz(\theta) = \begin{bmatrix} \cos\theta & \sin\theta & 0 & 0 \\ -\sin\theta & \cos\theta & 0 & 0 \\ 0 & 0 & 1 & 0 \\ 0 & 0 & 0 & 1 \end{bmatrix}$$

Translation along all three axes:

$$T(Dx,Dy,Dz) = \begin{bmatrix} 1 & 0 & 0 & 0 \\ 0 & 1 & 0 & 0 \\ 0 & 0 & 1 & 0 \\ Dx & Dy & Dz & 1 \end{bmatrix}$$

Scaling:

$$S(Sx,Sy,Sz) = \begin{bmatrix} Sx & 0 & 0 & 0 \\ 0 & Sy & 0 & 0 \\ 0 & 0 & Sz & 0 \\ 0 & 0 & 0 & 1 \end{bmatrix}$$

Multiple such processes will be required for converting from one coordinate space to another, and the various matrix transformations may be performed sequentially. It will be observed that translation is an additive process and that rotation and scaling are multiplicative. By the use of what are called homogeneous coordinates (as given above), it is possible to treat all three operations as multiplications, and in this way sequential transformations can be combined in a process referred to as concatenation or composition. A rigid-body transformation combining all of the above operations is thus represented:

$$T = R_x \cdot R_y \cdot R_z \cdot T_{xyz} \cdot S_{xyz}$$

Registration across multiple coordinate spaces may be similarly performed:

$$T_{AC} = T_{AB} \cdot T_{BC}$$

Given a point whose coordinates are known in coordinate space A, coordinates for that point in coordinate space C may be derived by matrix multiplication:

$$P_C = P_A \cdot T_{AC}$$

Although such formulation has the appeal of formulaic simplicity, in the actual computation of transformational processes, the mathematical operations are sometimes broken back down into addition and multiplication for the sake of greater efficiency in terms of the number of operations required. It should also be pointed out in this regard that there are alternative methodologies to matrices for such operations, for example, the use of direction cosines employed in early software for the Dartmouth microscope,[10] but these are mathematically equivalent.

The ability to move in the opposite direction between coordinate spaces—a desirable process in any truly interactive stereotactic system—is facilitated by the inverse transformation, represented symbolically by T^{-1}:

$$P_2 = P_1 \cdot T$$

$$P_1 = P_2 \cdot T^{-1}$$

Derivation of the transformation matrix required to move between patient-specific imaging coordinate spaces and stereotactic operating space can be achieved in a number of ways. The known geometry of specific stereotaxy frame superstructures visible in imaging space allows convenient determination of the necessary transformation. As previously alluded to, the simple hand calculation of Leksell x- and y-coordinates from a CT or MR console represents such a calculation, although a fairly constrained one; similarly, identification in image-space of so-called fiducial rods (or, in the two-dimensional image, points) of a Brown-Roberts-Wells frame enables formulaic calculation of selected targets in stereotactic operating space.

Fiducial Point Strategies

The simplest and most commonly used method at the present time of achieving co-registration of coordinate spaces with surgical navigation systems is that of matching a set of ordered points visible to both the imaging study and the intraoperative digitizer.[10,12-16] A minimum of three such noncolinear pairs of points is required for determination of the transformation, although many systems employ or allow additional pairs of points to improve registration accuracy. Such points may be markers that have been attached to the scalp prior to imaging (e.g., glass beads, staples, vitamin E capsules, or skull-embedded screws). Alternatively, such algorithms may be used with natural features such as the tragus, lateral canthi, or

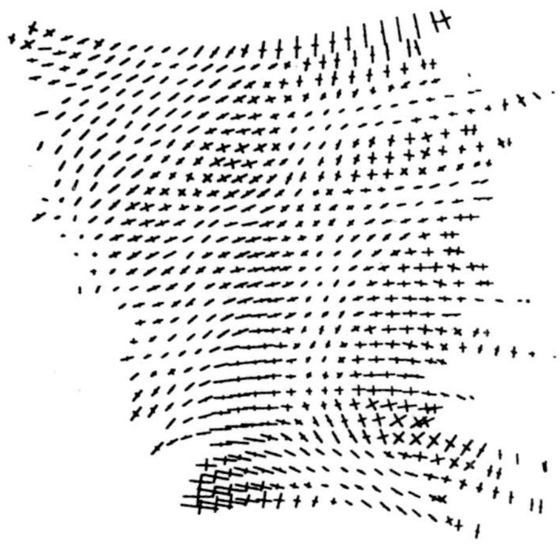

Figure 1-3. Feature maps of the scalp's surface, in this instance showing the inherent maximum and minimum curvatures at multiple points from a CT scan, have unique topographic features that can be used for matching. These maps can be derived from information obtained from an intraoperative sonic digitizer or from CT and MR imaging. The resulting feature maps, whose unique topography can be readily appreciated, can then be matched. (From Friets EM, Strohbehn JW, Roberts DW. Curvature-based nonfiducial registration for the frameless stereotactic operating microscope. IEEE Trans Biomed Eng 42:867-878, 1995.)

nasion. The less discrete nature of an anatomic feature may compromise accuracy, although such an approach has the advantage of not requiring a special imaging study. In either instance the algorithms used are the same.

Rather than matching readily apparent analogous points, one may derive a transformation using other features such as the intrinsic curvatures of the scalp surface to achieve alignment. By calculating from both imaging studies and from an intraoperative digitizer the mathematically defined curvatures over a sufficient portion of the scalp, it is possible to then align either points of maximum curvature or related features (such as ridge lines or saddle points) in a similar manner[17-19] (Fig. 1-3).

Given a set of ordered points whose coordinates are known in two different coordinate spaces, there are a number of approaches to the problem of determining the parameters of the rigid-body transformation relating those spaces. These include closed-form solutions such as singular value decomposition of a matrix, eigenvalue-eigenvector decomposition of a matrix, or unit quaternions as well as iterative solution techniques.[20] Given a set of reference features as described above, an iterative registration process requires two conceptual steps. The first is that of defining a disparity function, by which a measure of the correspondence between two sets of corresponding features can be determined. The most common such function is a least-squares criterion of the following type:

$$D = \sum_i w_i \{\text{distance}[F_{Ai}, \mathbf{T}(F_{Bi}, t)]\}^2$$

In this function D is equal to the sum of squares of the distances between each of i corresponding points (w is a weighting factor related to the noise of the mea-

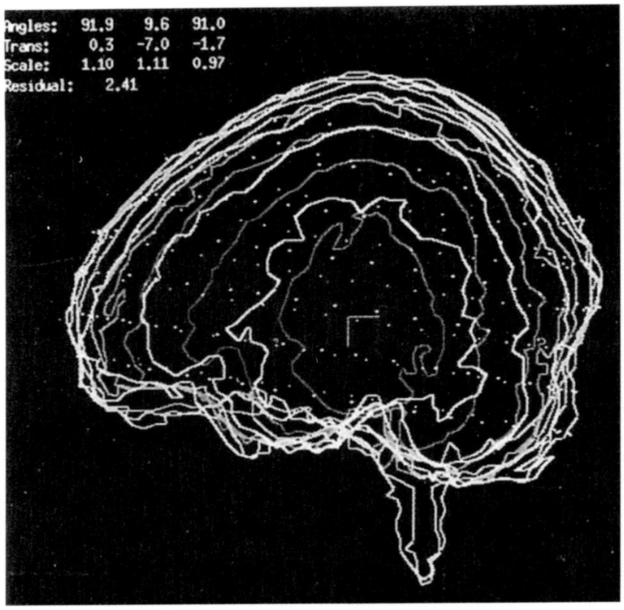

Figure 1-4. Two surfaces, represented by discrete points and contour lines, may be matched, much like a hat and a head, using algorithms such as that of Pelizzari and Chen. (From Pelizzari CA, Levin DN, Chen GTY, Chen C-T. Image registration based on anatomic surface matching. In Maciunas RJ, ed. Interactive Image-Guided Neurosurgery. Park Ridge, Ill.: American Association of Neurological Surgeons, 1993, pp 47-62.)

surements).[21] The second step is that of optimization of the disparity function, by which is meant the adjustment of various transformation parameters such that a usable value of the function is achieved. In the above example minimization of the function is desired, and when this is achieved, the registration process is complete. There are numerous optimization strategies, and when there is not a direct solution, nonlinear iterative methods are required. A frequently used method is that of gradient descent.[21]

Surface Matching Strategies

In the registration strategy described using three or more reference points, the ordering of those corresponding points in both coordinate spaces is known. There are alternative strategies, however, in which unordered sets of points may be used, as in matching the surface of the head as imaged by CT, MR, or PET scanning with the surface of the scalp as digitized in the operating room. This surface-to-surface matching has the advantage of using a natural feature of the head (so that additional, prospective imaging is not required) whose segmentation can be automated.

A number of such techniques have been developed, the best known of which is the "hat-and-head" matching algorithm of Pelizzari and Chen[22-25] (Fig. 1-4). In their method the distance between intraoperatively digitized surface points and the preoperatively imaged surface along rays extending from the centroid of that

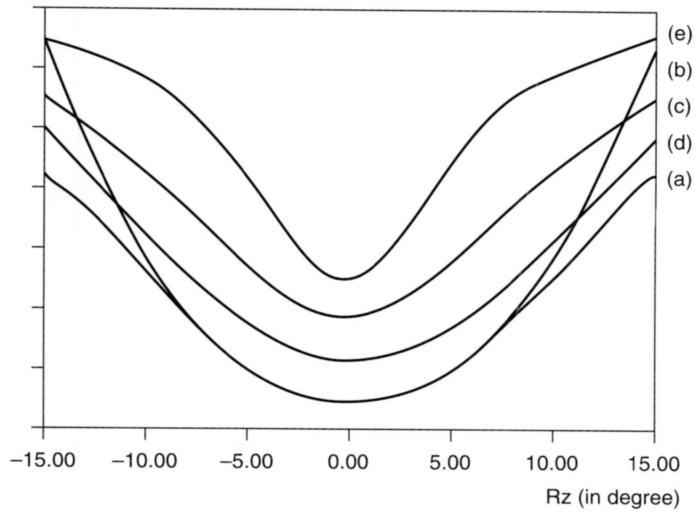

Figure 1-5. The shapes of various cost functions using simulated data; only a variation in rotation about the z-axis is shown. (From Cuchet E, Knoplioch J, Dormont D, Marsault C. Registration in neurosurgery and neuroradiotherapy applications. J Image Guided Surg 1:198-207, 1995. Reprinted by permission of Wiley-Liss, Inc., a subsidiary of John Wiley & Sons, Inc.)

surface to each point is computed, and the sum of these squared distances is then minimized. It will be appreciated that an iterative optimization process may inopportunely appear to have become optimized when it actually is not (the problem of local minima), and either initial guidance or later user intervention may be required to reduce this possibility. Numerous other surface-to-surface matching methodologies such as those of Jiang et al.,[26] Mangin et al.,[27] and Hemler et al.[28] have respective advantages and disadvantages in terms of ease of automation and computational efficiency, and although they vary in the details of their algorithms, all conceptually share the component steps of definition of a disparity function and optimization of that function.[21]

The accuracy, efficiency, and speed of various strategies using different functions and optimizations are understandably areas of considerable current attention[29,30] (Fig. 1-5). Further development of these more sophisticated registration strategies based on inherent anatomic features (i.e., not requiring placement of artificial fiducial markers on special scans) and fully automated segmentation and matching algorithms will make co-registration of multimodality and sequential imaging studies of a given patient a standard practice. The extension of these methods into the operating room using three-dimensional digitizers will render nearly all procedures stereotactic in a manner transparent to the operating surgeon.

SUMMARY

Co-registration, relating two or more coordinate spaces, is the process by which stereotactic operating systems achieve accurate integration of one or more databases into the operative field. Established mathematical methods for accomplishing this linkage have long been available, but newer algorithms adapted to the needs of the clinician are being developed and are better characterized. The availability of powerful computational resources within the operating room allows the use of more sophisticated algorithms that have eliminated the need for a stereotaxy frame, that have become increasingly more efficient and more accurate, and that have the potential to automate co-registration. Although the mathematical and computer skills enabling these latter developments have become more sophisticated, the fundamental mathematical principles remain accessible to all. Understanding these principles will lead to reduction of potential error in clinical practice and will facilitate further developments.

References

1. West BH, Griesbach EN, Taylor JD, Taylor LT. The Prentice-Hall Encyclopedia of Mathematics. Englewood Cliffs: Prentice-Hall, 1982, pp 119-126.
2. Clapham C. A Concise Dictionary of Mathematics. Oxford: Oxford University Press, 1990.
3. Lemieux L, Henri CJ, Wootton R, Collins DL, Peters TM. The mathematics of stereotactic localization. In Thomas DGT, ed. Stereotactic and Image Directed Surgery of Brain Tumors. Edinburgh: Churchill Livingstone, 1993, pp 193-216.
4. Kelly PJ, Goerss SJ, Kall BA. Modification of Todd-Wells system for imaging data acquisition. In Lunsford LD, ed. Modern Stereotactic Neurosurgery. Boston: Martinus Nijhoff, 1988, pp 79-97.
5. Lunsford LD, Kondziolka D, Flickinger JC, Bissonette DJ, Jungreis CA, Maitz AH, Horton JA, Coffey RJ. Stereotactic radiosurgery for arteriovenous malformations of the brain. J Neurosurg 75:512-524, 1991.
6. Grzeszczuk R, Tan KK, Levin DN, Pelizzari CA, Hu X, Chen GTY, Beck RN, Chen C-T, Cooper M, Milton J, Spire J-P, Towle VL, Dohrmann GJ, Erickson RK. Retrospective fusion of radiographic and MR data for localization of subdural electrodes. J Comput Assist Tomogr 16:764-773, 1992.
7. Mundinger F, Birg W. The imaging-compatible Reichert-Mundinger system. In Lunsford LD, ed. Modern Stereotactic Neurosurgery. Boston: Martinus Nijhoff, 1988, pp 13-25.
8. Brown RA. A computerized tomography-computer graphics approach to stereotaxic localization. J Neurosurg 50:715-720, 1979.
9. Apuzzo MLJ, Fredericks CA. The Brown-Roberts-Wells system. In Lunsford LD, ed. Modern Stereotactic Neurosurgery. Boston: Martinus Nijhoff, 1988, pp 63-77.
10. Friets EM, Strohbehn JW, Hatch JF, Roberts DW. A frameless stereotaxic operating microscope for neurosurgery. IEEE Trans Biomed Eng 36:608-617, 1989.
11. Foley JD, Van Dam A. Fundamentals of Interactive Computer Graphics. Reading, Mass.: Addison-Wesley, 1984, pp 245-266.
12. Roberts DW, Strohbehn JW, Hatch JF, Murray W, Kettenberger H. A frameless stereotaxic integration of computerized tomographic imaging and the operating microscope. J Neurosurg 65:545-549, 1986.
13. Galloway RL Jr, Maciunas RJ, Edwards CA. Interactive image-guided neurosurgery. IEEE Trans Biomed Eng 39:1226-1231, 1992.
14. Maciunas RJ, Fitzpatrick JM, Galloway RL, Allen GS. Beyond stereotaxy: Extreme levels of application accuracy are provided by implantable fiducial markers for interactive image-guided neurosurgery. In Maciunas RJ, ed. Interactive Image-Guided Neurosurgery. Park Ridge, Ill.: American Association of Neurological Surgeons, 1993, pp 259-270.
15. Day R, Heilbrun MP, Koehler S, McDonald P, Peters W, Siemionow V. Three-point transformation for integration of multiple coordinate systems: Applications to tumor, functional, and fractionated radiosurgery stereotactic planning. Stereotact Funct Neurosurg 63:76-79, 1994.
16. Heilbrun MP, Koehler S, MacDonald P, Siemionow V, Peters W. Preliminary experience using an optimized three-point transformation algorithm for spatial registration of coordinate systems: A method of noninvasive localization using frame-based stereotactic guidance systems. J Neurosurg 81:676-682, 1994.
17. Friets EM, Strohbehn JW, Roberts DW. Curvature-based nonfiducial registration for the frameless stereotactic operating microscope. IEEE Trans Biomed Eng 42:867-878, 1995.
18. Gueziec A, Ayache N. Smoothing and matching of 3-D space curves. Visualization in Biomedical Computing 1992. Proc SPIE 1808:259-273, 1992.
19. Balter JM, Pelizzari CA, Chen GTY. Correlation of projection radiographs in radiation therapy using open curve segments and points. Med Phys 19:329-334, 1992.

20. Maurer CR, Fitzpatrick JM. A review of medical image registration. In Maciunas RJ, ed. Interactive Image-Guided Neurosurgery. Park Ridge, Ill.: American Association of Neurological Surgeons, 1993, pp 17-44.
21. Lavallée, S. Registration for computer-integrated surgery: Methodology, state of the art. In Taylor RH, Lavallée S, Burdea GC, Mösges R, eds. Computer-Integrated Surgery. Cambridge, Mass.: MIT Press, 1996, pp 77-97.
22. Levin DN, Pelizzari CA, Chen GTY, Chen CT, Cooper MD. Retrospective geometric correlation of MR, CT, and PET images. Radiology 169:817-823, 1988.
23. Pelizzari CA, Chen GTY, Spelbring DR, Weichselbaum RR, Chen C. Accurate three-dimensional registration of CT, PET, and/or MR images of the brain. J Comput Assist Tomogr 13:20-26, 1989.
24. Tan KK, Grzeszczuk R, Levin DN, Pelizzari CA, Chen GTY, Erickson RK, Johnson D, Dohrmann GJ. A frameless stereotactic approach to neurosurgical planning based on retrospective patient-image registration. Technical note. J Neurosurg 79:296-303, 1993.
25. Pelizzari CA, Levin DN, Chen GTY, Chen C-T. Image registration based on anatomic surface matching. In Maciunas RJ, ed. Interactive Image-Guided Neurosurgery. Park Ridge, Ill.: American Association of Neurological Surgeons, 1993, pp 47-62.
26. Jiang H, Robb RA, Holton KS. A new approach to 3-D registration of multimodality medical images by surface matching. In Proceedings of the Second Conference on Visualization in Biomedical Computing. Chapel Hill, N.C., 1992, pp 196-213.
27. Mangin JF, Frouin V, Bloch I, Lopez-Krahe J, Bendriem B. Fast nonsupervised 3D registration of PET and MR images of the brain. Paris: Telecom Paris, 1993.
28. Hemler PF, Sumanaweera TS, van den Elsen P, Napel S, Adler J. A versatile system for multimodality image fusion. J Image Guided Surg 1:35-45, 1995.
29. Simon DA, Hebert M, Kanada T. Techniques for fast and accurate intrasurgical registration. J Image Guided Surg 1:17-29, 1995.
30. Cuchet E, Knoplioch J, Dormont D, Marsault C. Registration in neurosurgery and neuroradiotherapy applications. J Image Guided Surg 1:198-207, 1995.

2

Surgical Navigation System Technologies

Gene H. Barnett, M.D. • Charles P. Steiner, B.S. • David W. Roberts, M.D.

Perhaps the most confusing aspect of surgical navigation systems (SNSs) is the wide array of technologies used to determine the location of the pointing device in space.[1-20] The location of the pointing device, whether a wand, instrument, or microscope, must be accurately conveyed to the computer so that its position can be related to the imaging data. Typically this localization process is performed by some type of three-dimensional digitizer that spews out a set of coordinates (e.g., x, y, and z) that defines the location(s) of references point(s) that determine where the object is in space. This three-dimensional digitizer is commonly referred to as the front end of the SNS.

When assessing the merits of an SNS, the uninitiated are confronted with unfamiliar terms such as arms, sonic, optical, active, passive, machine vision, electromagnetic, direct current, alternating current, linear charge-coupled device, and two-dimensional charge-coupled device, each claimed by their respective manufacturers or developers to be superior to the competition.

As with most choices in life, each of these technologies has distinct advantages and liabilities that affect their use, the best choice may differ depending on the individual, and each SNS may uniquely dictate the way a surgeon must modify his or her operative style to use the system most effectively and accurately. This chapter is a primer on front-end units for SNSs, describing how they work, when they don't work, and constraints they may impose by virtue of their engineering. Although a complete review of all technologies is impossible, our goal is to present a balanced overview of the most common and promising systems.

MULTIARTICULATED ARMS

Among the first three-dimensional digitizers adapted for use with an SNS were articulated arms that identified the orientation of the distal segment and location of its tip[5,12,15-17,20] (Fig. 2-1). The base of the arm is rigidly fixed, typically to the head immobilizer, thereby allowing head tracking (see below). Several arm segments of known length are attached at joints where sensors are fitted that determine the angle of the joint. When all the angles are known, the calculation of the location and orientation of the tip is determined by a computer. Sensors are

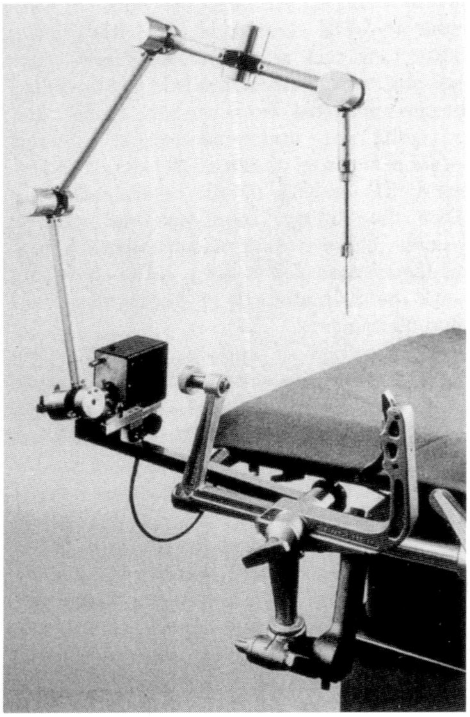

Figure 2-1. Mechanical stereotactic arm. These linked technologies use analog or digital sensors at each joint to deduce the location of the wand at its tip. Low cost and lack of line-of-sight constraints are among its benefits. These mechanically linked digitizers, however, tend to be cumbersome, analog sensors may drift, and the reach may be too limited.

usually potentiometers (analog) or digitizers (digital). The former are small and inexpensive but are subject to electrical "drift" that may result in erroneous localization information and require recalibration during the procedure. Digital sensors are not subject to drift, but greater accuracy requires larger, more expensive digitizers.

The principal advantages of these arms are that they are simple; do not require line-of-sight (see below), which is advantageous when using the surgical microscope; are an established technology; and some are approved for use as part of an SNS by the FDA. Unfortunately, they tend to be awkward to use since they drape over the surgeon's arm and are conceptually foreign as there is not a comparable instrument mechanically tethered to a point that is familiar to surgeons. If used in a sterile field, they must be covered with a sterile drape. Further, they are not readily adaptable for use with surgical instruments (bipolar, forceps, etc.) as the pointing device. Also, since these devices have limited length and orientations, it may not be possible to get the tip of the wand (especially along a desired trajectory) to a desired point in the surgical field during intracranial or spinal surgery. For these reasons, some investigators have switched to devices that do not rely on mechanical linkage.

SONIC SYSTEMS

A discussion of sonic SNSs is primarily of historic value since they represented one of the earliest technologies for surgical navigation.[4,10,11] One or more emitters were applied to a probe,[1-3] endoscope,[9] or microscope[4,10,11] to produce an

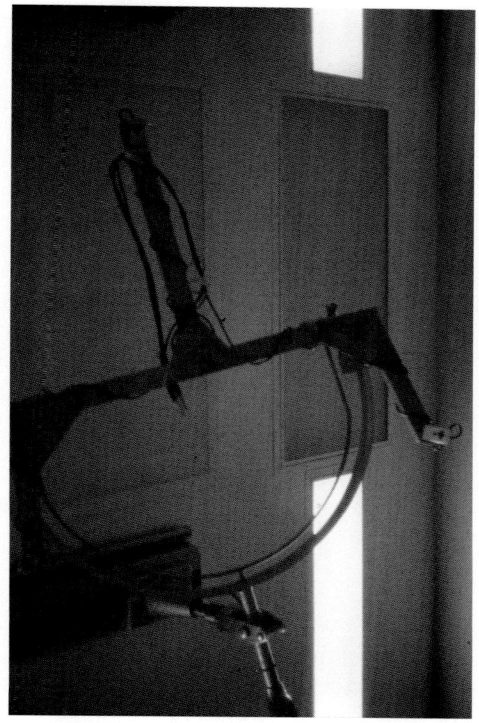

Figure 2-2. The stereotactic surgical microscope used three-dimensional sonic digitizers to determine the location of the operating microscope in space. This system was not mechanically linked, accurate, or inexpensive. It was subject to error from drafts and echoes and required line-of-sight between sources and receivers.

ultrasonic pulse that could be detected by an array of microphones fixed in a known configuration (Fig. 2-2). If the speed of sound was known, the time delay between production of the pulse and its detection by each microphone allowed the distances between emitter and microphones to be calculated.

The first such system used emitters fixed to a surgical microscope and a detector array fixed near the ceiling of the operating room.[4,10,11] Because of the long distances ("slant ranges") involved, prolonged sampling was necessary to achieve reasonable accuracy. This was possible, however, because the emitters were on a fixed object. Since the speed of sound varies with local temperatures as well as other factors, a direct determination was performed by firing a "pilot emitter" that had a known relationship to the microphone array. Echoes or reflections proved to be a source of spurious localization in some cases.

Development of a hand-held wand required several modifications to the stereotactic microscope schema[1-3] (Fig. 2-3). Long data acquisitions were not feasible, but this was found to be unnecessary if the detector was brought to within a meter of the wand. Although pilot emitters were used on early prototypes, using the inter-emitter distances on the wand itself produced an accurate determination of the local speed of sound. False echoes were eliminated by limiting the rate of firing so that all echoes dissipated by the time the next acquisition was made. Variations of wand systems include those with emitters on the wand and a microphone array near or mounted to the table and one with the microphones on the wand and the emitters on an array.

Sonic systems require line-of-sight between the emitters and all detectors. The principal advantages of sonic systems are that they are inexpensive, simple,

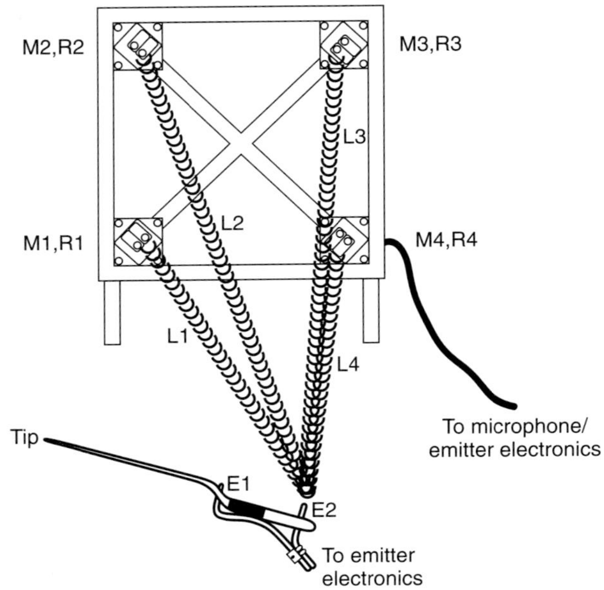

Figure 2-3. Adaptation of sonic technology to hand-held instruments required close placement of the receiving microphones and redesign of system electronics to minimize environmental factors except for drafts and ultrasonic noise. These systems still required line-of-sight and would fail if emitters got wet.

and robust. Compared to most front-end technologies, the cost of sonic digitizers is one half to one fourth of the cost for light-emitting diode three-dimensional digitizers. They require no alignment, have very large working volumes (typically 27 cubic feet), and can be set up rapidly, typically in 5 minutes or less. Also, since alignment is not critical and fragile cameras are not required, they are portable and hold up well in the operating room environment. Since the emitters are true point sources, localization of the source is accurate throughout a wide range of orientations (with respect to the microphone array) and precision can be improved by extending the duration of sampling. Emitters can be mounted on a wide array of instruments, making the localization process more natural.

Disadvantages of sonic systems include susceptibility to environmental noise and drafts. Although audible sounds (e.g., conversations and music) have no effect on sonic localization, ultrasonic interference from suction devices poses a problem and usually requires temporary occlusion of suction lumens in the operative field to optimize accuracy. Also, as noted earlier, the detector array must be in close proximity to the pointing instrument. Although table mounting the array may preclude use of scrub tables over the patient, the proximity of the detector has not been found to violate sterility of the operative field. The emitters currently in use are spark gaps and must not get wet during the procedure or they will fail to fire. Finally, although sonic systems are capable of uninterrupted firing, they emit an audible click when fired, which is annoying when used continuously. Therefore a point-and-shoot mode is typically used. At least one sonic SNS has

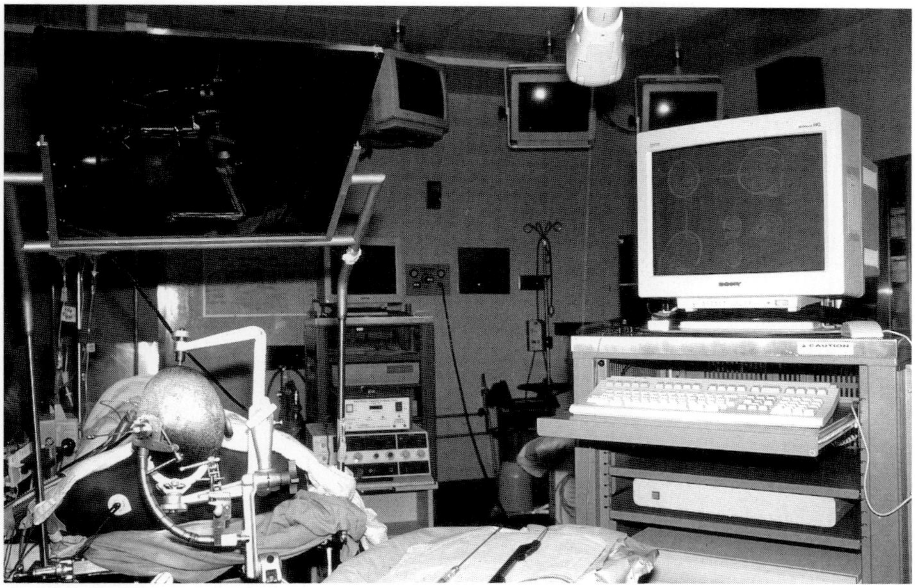

Figure 2-4. A commercially available SNS using sonic technology approved for cranial and spinal procedures. Head tracking is performed via a mechanical linkage between the patient's head and the detector array. The local speed of sound correction was based on the known distance between emitters on the wand.

received FDA approval for cranial and spinal use (Fig. 2-4). Most commercial sonic systems have converted to the optical technologies described below.

OPTICAL SYSTEMS

Light-Emitting Diode Systems

The light-emitting diodes (LEDs) typically used in SNSs emit near-infrared light that is invisible to the human eye but is detected by solid-state cameras, usually composed of linear or two-dimensional charge-coupled devices (CCDs) (similar in concept to those used in commercial camcorders).[7,14,18] These line-of-sight systems work silently and almost magically compared with mechanical arms or sonic systems. The emitters are usually pulsed or strobed to conserve emitter life, to identify which emitter is where, and to help differentiate the emitter from background light.

CCDs are quite sensitive to infrared energy and ideally suited as detectors for such systems. As with any optical camera, direct and reflected light is refracted and focused to form an image within the CCD camera. Instead of film, however, a multiplicity of tiny CCD sensors detect the infrared energy, which is then converted to electrical impulses that may remain digital for further signal processing or be converted to analog signals. CCD elements are arranged in either a single line (Fig. 2-5) or a two-dimensional array (Fig. 2-6).

CCD cameras in the operating room should be placed to avoid potential

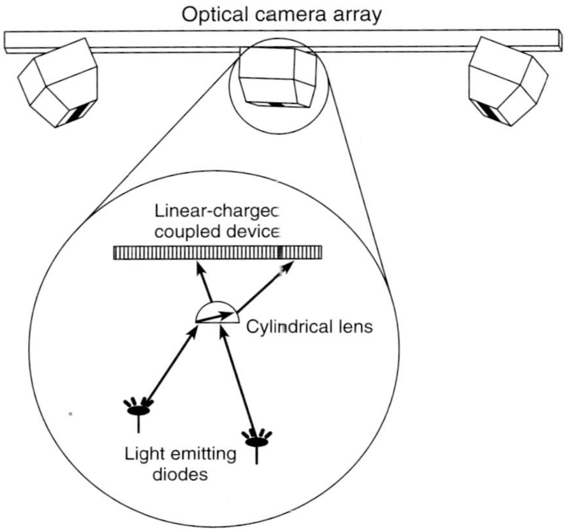

Figure 2-5. Diagram of an infrared optical system using three linear CCD cameras. These systems are silent and can readily provide continuous tracking of instruments equipped with LEDs. They require line-of-sight, are susceptible to interference from light sources, and linear cameras tend to be large and provide only the minimum information to localize an LED in space.

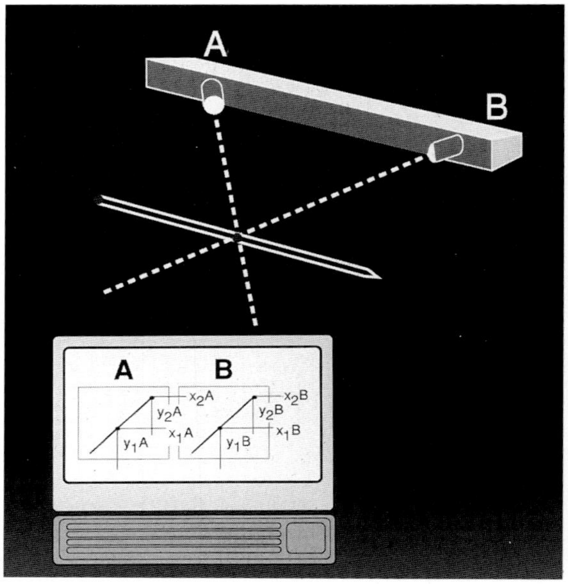

Figure 2-6. Emitters or reference points are viewed stereoscopically in optical systems using a pair of two-dimensional CCDs (passive or active infrared and machine vision). The principal advantages over linear systems are that they tend to be smaller, require a smaller line-of-sight corridor, and provide redundancy that may detect misalignments.

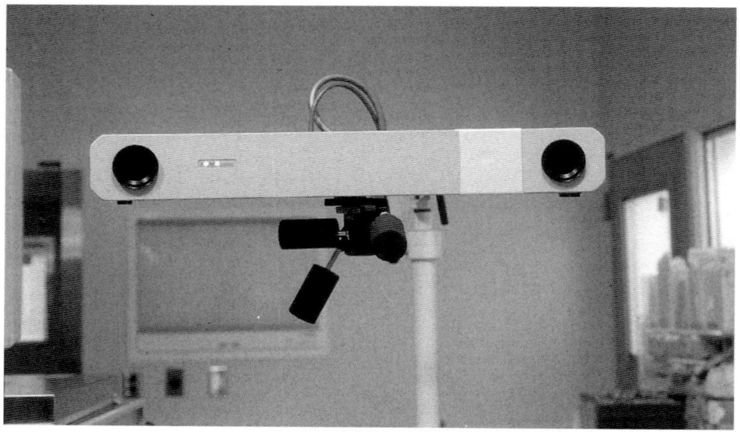

Figure 2-7. Commercially available camera using a pair of two-dimensional CCDs.

sources of interference from light sources. They are probably best situated so that they do not "look" directly at illuminated view boxes, sunlight, or the surgeon's headlight. At times intense operating room lights illuminate the operative field and may induce reflections that can also confuse the detection system.

Linear CCDs

One type of CCD camera for LED SNSs relies on tens of thousands of CCD elements situated in a linear arrangement for each sensor. A lens focuses infrared light from the LED on a limited number of these elements (see Fig. 2-5). Localization may then be accomplished in several ways, including picking the element with the strongest illumination, digital signal processing to minimize the effect of reflections, and conversion to an analog signal. Three or more of these linear CCD sensors are required to determine the three-dimensional coordinate of each emitter. Clearly, precise and stable alignment of cameras is a prerequisite of such systems.

Advantages of one-dimensional CCD systems include high resolution and precision although at considerable expense because of their limited production compared with their two-dimensional counterparts. Several commercially available FDA-approved SNSs use linear CCDs.

Two-Dimensional CCDs

In two-dimensional CCDs the CCD elements are positioned in a rectangular arrangement. Again, a lens distributes the LED emissions but in this case across the two-dimensional sensor. Similar detection techniques are used as described above (see Fig. 2-6). Only two sensors are required for this arrangement but alignment is again critical.

Commercially available sensors are relatively inexpensive and even consumer camcorders can be used. Resolution is poorer than with comparably priced linear devices unless special processing techniques are used that can provide better resolution. High-resolution two-dimensional CCDs are expensive, but the price is decreasing, even for those with digital transmission. Precise stable alignment remains critical unless on-site realignment capability is available. Several commercially available FDA-approved SNSs use two-dimensional CCDs (Fig. 2-7).

Position Sensing Device

Rather than using the discrete elements of two-dimensional CCDs, these are two-dimensional analog devices. Emitter position is determined by assuming that the electrical output in either dimension is proportionate to the location on that axis. Unfortunately, reflections severely distort the real vs. apparent position. Our experiments suggest that this is not a commercially viable device.

Passive Infrared Light

Similar cameras (linear or two dimensional) can be used, but instead of active emitters, an infrared light source illuminates the operative field and reflective spheres are mounted on the pointing device(s). The principal advantages of such a system are that instruments tagged with these spheres are wireless and in theory autoclavable, whereas some LED instruments require gas sterilization. By virtue of this design in which individual emitters cannot be strobed, passive reflectors all appear simultaneously to the cameras and thus large numbers of these devices can confuse the system; even probe orientation (i.e., pointing toward or away from the head) may not be easily determined. Sophisticated machine vision techniques may obviate these problems. Nonetheless, such systems are commercially available and have received FDA approval.

Passive Ultraviolet Light

Near-ultraviolet light can also be used to illuminate the surgical site. Fluorescent markers can then be used to absorb these frequencies of illumination and reradiate energy at visible frequency levels above ambient reflected visible light. The advantage is the markers are more easily distinguished from background data, the frequency (i.e., color) of re-irradiated light can be coded to define what marker is being imaged, and inexpensive color cameras can be used as detectors. Aside from alignment issues discussed above, work in our laboratory indicates that the major limitation of this approach is that ultraviolet radiation in this range is extremely fatiguing on the human eye and may be potentially dangerous.

Machine Vision

This system is entirely passive in the sense that pointing devices are passively detected by some type of camera system and special illumination systems are not required, although they are not specifically excluded.[6,19] In its purest sense, two or more video cameras (analog or digital) (Fig. 2-8) in a known geometric configuration are aimed at the surgical field. Surgical tools and even the surgical microscope are compared to a reference set of surgical tools of known geometries. Special passive markers may be used to assist recognition at strategic locations (Fig. 2-9). Once identified, best-fit calculations can be performed to determine the location and orientation of the instrument in space, even if partially obscured by the surgeon's hand

Still in the development stage, this system is probably the line-of-sight system of the future. In theory, any instrument could be used with minimal if any adaptation once geometries are entered into the computer's database. Front-end hardware is inexpensive unless extremely high-resolution color systems are used. Software development, however, is the most complex of any SNS front end and is typical of that used in sophisticated military applications.

MAGNETIC SYSTEMS

These systems use magnetic gradients or waves to provide localization information to appropriate sensors.[8,13] Aside from mechanical arms, this is the only other commercially available device not requiring line-of-sight (Fig. 2-10). In theory, these systems are not hampered by acoustic and optical obstructions such

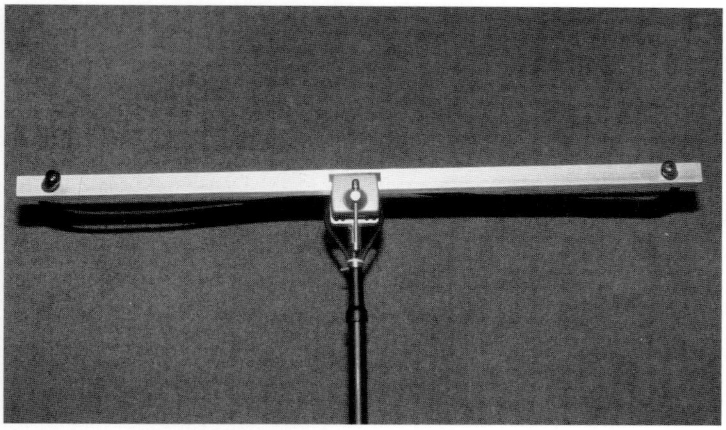

Figure 2-8. Prototype machine vision camera developed in our laboratory.

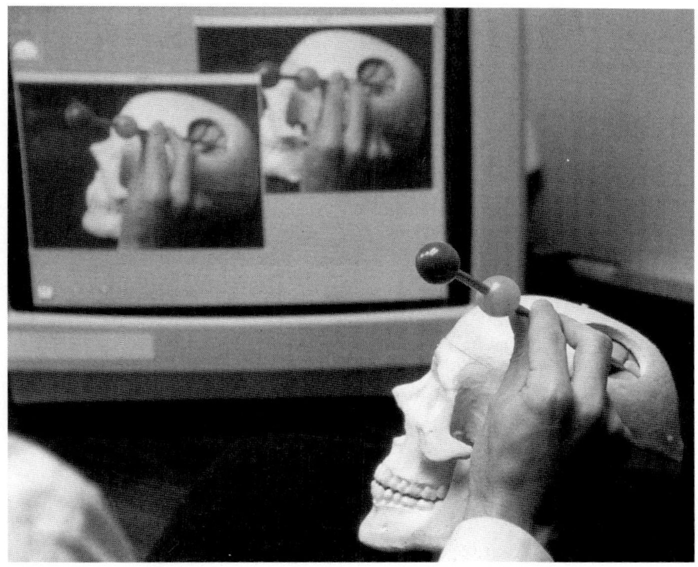

Figure 2-9. Images delivered by the machine vision camera shown in Fig. 2-8. Both windows provide real-time visualization of an image provided by the respective cameras.

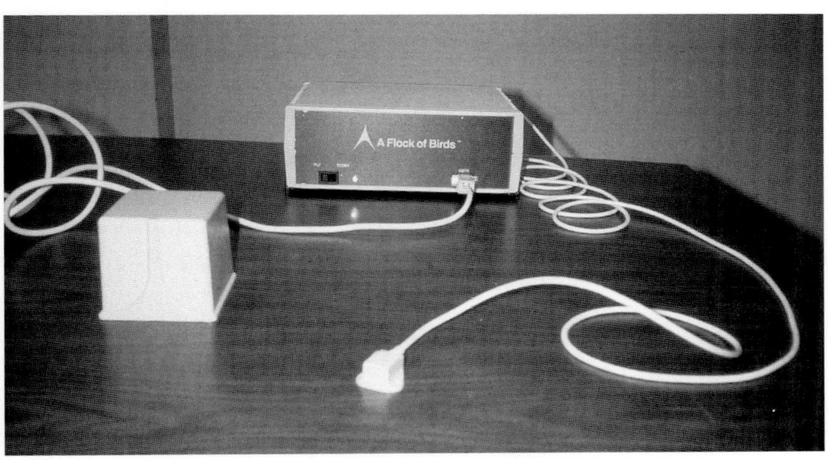

Figure 2-10. Commercially available magnetic three-dimensional digitizer. The smallest device is the transmitter and the white cube is the detector. These systems do not require line-of-sight, but accuracy may be distorted by movement of metal objects near the surgical field.

as drapes and even human limbs. Metal objects common to the surgical field, however, can prove formidable obstacles to optimal use of these systems, although optimization of frequencies may minimize this problem. At least one commercially available system in the United States uses magnetic technology in conjunction with a stereotaxy frame.

Direct Current

Once again, a linear relationship exists between what is detected and the assumed location. Unfortunately, metallic objects in or near the line-of-sight may result in spurious localization of the emitter. Electrical drift is also a consideration. This system is not commercially available at this time in the United States.

Alternating Current

By producing a magnetic field that alternates, interference from magnetic objects and drift can be minimized, but not eliminated. The one commercial version of this system available in the United States is restricted to use with a specific stereotaxy frame that results in both relative predictability of perturbations of the magnetic field and corroboration of results with frame guidance. Use of only nonmetallic surgical instruments would improve the feasibility of such systems substantially. If used in an MR imager, a complex integration of systems would be necessary unless the magnet was off, such as is feasible with resistive magnet systems.

FUTURE TECHNOLOGIES

A host of new front-end systems may result in improved SNS localization technologies. Among these, robotic applications using integrated sensors and/or external sensors to determine patient or probe position are undergoing development.

Robotics

The integration of robotic technology into the neurosurgical operating room began with the adaptation of industrial robots to stereotactic tasks. Kwoh et al.[21,22] and Young and Kwoh[23,24] coupled a conventional stereotactic base ring with a PUMA 260 robot, using the latter to replace the stereotactic arc in more efficiently positioning an end-effector probe. A similar implementation was used by Drake et al.[25-27] in a small series of children with deep benign astrocytomas.

Development of robotic instrumentation specifically designed for operative tasks has been the focus of both the Grenoble team led by Benabid et al.[28-33] and the Minerva project based in Lausanne.[34-37] These investigators have demonstrated the feasibility, reliability, and efficiency of robotic assistance, and the former system has been used extensively in clinical use, principally for stereotactic biopsies.

The most recent robotic development has been in microscope support sys-

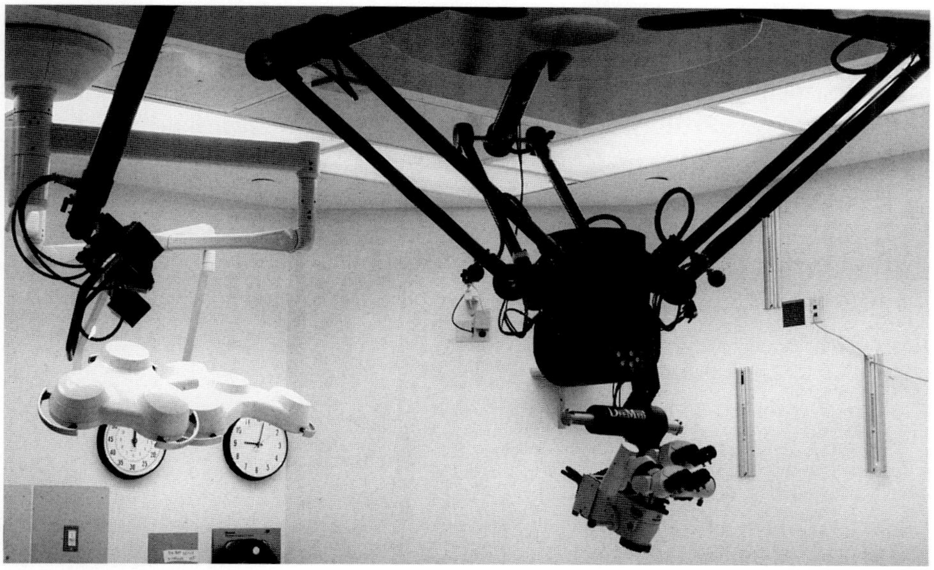

Figure 2-11. The SurgiScope system (Elekta AB, Stockholm) is a ceiling-mounted, robotic microscope holder, efficiently combining the functionalities of stereotactic guidance and instrument manipulation. (From Maciunas RJ, Alexander E III, eds. Advanced Neurosurgical Navigation. New York: Thieme Medical Publishers [in press].)

tems. The merging of the roboticized microscope holder developed in Grenoble (Dee Med MSS) with frameless coregistration methodology has produced the SurgiScope stereotactic system (Elekta AB, Stockholm, Sweden)[31,38,39] (Fig. 2-11). The MKM microscope system (Carl Zeiss, Inc., Oberkochen, Germany)[40,41] and the Telerobot system described by Giorgi et al.[42] are similar robotic devices. All of these have both the navigational capabilities of non-robotic "frameless" devices and the capability of micromanipulating a surgical tool. These combined functionalities have the potential to some day automate certain surgical tasks, filter out unwanted physiologic movement, enable movement at otherwise unachievable scale, and even manipulate tissue remotely.

Others

Accelerometers, similar to those used in automobile air bag systems, could provide location information without line-of-sight or magnetic constraints if users were willing to place it back in a reference holder after a few minutes of use. Other techniques using radio waves and even the global positioning system are being considered.

COMMON PITFALLS

Head Tracking

Virtually all SNSs allow the surgeon to change the position of the patient after initial registration (i.e., raise-lower, rotate, or pitch the head of the bed). To do this without necessitating reregistration, which may be tedious or impossible, some means of keeping track of the position of the head with respect to the detection mechanism is required. Common strategies include a reference directly affixed to the head or to the head-holder or by a mechanical linkage of the primary sensor to the head-holder or the operating table. Unfortunately, none of these systems is without fault, either in terms of inconvenience or accuracy.

The ideal head tracking system accurately and continuously follows all subtle movements of the head, transparently adjusting the initial registration throughout the entire surgical procedure in a noninvasive fashion, requiring no special head fixation device, and posing no health risk to personnel in the room. To date, such a system does not exist.

Table-Mounted Detectors

The principal disadvantage of table-mounted detectors is maintaining rigid mechanical coupling of the head to the operating room table and in turn the detector. Detectors mounted to the operating room table do move by virtue of their own weight, although well-designed systems move very little.

The obvious rule of "the more bracing the better" seems to hold. Our laboratory experiments show that detectors of identical weight are more accurate if two supports are used to span the bed rather than a single support. Extreme bracing seems to provide nearly perfect registration but precludes use of common three-point head fixation devices. Also, since the detector must be mounted to the head segment, a nonsterile device is close to the head. For various reasons, this detector location may not be optimal for accurate sensitivity.

The primary advantage of table-mounted detectors is that they do not require secondary transformations or calculations that may limit accuracy, and a head tracking device to be monitored by a detector does not restrict head position. They are also simple and inexpensive. Such systems are currently used with sonic, optical, and electromagnetic systems.

Surgical style must be modified so that forces that may displace the head with respect to the table are avoided. For this reason, only self-retaining scalp retractors should be used that do not pull the head and draping must not be under tension when using table-mounted detectors.

Table-Mounted References

A lightweight reference can be mounted to the table with a remote sensor. The disadvantages are head-to-table-to-reference coupling along with the need for secondary transformations in some systems. Table-mounted references offer little advantage over fixation-mounted reference systems aside from some increased flexibility in reference placement.

Head-Holder Mounts

This approach removes several linkages that are assumed to be rigid (but may not be) for table-mounted systems, specifically joints between the head-holder

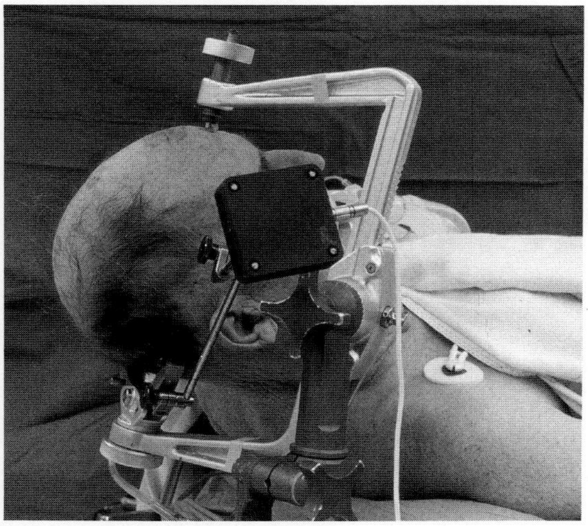

Figure 2-12. Optical head reference mounted to the C-arm of a Mayfield head clamp. Other means of tracking head movement include mounting reference to body of clamp or patient table or mounting the detector itself to one of these structures. Accuracy relies on ongoing lack of movement between head and these references so as to avoid drift. The farther away from the head the more likely there may be movement.

and its table attachment, the junction with the table, and the junction between the table and the detector or reference. By directly attaching to the head-holder most, but not all, potential movement between the head and the front-end system is eliminated, making head tracking generally more accurate. Common three-point fixation devices, however, still allow head movement with respect to the main structural frame. As such, the caveats about scalp retraction and draping mentioned above should still be observed even when using these systems. Head-holder mounts are most commonly used for some arms and electromagnetic systems.

Head-Holder References

This approach provides the advantages of head-holder mounting for systems that require the detector to be placed remotely, such as sonic and most optical systems. When using the popular Mayfield head fixation device, however, most systems mount to the body or attachment portions of the device, which may allow some head movement (principally rotational) with respect to the tracker. One commercial system attaches the head tracking device directly to the C-arm portion of a Mayfield fixation device. This approach virtually eliminates issues of head movement (Fig. 2-12). The principal disadvantages are that line-of-sight must be maintained between the detector and the pointing device as well as the detector and the reference and a second mathematical transformation is required that may reduce accuracy.

LINE-OF-SIGHT

Sonic and optical systems require an unimpeded line-of-sight between emitters or, for passive systems, the object(s) to be detected and the detectors (e.g., microphones and cameras). For sonic systems, this means no obstruction at all, whereas for optical systems, thin transparent materials may be acceptable unless they introduce refraction or reflections. This requirement imposes several constraints that some surgeons find objectionable, such as restricted positioning of the patient, detectors, and references and arrangement of other equipment or personnel that may eclipse the view of the detector to the tracked object(s).

Detectors may be placed overhead, but this arrangement often minimizes accuracy when using a vertical surgical trajectory. Typically it is best to have the long axis of the reference points (e.g., emitters) parallel to that of the plane of the detectors. Horizontally mounted detectors have similar problems with horizontal trajectories as well as frequent obstructions by drapes, limbs, and other objects moving through or near the surgical field. Probably the best arrangement is for the detectors to be elevated and horizontally displaced, thereby having reasonable accuracy from most applications and adjusting the detector for its best "view" of the surgical field and head tracking reference. However, some systems can only view from a horizontal or vertical position, which may impose serious constraints on the surgical approach for best system accuracy.

An extreme but valid example of how line-of-sight can limit orientation options occurs in optical SNSs with two detectors and two or three colinear reference points on the probe in the special circumstance when the probe's reference points are in line with one of the cameras. There is ambiguity as to whether the emitters are truly eclipsing each other or whether detection of the eclipsed point(s) is due to obstruction of the line-of-sight by some other object. The only safe option is for the SNS to declare a failure to localize.

SUMMARY

SNS technology continues to evolve. The systems commonly used today will likely evolve into totally different technologies in the near future. All present systems and those under development have limitations and advantages that potential users should be aware of to ensure the greatest surgical benefit.

References

1. Barnett GH, Kormos DW, Steiner CP, Piraino D, Weisenberger J, Hajjar F, Wood C, McNally J. Frameless stereotaxy using a sonic digitizing wand: Development and adaptation to the Picker ViStar medical imaging system. In Maciunas RJ, ed. Interactive Image-Guided Neurosurgery. Park Ridge, Ill.: American Association of Neurological Surgeons, 1993, pp 113-119.
2. Barnett GH, Kormos DW, Steiner CP, Weisenberger J. Intraoperative localization using an armless, frameless stereotactic wand. J Neurosurg 78:510-514, 1993.
3. Barnett GH, Kormos DW, Steiner CP, Weisenberger J. Use of a frameless, armless stereotactic wand for brain tumor localization with 2-D and 3-D neuroimaging. Neurosurgery 33:674-678, 1993.
4. Friets EM, Strohbehn JW, Hatch JF, Roberts DW. A frameless stereotaxic operating microscope for neurosurgery. IEEE Trans Biomed Eng 36:608-617, 1989.
5. Guthrie BL, Adler JR. Frameless stereotaxy: Computer interactive neurosurgery. Perspect Neurol Surg 2(1):1-19, 1991.
6. Heilbrun MP, Koehler S, McDonald P, Peters W, Sieminow V, Wiker C. Implementation of a machine vision method for stereotactic localization and guidance. In Maciunas RJ, ed. Interactive Image-Guided Neurosurgery. Park Ridge, Ill.: American Association of Neurological Surgeons, 1993.
7. Maciunas RJ, Galloway RL Jr, Fitzpatrick JM, Mandava VR, Edwards LA, Allen GS. A universal system for interactive image-directed neurosurgery. Stereotact Funct Neurosurg 58:108-113, 1992.
8. Manwaring KH. Magnetic field guided endoscopic dissection through a burr hole may avoid more invasive craniotomies—A preliminary report. Acta Neurochir Suppl 61:34-39, 1994.

9. Rhoten RP, Luciano M, Barnett GH. Computer-assisted neuro-endoscopy (CANE). Neurosurgery 40: 635-638, 1996.
10. Roberts DW, Strohbehn JW, Friets EM, Kettenberger J, Hartov A. The stereotactic operating microscope: Accuracy refinement and clinical experience. Acta Neurochir Suppl 46:112-114, 1989.
11. Roberts DW, Strohbehn JW, Hatch JF, Murray W, Kettenberger H. A frameless stereotaxic integration of computerized tomographic imaging and the operating microscope. J Neurosurg 65:545-549, 1986.
12. Watanabe E, Watanabe T, Manaka S, Mayanagi Y, Takakura K. Three-dimensional digitizer (neuronavigator): New equipment for computed tomography-guided stereotaxic surgery. Surg Neurol 27:543-547, 1987.
13. Kato A, Yoshimine T, Hauakawa T, Tomita Y, Ikeda T, Mitomo M, Harada K, Mogami H. A frameless, armless navigational system for computer-assisted neurosurgery [Technical note]. J Neurosurg 74:845-849, 1991.
14. Ryan MJ, Erickson RK, Levin DN, Pelizzari CA, Macdonald RL, Dohrmann GJ. Frameless stereotaxy with real-time tracking of patient head movement and retrospective patient-image registration. J Neurosurg 85:287-292, 1996.
15. Golfinos JG, Fitzpatrick BC, Smith LR, Spetzler RF. Clinical use of a frameless stereotactic arm: Results in 325 cases. J Neurosurg 83:197-205, 1995.
16. Olivier A, Germano IM, Cukiert A, Peters T. Frameless stereotaxy for surgery of the epilepsies: Preliminary experience. J Neurosurg 81:629-633, 1994.
17. Doshi PK, Lemieux L, Fish DR, Shorvon SD, Harkness WH, Thomas DG. Frameless stereotaxy and interactive neurosurgery with the ISG viewing wand. Acta Neurochir Suppl 64:49-53, 1995.
18. Smith KR, Frank KJ, Bucholz RD. The NeuroStation—A highly accurate, minimally invasive solution to frameless stereotactic neurosurgery. Comput Med Imaging Graph 18:247-256, 1994.
19. Heilbrun MP, McDonald P, Wiker C, Koehler S, Peters W. Stereotactic localization and guidance using a machine vision technique. Stereotact Funct Neurosurg 58:94-98, 1992.
20. Guthrie BL, Adler JR Jr. Computer-assisted preoperative planning, interactive surgery, and frameless stereotaxy. Clin Neurosurg 38:112-131, 1992.
21. Kwoh YS. Special stereotactic technique: Robotic methods applied to stereotactic surgery. In Heilbrun MP, ed. Stereotactic Neurosurgery. Baltimore: Williams & Wilkins, 1988, pp 219-226.
22. Kwoh YS, Hou J, Jonckheere EA, Hayati S. A robot with improved absolute positioning accuracy for stereotactic brain surgery. IEEE Trans Biomed Eng 35:153-160, 1988.
23. Young RF. Application of robotics to stereotactic neurosurgery. Neurol Res 9:123-128, 1987.
24. Young RF, Kwoh YS. Robotic-aided surgery. In Kelly PJ, Kall BA, eds. Computers in Stereotactic Neurosurgery. Boston: Blackwell, 1992, pp 320-329.
25. Drake JM, Joy M, Goldenberg A, Kreindler D. Computer- and robot-assisted resection of thalamic astrocytomas in children. Neurosurgery 29:27-31, 1991.
26. Drake JM, Prudencio J, Holowka S. A comparison of a PUMA robotic system and the ISG Viewing Wand for neurosurgery. In Maciunas RJ, ed. Interactive Image-Guided Neurosurgery. Park Ridge, Ill.: American Association of Neurological Surgeons, 1993, pp 121-133.
27. Drake JM, Prudencio J, Holowaka S, Rutka JT, Hoffman HJ, Humphreys RP. Frameless stereotaxy in children. Pediatr Neurosurg 20:152-159, 1994.
28. Benabid AL. A routine stereotactic procedure in 2003. Neurosurgery 33:660-662, 1993.
29. Benabid AL, Cinquin P, Lavallée S, Le Bas JF, Demongeot J, Rougemont J. Computer-driven robot for stereotactic surgery connected to CT scan and magnetic resonance imaging: Technological design and preliminary results. Appl Neurophysiol 50:153-154, 1987.
30. Benabid AL, Hoffman D, Lavallée S, Cinquin P, Demongeot J, Le Bas JF, Danel F. Is there any future for robots in neurosurgery? In Symon L, ed. Advances and Technical Standards in Neurosurgery. Wien: Springer, 1991, pp 3-45.
31. Benabid AL, Hoffmann D, Munari C, Le Bas JF. Surgical robots. In Cohen AR, Haines SJ, eds. Minimally Invasive Techniques in Neurosurgery. Baltimore: Williams & Wilkins, 1995, pp 85-97.
32. Benabid AL, Lavallée S, Hoffman D, Cinquin P, Demongeot J, Danel F. Computer-driven robot for stereotactic neurosurgery. In Kelly PJ, Kall BA, eds. Computers in Stereotactic Neurosurgery. Boston: Blackwell, 1992, pp 330-342.
33. Benabid AL, Lavallée S, Hoffman D, Cinquin P, Demongeot J, Danel F. Potential use of robots in endoscopic neurosurgery. Acta Neurochir Suppl (Wien) 54:93-97, 1992.
34. Fankhauser H, Glauser D, Flury P, Piguet Y, Epitaux M, Favre J, Meuli RA. Robot for CT-guided stereotactic neurosurgery. Stereotact Funct Neurosurg 63:93-98, 1994.
35. Glauser D, Flury P, Durr PH, et al. Configuration of a robot dedicated to stereotactic surgery. Stereotact Funct Neurosurg 54,55:468-470, 1990.

36. Glauser D, Fankhauser H, Epitaux M, Hefti J-L, Jaccottet A. Neurosurgical robot Minerva: First results and current developments. J Image Guided Surg 1:266-272, 1995.
37. Koyama H, Uchida T, Funakubo H, Takakura K, Fankhauser J. Development of a new microsurgical robot for stereotactic neurosurgery. Stereotact Funct Neurosurg 54,55:462-467, 1990.
38. Marinov M, Roberts D. Interactive image-guided cranial neurosurgery using the SurgiScope. Bulg Neurosurg 4:9-18, 1996.
39. Roberts DW, Darcey TM. The evaluation and image-guided surgical treatment of the patient with a medically intractable seizure disorder. In Maciunas RJ, ed. Clinical Frontiers of Interactive Image-Guided Neurosurgery. Philadelphia: WB Saunders, 1996, pp 215-227.
40. Pillay PK. Image-guided stereotactic neurosurgery with the multicoordinate manipulator microscope. Surg Neurol 47:171-177, 1997.
41. Wirtz CR, Bonsanto MM, Knauth M, Tronnier VM, Albert FK, Staubert A. Intraoperative magnetic resonance imaging to update interactive navigation in neurosurgery: Method and preliminary experience. Comp Aid Surg 2:172-179, 1997.
42. Giorgi C, Eisenberg H, Costi G, Gallo E, Garibotto G, Casolino DS. Robot-assisted microscope for neurosurgery. J Image Guided Surg 1:158-163, 1995.

3

Target and Trajectory Guidance

Charles P. Steiner, B.S. • Gene H. Barnett, M.D. • Joseph P. Weisenberger, R.T.

Image-guided frame stereotaxy permits accurate guidance to image-derived targets and can readily do so along predefined surgical trajectories.[1-3] Frame stereotaxy systems have had limited application in procedures such as craniotomy[4-9] because many neurosurgeons find these devices cumbersome and logistically difficult to use for surgical guidance. Additionally, the ability of frame stereotaxy systems alone to provide localization and orientation information in real time is, at best, limited.

In contrast, interactive surgical navigational systems (SNSs) are adept at showing the location and orientation of an instrument during surgery on image data obtained preoperatively.[10-13] Unlike image-guided frame stereotaxy, however, the ability of SNSs to guide the surgeon to predefined targets along prescribed trajectories has been typically limited and awkward.

Although most SNSs readily identify tip position and orientation of a pointing device (e.g., wand), they do not readily provide intuitive access to a predefined target or replicate a desired trajectory. The development of a target and trajectory guidance system should help extend the applications of SNSs beyond craniotomy since it facilitates guidance to small, deep intracranial structures.[14] A method of target and trajectory guidance will be presented that has been proved to be simple, reliable, and accurate.

SYSTEM DESCRIPTION AND REQUIREMENTS

Target and trajectory guidance routines were developed as enhancements for the prototype computer-assisted minimally invasive surgery (CAMIS) system at The Center for Computer-Assisted Surgery in The Cleveland Clinic Foundation's Department of Neurosurgery. This SNS has a modular design and presently uses an infrared optical three-dimensional digitizer with dual two-dimensional charge-coupled device cameras and DEC Alpha Station 5000 workstation. The image is displayed on 20-inch RGB monitors and a prototype head-mounted display.

The software architecture of CAMIS incorporates an open toolkit methodology that allows for rapid prototyping of new features, typically on the order of hours as opposed to weeks. The fine tuning of new techniques can be performed on a large collection of phantoms or in the operating room while providing adequate backup mechanisms.

The target and trajectory guidance system design concept was to create a methodology that fulfilled the following criteria:

- The ability to select one or more targets
- The option to predefine one or more trajectory(ies) to reach the target
- The ability to select the entry point from image data or wand location
- Will provide depth information from wand tip to target slice
- Will visually provide reorientation information
- Will have automatic operation capabilities at surgery
- Can be portable to any SNS

Our approach to target guidance was to logically extend a previously designed method[10,11] to "look beyond" the physical limits of a navigational probe to the view(s) at a defined depth. This would require a mechanism to select targets and entries in three-dimensional space as well as a display interface to correctly describe one's current orientation relative to the preselected target.

LOCALIZATION AND ORIENTATION

The CAMIS system provides two display motifs. A triplanar display simultaneously shows three orthogonal images with a common vertex (i.e., images parallel to coronal, sagittal, and transverse planes) and is typically used at surgery for purposes of real-time localization (Fig. 3-1). The manual selection of this vertex can be accomplished through the use of a mouse cursor, the localizing wand, or slider controls on screen. Placing the cursor over a point on any of the three orthogonal images and pressing a mouse button cause the system to extract and display the two other images that are perpendicular to the current image and parallel to the principal axis of the data set. This process can also be used to browse through the image data and to select voxel coordinates for storage, such as target and/or entry point selection.

The second display mode of the CAMIS system is where images are extracted based on the orientation of the pointing device (typically a hand-held wand). The primary image obtained is perpendicular to the axis of the pointing device with the position of the pointer displayed in the center of this image (surgeon's view). The rotation corresponds to the view of the operator down the wand axis, and the default depth is at the tip of the localizing wand. The distance or depth from the tip of the wand to the surgeon's view can be "pushed" deeper or "pulled" more superficial by the surgeon using either a mouse or foot pedals. Two other images, both containing and displaying the localizing axis of the pointing device and perpendicular to each other, are generated in real time, thereby creating a display with three mutually orthogonal images ("multiplanar obliques," or MPO) although usually not parallel to the principal axis of the data set (Fig. 3-2).

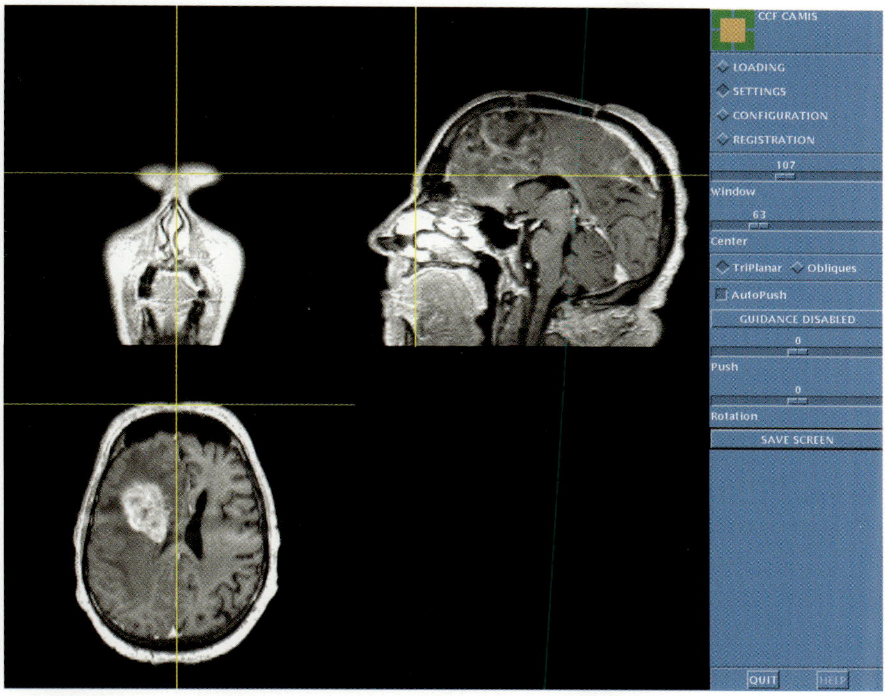

Figure 3-1. Triplanar display of coronal, sagittal, and transverse planes with a common vertex.

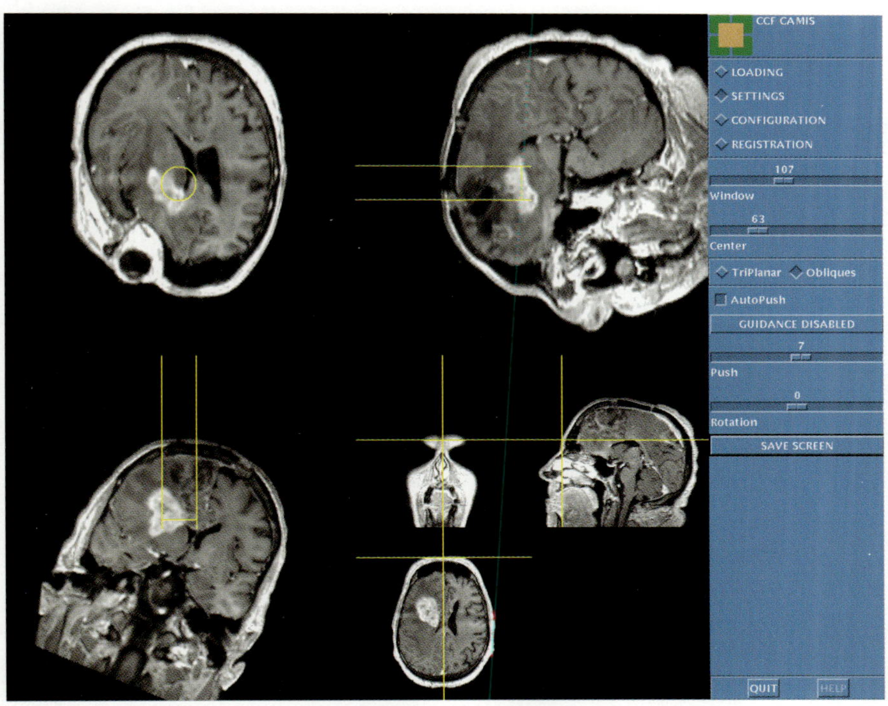

Figure 3-2. MPO display with mutually orthogonal images oriented based on the pointing device.

TARGET GUIDANCE
Target-Push

Target guidance on the CAMIS system uses this MPO display to show the relationships between predefined targets and/or trajectories with the actual wand trajectory (AWT). Once the AWT is determined by performing a localization, one of an indefinite number of parallel images must be reformatted to provide the surgeon's view image. The target-push feature of target guidance selects the one image that is perpendicular to the viewing axis and contains the predefined target (Fig. 3-3). The distance from the wand tip to the plane along the present wand trajectory is also calculated and presented.

Concentric Circles

Conceptually the target can be considered a 4 mm sphere centered at the predefined location. The intersection of any target-push plane with this sphere results in a circle with a 4 mm diameter. Similarly, the wand can be considered a cylinder of larger diameter, and its projection along the AWT necessarily results in another circle where it intersects the auto-push plane (Fig. 3-4). On this image the projected position of the pointing device is fixed as the center of the frame and is shown as a small circle in a user-selectable color. The position of the target is also shown on this image as a smaller circle in a different color. Should the boundaries of these circles overlap, the smaller circle is presented on top of the larger one.

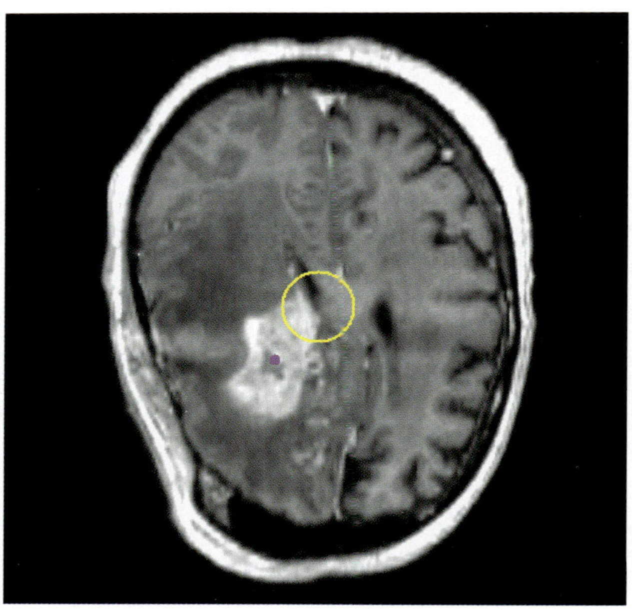

Figure 3-3. Surgeon's view oblique image perpendicular to the viewing axis containing the predefined target depicted as a solid circle.

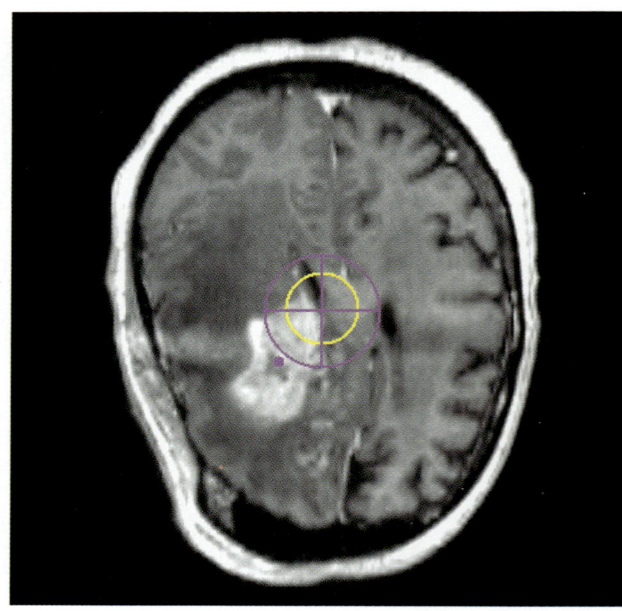

Figure 3-4. Surgeon's view oblique image perpendicular to the viewing axis containing the predefined target and probe position as two open circles.

Reorientation of the wand simply requires rotating or translating the wand to move the larger circle in a direction that will result in the two circles being concentric. Together, target-push and concentric circles are sufficient to provide guidance to a target when it is not necessary to follow a predefined trajectory.

TRAJECTORY GUIDANCE

Colinear Spheres and Concentric Circles

The addition of a trajectory guidance function provides information about the position and orientation of the pointing device with respect to a predefined surgical trajectory. Creation of the surgical trajectory requires the same tools discussed earlier for target selection for definition of an entry point. Together, target and entry points define a linear surgical trajectory. In theory, nonlinear trajectories could be approximated by a series of linear surgical trajectories.

The target is once again represented by a small sphere, and the intersection of the target sphere with the target-push plane generates a small circle. Although the previous paradigm for generating the AWT circle remains valid, an alternative mechanism is to create a virtual sphere at the tip of the wand. Its projection down the AWT such that its center is in the target-push plane will also result in a circle where sphere surface and plane intersect. Finally, a virtual sphere of larger diameter is envisioned at the entry point and is projected onto the target-push plane along a line parallel to the AWT, the intersection of which results in a third circle.

Appropriate wand rotations and translations of the wand are performed to make the three circles concentric. This is most easily achieved by first aligning the target circle with the entry circle using a series of rotations followed by wand translations to achieve concentricity. When the wand is appropriately oriented to access the target along this predefined trajectory, not only are the three auto-push circles concentric, but the three virtual spheres are colinear.

Trajectory Projection

Since some users find it difficult to align the circles to replicate a desired trajectory, an additional method of trajectory guidance called trajectory projection was devised. The MPO images contain the AWT, and as a result the surgical trajectory can be projected onto these images to provide information as to the necessary translations and rotations required to orient the pointing device along the surgical trajectory. When the pointing device is properly oriented, the image perpendicular to the pointing device will show three concentric circles, and the other two MPO images will show vectors aligned parallel and colinear with the pointing device's orientation (Fig. 3-5).

The alignment method used by most surgeons is to first rotate (tilt) the wand such that the AWT is parallel to the predefined surgical trajectory. Final alignment is achieved by wand translations until the AWT and surgical trajectory are colinear. The amount and direction of translation required is depicted by the separation of the parallel vectors displayed on the alternate images.

A

B

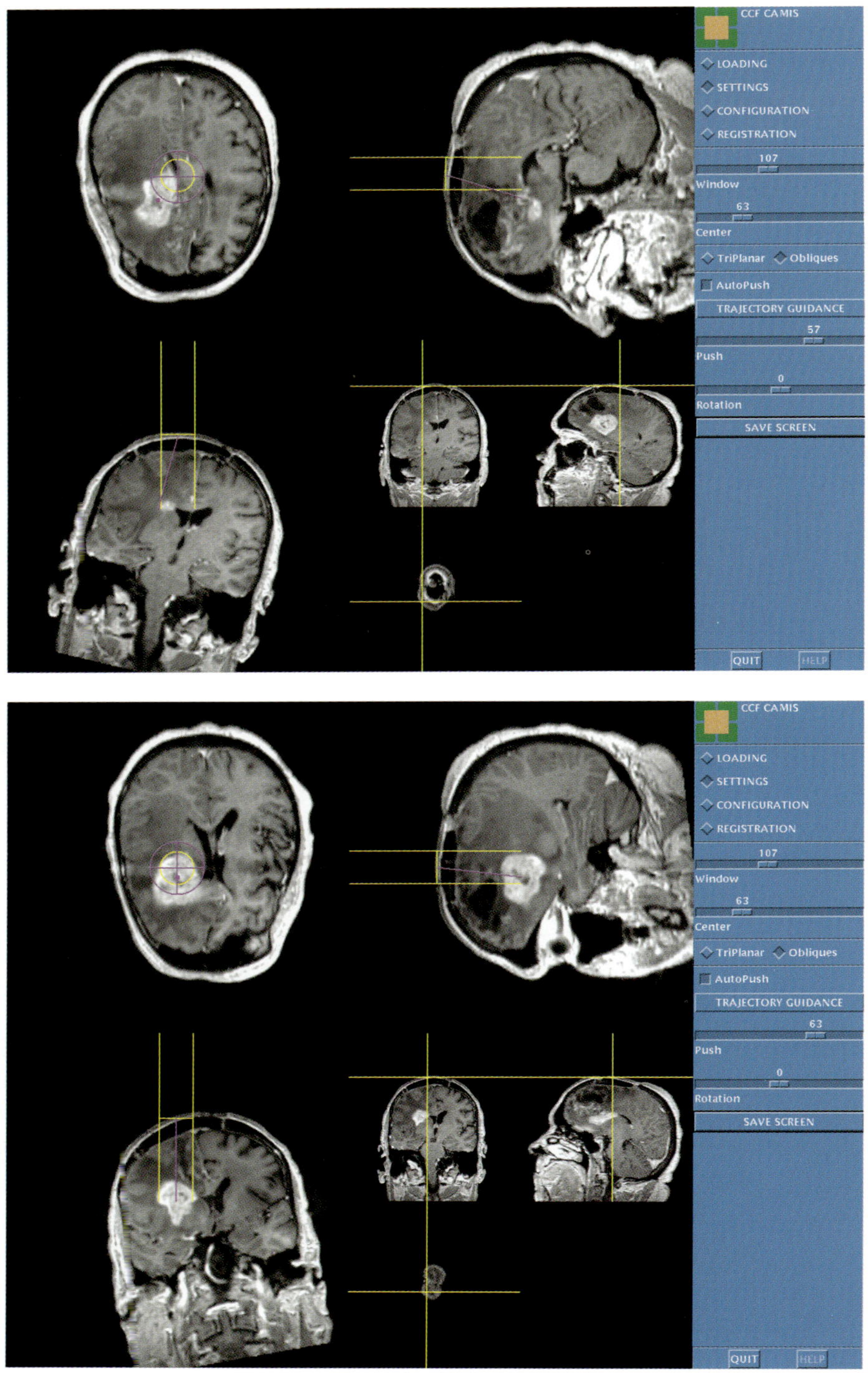

Figure 3-5. A, MPO display showing three concentric circles and alignment vectors, yellow indicating AWT and violet the intended trajectory. **B,** The initial alignment step is to make vectors parallel by vand rotations.

Continued.

C

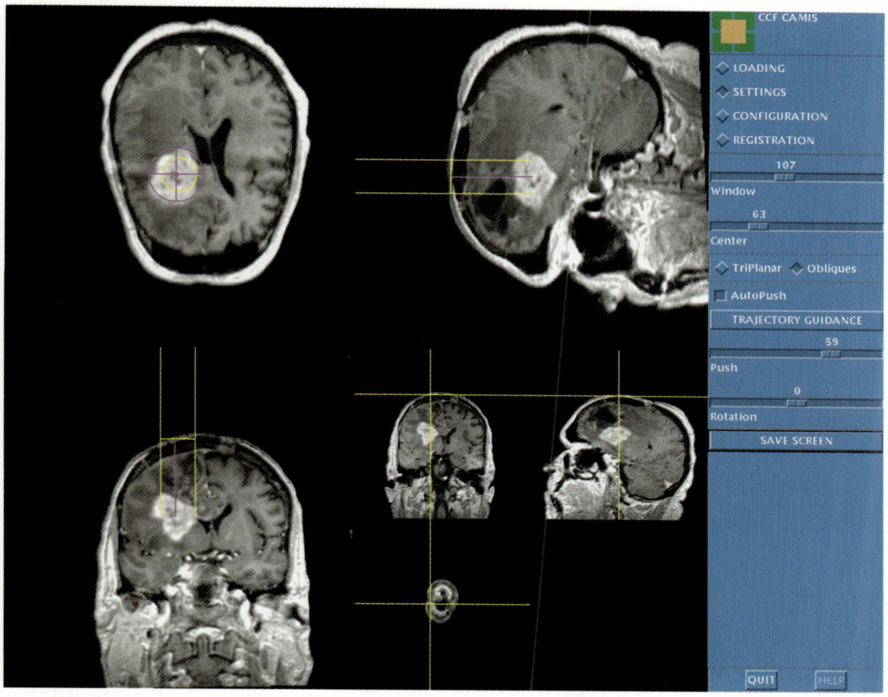

Figure 3-5, cont'd. C, The wand is then translated while maintaining the same rotational orientation. Colinear vectors result in concentricity of all circles, indicating correct surgical trajectory.

DISCUSSION

It became clear that virtually all of the design goals for this target and trajectory target system were easily met except for devising a simple, intuitive form of presentation to reorient the surgeon. Certainly the most direct approach would be to have robotic manipulation of the wand.[15-17] Although promising work on bringing robotic technology to the surgical arena has been reported, such a solution was beyond the scope of this project. Another approach considered was to create volume cutaways oriented such that one is looking down the AWT. This proved excessively computer intensive and to some confusing. An alternative was to represent the target as a solid seen through a semitransparent three-dimensional surface (Fig. 3-6, *A*). Similarly, an idealized trajectory could be projected and compared to the AWT. Unless the images were presented stereoscopically or from orthogonal views, however, it was difficult to visually interpret the depth of the object or even which side of the brain it was on (Fig. 3-6, *B*). Finally, this technique also proved too computationally intensive to provide useful information in a near real-time fashion. Instead of projecting the entry point onto the target-push plane, we attempted to show the entry point in a semitransparent plane parallel to the target-push plane. Although less computer intensive, this method proved too confusing to be reliably helpful.

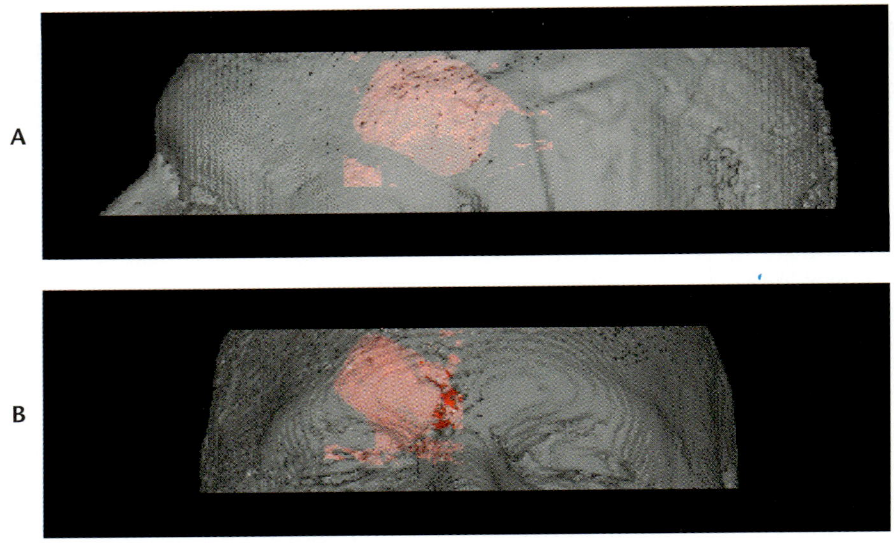

Figure 3-6. A, Three-dimensional representation of patient with the target depicted as a solid object viewable through a semitransparent surface (lateral view). **B,** Three-dimensional representation of patient with the target depicted as a solid object viewable through a semitransparent surface (anteroposterior view).

After seeing the MPO display of a CAMIS-derived system, Dr. M. Peter Heilbrun (personal communication, 1993) suggested the use of vectors to help define the direction and magnitude of reorientation for target and trajectory guidance. Initial results appeared promising since vectors could visually represent the necessary modifications to the AWT for target and/or trajectory guidance under most circumstances (Fig. 3-7). However, as the AWT approached the target or surgical trajectory, the vectors became so small that magnitude and direction of correction became unclear.

It became apparent that a similar visually intuitive display for target guidance could be achieved by representing the target and AWT as circles, the space and orientation between them providing the same information as the vector display. However, unlike vectors, as the AWT approaches the target, the reorientation information remains robust, aiding final reorientation of the wand resulting in concentric circles that denote being "on target." Although other shapes (triangles, squares, etc.) could have been used, rotational alignment of the vertices adds further computations but conveys no further information than that derived from circles. A similar paradigm developed to replicate trajectories with concentric circles and a triad of virtual colinear spheres proved less intuitive to some users while adopted easily by others. The use of trajectory projection onto the MPO planes serves as an additional or alternate guide when attempting to duplicate a predefined trajectory.

The purpose of any surgical tool is to provide function with ease of use. Computer interfaces suitable for operation by a programmer may be far too cumbersome to be used in the operating room.[16] This implementation of a surgical guidance tool incorporates the sophisticated features of a flight simulator while limiting the controls and configuration to those needed for surgery.[18,19]

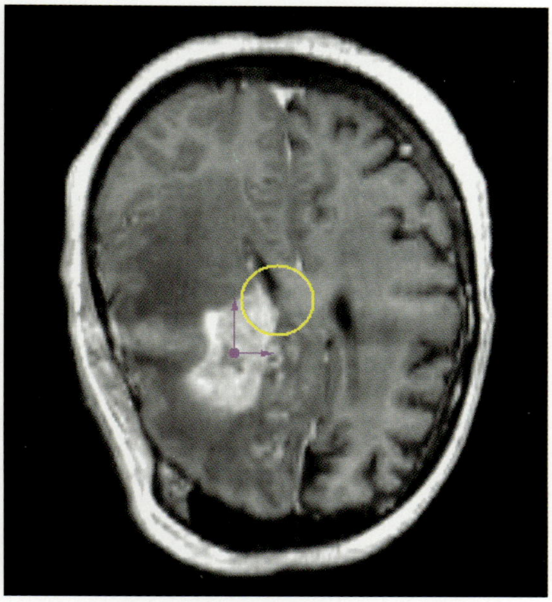

Figure 3-7. Surgeon's view oblique image perpendicular to the viewing axis containing direction vectors indicating the direction and magnitude of correction necessary to position the AWT along the idealized surgical trajectory.

Target guidance is the simplest function of this system, providing the information necessary to orient a pointing device in space such that it will intersect a predetermined target. The distance from the tip of the pointing device to the intersection of this target is displayed, information that is useful when approaching a subcortical lesion during craniotomy, and also allowing appropriate depth setting of instruments used for biopsy, cyst aspiration, depth electrodes, and similar applications. The use of trajectory guidance may refine the surgical approach such as when it is desired to avoid eloquent areas or it is necessary to pass through an identifiable structure en route to the target (e.g., foramen of Munroe for third ventriculostomy).

This implementation of target and trajectory guidance has been used in over 200 neurosurgical procedures and has proved a simple and accurate solution to the problem of guidance in surgery.

We wish to thank Dr. M. Peter Heilbrun for his insightful suggestions and Picker International for material support of this research.

References

1. Abernathy CD, Camacho A, Kelly PJ. Stereotactic suboccipital transcerebellar biopsy of pontine mass lesion. J Neurosurg 70:195, 1989.
2. Brown RA. A computerized tomography–computer graphics approach to stereotaxic localization. J Neurosurg 50:715-720, 1979.
3. Galloway RL, Maciunas RJ, Latimer JW. The accuracies of four stereotactic frame systems: An independent assessment. Biomed Instrum Technol 25:457-460, 1991.
4. Barnett GH, McKenzie RL, Ramos L, Palmer J. Nonvolumetric stereotaxy-assisted craniotomy. Results in 50 consecutive cases. Stereotac Funct Neurosurg 61:80-95, 1993.
5. Gomez H, Barnett GH, Estes ML, Palmer J, Magdinec M. Stereotactic and computer-assisted neurosurgery at the Cleveland Clinic. Review of 501 consecutive cases. Cleve Clin J Med 60:399-410, 1993.
6. Hassenbusch SJ, Anderson JS, Pillay PK. Brain tumor resection aided with markers placed using stereotaxis guided by magnetic resonance imaging and computed tomography. Neurosurgery 28:801-806, 1991.

7. Kelly PJ. Volumetric stereotactic surgical resection of intra-axial brain mass lesions. Mayo Clin Proc 63:1186, 1988.
8. Kelly PJ, Kall BA, Goerss S, Earnest F IV. Computer-assisted stereotaxic laser resection of intra-axial brain neoplasms. J Neurosurg 64:427, 1986.
9. Moore MR, Black PM, Ellenbogen R, Gall CM, Eldredge E. Stereotactic craniotomy: Methods and results using the Brown-Roberts-Wells stereotactic frame. Neurosurgery 25:572-577, 1989.
10. Barnett GH, Kormos DW, Steiner CP, Piraino D, Weisenberger J, Hajjar F, Wood C, McNally J. Frameless stereotaxy using a sonic digitizing wand: Development and adaptation to the Picker ViStar Medical Imaging System. In Maciunas RJ, ed. Interactive Image-Guided Neurosurgery. Park Ridge, Ill.: American Association of Neurological Surgeons, 1993, pp 113-119.
11. Barnett GH, Kormos DW, Steiner CP, Weisenberger J. Intraoperative localization using an armless, frameless stereotactic wand [Technical note]. J Neurosurg 78:510-514, 1993.
12. Guthrie BL, Adler JR. Frameless stereotaxy: Computer interactive neurosurgery. Perspect Neurol Surg 2(1):1-19, 1991.
13. Maciunas RJ. Yesterday's tomorrow: The clinical relevance of interactive image-guided surgery. Neurosurg Top 1:3-8, 1993.
14. Barnett GH, Steiner CP, Weisenberger J. Target and trajectory guidance for interactive surgical navigation systems. Stereotact Funct Neurosurg 66:91-95, 1996.
15. Buckingham R. Robotics in surgery. IEEE Rev 40:193-196, 1994.
16. Cohn MB. Surgical applications of milli-robots. J Robotic Syst 12:401-416, 1995.
17. Glauser D, Fankhauser H, Epitaux M, Hefti JL, Jaccottet A. Neurosurgical robot Minerva. First results and current developments. J Image Guided Surg 1:266-272, 1995.
18. Beardsley T. A new view for surgeons. Sci Am 271:100, 1994.
19. Swenson HN, Jones RD. Combat automation for airborne weapon systems: Man/machine interface trends and technologies. AGARD N93-28850, 1993, pp 11-54.

4

Pitfalls

Robert J. Maciunas, M.D.

Recent technologic advances have initiated an ongoing revolution in surgical navigation.[1-3] Digital tomographic imaging modalities produce three-dimensional mosaics of patient data that are exquisite in sensitivity and detail and can be used as spatially accurate maps of patients' anatomy. Novel methods of registering, or mapping, these image data sets onto patient anatomy as it exists in physical space have made stereotaxy frames obsolete for this purpose. Interactive localization devices have provided a means of three dimensionally digitizing the surgical work space, relating the imaging data sets and the patients' anatomy to surgeons and their instruments. Computers enable us to manipulate enormous volumes of information and display this information in a visually compelling and clinically meaningful manner. The incorporation of real-time intraoperative data into our calculations is rapidly expanding. Further advances in visualization and robotics promise to further transform the neurosurgical process in our lifetimes. These technologic developments are sufficiently profound so that clinical optimism about what is possible to accomplish via neurosurgical intervention has reached new heights.

All is for the best in this best of all possible worlds.
—Voltaire, *Candide*

Before we are overcome by the hubris of technologic advance and submit ourselves to the uncritical optimism of Dr. Pangloss, we should consider the inherent risks and limitations—whether resulting from imperfect manifestations of what can be accomplished with this technology, inherent limitations of the technologic solutions themselves, or limitations of our own abilities and judgment. It behooves us to become cognizant of the pitfalls of using surgical navigation technologies so that we might more safely, efficiently, and effectively make use of them to the benefit of those under our care.

There lives more faith in honest doubt, believe me, than in half the creeds.
—Tennyson, *In Memoriam*

These new technologies for surgical navigation and image analysis have been termed *interactive image-guided neurosurgery*. A system is composed of five fundamental elements: a method for registration of images and physical space, an interactive localization device, a computer with its requisite software interface and video display system, the integration of real-time feedback, and robotics.

The pitfalls of interactive image-guided neurosurgery may be analyzed by sequentially discussing the following nine topics: definition of accuracy, image acquisition, registration techniques, computers and software interfaces, interactive localization devices and intraoperative use, integration of real-time data, tissue displacement, robotics, and, finally, judgment and clinical experience.

DEFINITION OF ACCURACY

In an article on three-dimensional digitizers, T. Wohlers wrote a sidebar commentary entitled "How Accurate is Accurate?" In his comments, he states:

> Comparing the accuracy of 3-D digitizers can be confusing. The terms "accuracy," "precision," "resolution" and "repeatability" are often misused, misunderstood, misleading or just plain omitted. Buyer confusion also occurs when digitizer suppliers publish numbers related to the specific parts . . . that make up the system. This can be misleading. The precision of the system's mechanics does not reflect the accuracy of the process. In fact, the precision of the mechanics is . . . always better than the accuracy of the process.[4]

Because a stereotactic surgical guidance system is essentially a three-dimensional spatial digitizer coupled with mapping image space onto physical space, Wohlers' caveats are appropriate. Although the terms "stereotactic" and "submillimetric accuracy" are usually closely associated in the literature, the neurosurgeon must exercise considerable caution when dealing with such assumptions. A considered approach to the subject of stereotactic accuracy requires attention to the definition of terms.

First, a clear distinction must be drawn between three commonly misused terms: "unbiasedness" (or lack of skew), "precision," and "accuracy." A series of observations that tend to the true value are *unbiased*, or without skew. If these observations have considerable spread, however, they lack *precision*. A series of observations with little spread among them indicate precision, although they are biased, or skewed, if the observations tend to center at a value displaced from the true value. *Accuracy* encompasses both unbiasedness and precision: accurate measurements are both unbiased and precise, although inaccurate measurements may be biased, imprecise, or both.

Because the mechanical precision of a stereotaxy frame system determines how well it can return to a point, it may be thought of as being, in effect, a measure of how finely incremented a relative ruler the apparatus is. Finer increments on the verniers or better machining tolerances can be expected to improve mechanical precision. Incidentally, it is often this number that is advertised for stereotactic devices When a system of interactive image-guided surgery demonstrates a tendency to consistently arrive at a wrong answer, this skew results from mechanical bias in a precise system. The mechanical accuracy of a surgical navigation apparatus is the accuracy with which it can bring the tip of a straight probe to a given coordinate within the stereotactic coordinate system. This requires both mechanical unbiasedness and mechanical precision but does not include the effects of imaging technologies on localization. The standard performance specifications for cerebral stereotactic instruments issued by the American Society for Testing and Materials state that the mechanical accuracy of a stereotaxy frame-based system shall be submillimetric.

In addition to the mechanical limitations of the stereotaxy frame, the error associated with the many steps of stereotaxy (including imaging techniques, point selection, vector calculation, vernier settings, mechanical couplings, and adjustments) contributes to the final clinically relevant error. Human operator error is outside the realm of this discussion, although tedious calculations or taxing calibrations imposed by a system will make these errors more likely.

It is in the interest of the neurosurgeon to go beyond assessment of the mechanical accuracy of various surgical navigation systems (SNSs) to assess what may be termed the *application accuracy* of these devices. This is a measure of the accuracy of these devices when they are used in their real-world setting. It is separate and distinct from any mere measurement of the unbiasedness, precision, or accuracy associated with the machinery of the interactive image-guided system or with the stereotaxy frame construction itself.

When the application accuracy of various stereotaxy frames was analyzed, it was demonstrated that these devices had a millimetric to centimetric level of accuracy, which was strongly dependent on scan slice thickness.[5] Furthermore, the method of reporting this number was itself reassessed. What is reported is the mean of the errors and not the mean for all erroneous coordinates, which may end up being closer to the correct value if two oppositely incorrect values cancel each other out. Most previous reports had offered a mean value as the only numeric statement, and some reported a mean with the standard error of the mean. The standard error of the mean, however, is not relevant to this discussion and is smaller than the standard deviation (SD), which is the value that should be reported. Therefore the mean ± SD is the standard for reporting the application accuracy, or target localization error, values. Finally, a 99% confidence interval may be reported, which is equal to the mean plus three times the SD. This allows the surgeon to understand how the system will perform 99 times out of 100, a situation more analogous to the calculation of surgical clinical risk.

When assessing accuracy, three separate, distinct, and not directly related numbers must be assessed. The first is fiducial localization error. This is the accuracy of the system in finding the fiducial in an image or in physical space. The next is fiducial registration error. This is the residual error after registration of two images or of an image with physical space as judged by the sum of the root mean square error for the mapping of fiducial markers in one image set onto fiducial markers in another image set. This is mathematically related to the fiducial localization error and is a larger number. The most clinically important value is the target localization error, which is not directly correlated with the fiducial registration error, although it does track along with it and is often a larger number. The clinician wants to know the target localization error; instead, the SNS usually reports the fiducial registration error as a number for his or her approval. It is also important to realize that eliminating fiducials to decrease the fiducial registration error may create a seemingly good registration but a very poor target localization error. This occurs when the fiducials eliminated are those farthest from the surgical field, leaving only a group clustered near one another; if the target is distant from these fiducials, then the target localization error may worsen when the distant fiducial is eliminated, and the registration will be inadvertently skewed.

Ultimately, we are left with an operational definition of accuracy for image-assisted and image-guided surgery: an SNS is accurate (precise and unbiased) when the surgeon observes that the anatomic structure localized in physical space always corresponds to an appropriate address in image space.

> *It's hard to define, but I know it when I see it.*
> —To paraphrase Justice Potter Stewart
> in Jacobelis vs. Ohio, 378 US 184, 197 (1964)

This aphorism holds true so long as the surgeon is independently secure with an alternative way of defining a target; once the system is guiding rather than assisting the surgeon, full reliance is placed on its accuracy without a realistic capability for cross-checking with an anatomic landmark. This is especially true for pedicle screw placement, where cross-checking is possible for surface anatomy but not for deep pedicular anatomy and intraoperative fluoroscopy is used as an independent, intraoperative, real-time imaging modality to cross-check the system and perhaps to update the registration.

IMAGE ACQUISITION

The ability of neurodiagnostic images to form a satisfactory basis for surgical navigation is dependent on the images' spatial fidelity and precision and on their gray scale depth of discrimination. The capacity to provide true, point-to-point maps relies on the images having a consistent, predictable, and finely resolved matrix of spatial addresses for each pixel. The surgeon must be certain that the presumed location of a specific anatomic detail corresponds to its displayed position in the image.

Without a clearly defined relationship that can be relied on in all the parts of an image, misregistration or mismatching of individual points between images and physical space will occur. The images will not serve as true maps but will, in effect, be cartoons that give the qualitative appearance of an anatomic structure without quantitatively providing a reliable address for each point. An example of this is digital angiography. Here, the photomultiplier tube generating the image will introduce a series of spatial distortions on the image that are variable, depending on the status of the tube, patient, and radiographic settings. These distortions are not consistent, predictable, or reproducible, thus preventing engineers from producing an algorithm to correct spatial misrepresentations a priori. For this reason, digital angiography is used with circumspection in stereotactic radiosurgery and image-guided surgery.

Maciunas et al.[4] definitively established that slice thickness is an overriding factor in determining the maximal level of localization accuracy with a given imaging data set. This understanding has resulted in increasing clinical reliance on thinner slice thickness for navigation scans. Although in the early pioneering work of Kelly[6] and Kelly et al.,[7] a slice thickness of 8 to 10 mm was used, routine clinical use now presumes slices of 1 to 4 mm in thickness. The overlapping of slices has been abandoned because thinner slices are a more effective means of improving resolution and the overlapping itself presents considerable complexities for the computerized reconstruction of a three-dimensional database from the slices. Similarly, spacing between slices has been eliminated in CT with the advent of rapid spiral acquisitions with parallel-slice reconstruction. Thus no imaging information is lost in the gaps between slices. In MR images, spacing between slices is favored by radiologists and technicians because it prevents interslice interference. When used, the slices should be handled as if they were simply that much thicker than the thickness imaged. With the advent of three-dimensional fast acquisitions, this is becoming less of an issue. Some MR image scanners and pulse sequences are particularly prone to geometric distortions and to "wrapping" artifacts, thus limiting their use for surgical navigation. This has to be carefully and individually assessed by the clinician for each machine used.

The soft tissue discrimination of MR imaging is superior to that of CT, but on the other hand, MR images manifest geometric distortions caused by many factors. Geometrically distorted MR images can lead to errors in fiducial localization, fiducial registration, and intracranial target localization. The causes of geometric distortion in MR images are multifactorial.[8] Those resulting from the machine itself include inhomogeneity of the main magnetic field (Bo), nonlinear magnetic field gradients, imperfect slice or volume selection pulses, eddy currents caused by switching of the gradients, and magnetic debris caught up in the equipment. Those resulting from the patient include magnetic field susceptibility variations, chemical shifts, flow-induced distortions, and eddy currents cause by metallic objects, including stereotaxy frames or fiducial markers.[9]

The correction of distortions in MR images requires attention to manufacturer design and construction, site preparation, shimming of the magnet, selection of appropriate compromises for field and gradient strength, incorporation of flow-corrected MR angiographic pulse sequences, and avoidance of chemical shifts when selecting fiducial markers. A joint task force composed of neurosurgery and radiology department representatives as well as other interested parties is necessary to properly deal with these concerns.

The rectification of distortions in MR images by universally applicable computer algorithms has been described by two groups of investigators from Vanderbilt and Stanford universities.[8,10-13] Both groups advocate postprocessing of additional scans. The technique used by the Stanford University group is elegant but limited because it requires considerable postprocessing time and is unable to rectify MR images of patients when standard stereotaxy frames are attached. The technique used by the Vanderbilt University group produces a significant improvement in localization accuracy by using 4 mm thick spin echo MR images ranging from 3.833 ± 0.992 to 1.986 ± 0.605 mm. Less than 1 minute of postprocessing time is required. Image quality is not adversely affected.

Chemical shifts in MR images can be induced by the chemicals used in fiducial markers. This is especially significant in fats or oils, causing vitamin E capsules to be unacceptable for use as fiducials, despite their bright signal characteristics. Additional spatial distortions are created by the flow of blood in MR angiographic images, and these distortions are not corrected for by any currently employed algorithm. The degree of shift is up to 5 mm, which represents a significant caution in the routine use of these images.

For CT, the greatest source of spatial inaccuracy is error in calibration of table movement between slices or of patient movement during a scan set. If the patient moves substantially between the time it takes to obtain two slices of a scan set but does not move during scanning, no movement artifact will be present, but the anatomic volumes imaged above and below the slice of movement will not be correlated with one another as a single volume. These issues of table movement and patient movement have been dramatically ameliorated by rapid scanning with spiral acquisitions and slice reconstructions. In my experience and that of my colleagues at Vanderbilt University, the average amount of error in CT has dropped from approximately 1.0 to 2.0 mm to 0.3 mm once these new scanners are used. Very pernicious indeed is the acquisition of a volumetric CT set with the gantry angled away from 0 degrees. When this data set is reconstructed in the computer as if the gantry angle were 0 degrees (the baseline assumption), the volume is dramatically and irreversibly skewed with the address for each successive slice offset in relation to the gantry angle. Equally subtle and devastating is the effect of "recentering" the slice image during slice acquisition, something that is done merely to improve the aesthetics of the picture. This has the similar effect of offsetting slices and destroying the spatial integrity of the image volume.

Every neurosurgeon who intends to employ neurodiagnostic images for surgical navigation must develop a close collaborative working relationship with colleagues in his or her institution's radiology department to effectively communicate the concerns and requirements to everyone involved. Because the accuracy of the system is based on the images used, these must be appropriate for the intended purpose. This never proves to be a simple, let alone an automatic transfer of data. Instead, an ongoing and close personal relationship is critical to ensure that all parties maintain quality in the use of images in a manner entirely different from that anticipated by previous clinical requirements. Furthermore, once understanding of goals and requirements and a consensus of methods have been achieved continual careful maintenance and servicing schedules must be observed to produce a consistently reliable source of clinical information.

Often factors outside the awareness and control of one party will have a radical impact on the ability of the other parties involved. For example, routine installation of a minor upgrade in one function of a PACS network software interface will suddenly render image transfer to an SNS highly problematic if steps have not been taken beforehand to rewrite the appropriate code to deal with this potential pitfall. Most MR imaging units need to be reshimmed and retuned on a weekly or monthly basis; when used for surgical navigation data acquisition, the system requirements may be sufficiently changed so as to require that weekly or even daily adjustments be made.

REGISTRATION TECHNIQUES

Registration is a method for the mapping of individual patient-specific image spaces to one another and to physical space by means of identifying corresponding points in each image and in physical space. Registration is a fundamental process underlying the ability of all SNSs to perform the task at hand, and it belongs to a different category than reformatting or rendering of images. Reformatting is the reslicing of a volumetric image data set along a new angle to approximate the orientation of another image set. Rendering is the segmentation and display of image information in such a way as to present the data set as if it were a photograph of a three-dimensional object seen from a given perspective. These latter two procedures are ways of manipulating images for display purposes and do not fundamentally affect the relationships between different images or physical space. Therefore, improvements in techniques for the pseudo–three-dimensional display of rendered image data cannot in any way affect the determination of corresponding points in two different views of the same object because this registration of those images logically precedes any manipulation of their display.

Alternative techniques of registration have consisted of point methods (including stereotaxy frames, fiducial markers, and anatomic landmarks), curve and surface methods, moment and principal axes methods, correlation methods, and atlas methods.[14] Extrinsic point methods using implantable fiducial markers provide the fastest and most accurate form of registration and can define the level of accuracy for each patient encounter. This has made them popular among investigators, despite their minimally invasive nature and their inability to retrospectively register image data sets obtained without markers already in place.

Surface-based registration has the attraction of being the only method currently available that potentially requires no special imaging and can instead use "retrospectively acquired" images, that is, images not intended for navigation but only for initial diagnosis.[15] This economic consideration may be significant, but it does not alter the highly variable ways in which these retrospectively acquired images might have been performed and collected. Their indiscriminate use is an invitation to introduce a variety of unpredictable sources of localization error about which nothing can be done post hoc. To say that bad images are better than expensive images or no images at all is an economic consideration, but not an engineering or medical consideration. On the other hand, most practitioners who attempt registration using surface-based algorithms do use carefully obtained prospectively acquired images to suit the needs of navigation accuracy. In these settings, the limitations of the registration technique become the most significant concern. Surface-based registration techniques are less accurate and less reliable than are fiducial marker-based registration techniques, and it takes considerably more technical support and operator time to make them work at all. Most typically, the level of application accuracy achieved by these techniques under optimal circumstances is on the order of 3 to 10 mm.[16]

Some investigators have preferred to use anatomic landmarks such as the bridge of the nose, tragi, or lateral canthus for registration.[17,18] These intrinsic landmarks are also readily available and allow retrospectively acquired images to be used for registration and navigation. Their successful use does, however, entail a considerable component of individual operator skill and experience. Thus their use has been limited to those centers with skilled practitioners who prefer them to surface registration techniques or to skin-mounted fiducial markers. The ideal intrinsic anatomic fiducial markers are as small as possible to minimize the inherent definitional challenge of finding them on CT or MR images and in physical space. Very few structures satisfy these criteria; instead, different landmarks may be chosen for different scans and vice versa. Bony foramina, joints, or spicules have been used to great advantage by some for CT-based registration during skull base surgery and pedicle screw placement surgery.

Extrinsic fiducial markers may be attached to soft tissue (such as the skin or scalp) or to bony tissue (such as the skull or spinous process).[19] The movement of skin, especially of the scalp during prone positioning for suboccipital craniectomies, is a variable source of error that degrades both fiducial registration error and target localization error. Also, fiducials can fall off the skin if adhesives do not stick. To overcome the inadequacies of skin-mounted fiducials, most practitioners place many markers, often 5 to 10, for a given case. A minimum of three noncolinear points defines a volume; any more are redundant but serve to improve the chances of adequate registration. Imaging limitations of fiducial markers must be kept in mind. Some markers such as titanium pellets or screws are useful only with CT. Some skin-mounted fiducials using hydrogel compounds do not show up well in T2-weighted spin echo MR images, limiting their use for low-grade glioma resectional surgery.

The distribution of markers is also an important consideration. Clustering of the markers is suboptimal. The markers should be spread out as far over the cranial surface as possible, especially on the contralateral side. Clustering may produce less fiducial registration error, but this is misleading because target registration error rapidly degrades the farther away from the fiducials one gets. On the other hand, widely spaced fiducials are less convenient for the patient preoperatively and for the surgeon intraoperatively during registration. Obviously, markers placed in the field of the craniotomy itself will need to be removed during surgery, preventing reregistration in the event of a registration failure.

Bone-anchored fiducial markers provide the most reliable and accurate method of surgical registration and navigation.[19-21] Under ideal circumstances, their application accuracy equals or exceeds that of stereotaxy frame systems. Their implantation involves an invasive surgical procedure that carries potential risks, and this fact must be balanced against their ease of implantation and their benefit to the surgery being planned. Four bone-implanted fiducial markers are typically used in a given patient to provide some redundancy to the system. The larger the imaging fiducial marker is, the more accurate is the registration of images because the centroid can be better calculated. This fact must be balanced against the surgeon's desire for a minimally invasive marker. The closer to a sphere the fiducial marker is, the easier are the calculations for identifying the centroid of the marker. Any shape known a priori can be used satisfactorily.

Infection or local trauma has not been a significant observation to date. Perhaps the greatest risk from fiducial markers is their potential for contributing to an uncritical attitude regarding the results of a given registration value intraoperatively should that value prove misleading. For the most part, however, fiducial markers appear to increase the level of reliability of SNSs.

COMPUTERS AND SOFTWARE INTERFACES

Trifles make perfection, and perfection is no trifle.
—Michelangelo, *Lacon*

The clinically relevant display of registered imaging data to the surgeon requires appropriate imaging data input, computer hardware and software integration, and video display capabilities. Rapid advances in this field have produced a kaleidoscopic pattern of rapidly evolving attempted solutions to these system requirements. Because medicine is a "niche" market for the manufacturers involved, this field is largely driven by external forces of technology development and transfer. The anatomic detail provided by thin-slice gradient echo-planar MR images mapped onto the information derived from functional MR imaging or positron emission tomography studies, perhaps in combination with digitized stereotactic atlases, shows promise for optimal definition of these target volumes.

The greatest pitfalls in the use of SNSs have involved the inability to translate a given scanner's file format or header information into the form understood by the navigation system's computer. Although DICOM3 compatibility promised by manufacturers of scanners and PACS systems has the potential to clear this unnecessarily painful interface incompatibility thicket, it will not make these problems disappear altogether in the near future. Working in collaboration with radiologists and their technicians and corporate representatives, the surgeon must be prepared to expend a significant amount of time and capital to provide a solution for clinical use and maintenance. Once images have been successfully entered into the system, the surgeon must familiarize himself with the software architecture and menu structure of the navigation software. This must be done systematically and "off-line," before any patient is operated on. The operating room during a surgical procedure is an unforgiving environment in which to learn nuances of menu-driven program structure and function. If at all possible, the presence of a dedicated computer-literate technician in the operating room will reinforce the utility and benefit of these systems for the surgeon.

The software used may have varying levels of robustness, transparency, or flexibility for the clinical situation at hand. Preoperative treatment planning and simulations can often speed the actual surgery along by offering those involved the opportunity to rehearse the desired procedures and anticipate common distractions or complications.

Every system has its own dedicated computer hardware with its own peculiarities, requirements, and limitations. These must be appreciated to maintain functionality in the operating room. An uninterruptible power supply should be standard equipment in each system to prevent the loss of registration data in the event of disconnection and power loss. Although most hardware is well shielded against radiofrequency currents, the simple physical assault of being bumped, dropped, or turned upside down must be anticipated. The violation of operating field sterility is always a potential hazard with large computer monitors situated nearby.

The two-dimensional video display of three-dimensional information introduces an inevitable layer of graphics interface distortion and misrepresentation of reality. Each surgeon must determine which type of image display is the most meaningful and least confusing for a given operation. Triplanar orthogonal views of anatomy are extremely helpful in orienting the surgeon during complex surgery. Oblique views have limited benefit for craniotomies to resect tumors, although they can be very helpful during stereotactic biopsies and pedicle screw placements. Rendered information is of some benefit during cortical localization and superficial resective surgery but is less helpful when dealing with subcortical or intraventricular anatomy. The solid tumor tissue component of a malignant brain tumor is often best appreciated on contrast-enhanced CT, although it is clearly seen but occasionally overreported on contrasted T1-weighted MR images. Rendered outlines of lesions seen through a microscopic navigation system are subject to misregistration and are confusing to some surgeons.

Ultimately, when a disagreement arises between the graphics display and what the surgeon visualizes directly, the surgical procedure should be stopped for a moment of reflection and analysis to resolve the conflict. Although the navigation system must be treated skeptically at times, the surgeon must also reassess how much has actually been accomplished at any given point during the surgery in light of conflicting information. This represents a critical moment during the operation, demanding the highest levels of concentration and using the surgeon's knowledge base and judgment for correlation, skepticism, and resolution.

INTERACTIVE LOCALIZATION DEVICES AND INTRAOPERATIVE USE

A fool with a tool, is a fool.
—Aphorism attributed to Lars Leksell

An interactive localization device is necessary to define the spatial coordinates of physical space in the operating room. Alternative technologies used to date may be categorized as either tethered or untethered systems. Tethered systems are conceptually and technically simpler from an engineering point of view but have the disadvantages of drag and tethering of the device in the surgeon's hand. Untethered devices are more acceptable as surgical instruments because they are less intrusive and do not have physical links or tethers, but they introduce a number of clinical and engineering concerns such as line-of-sight issues. The individual surgeon must evaluate which system is best suited to the operative procedure planned and the clinical setting available.

Tethered interactive localization systems include stereotaxy frame systems,[6,22] active robotic arms,[23] passive localization arms with joint-position sensors using potentiometers or optical encoders,[24] and intraoperative CT or MR imaging scanners. Nontethered systems include spark-gap emitters with microphone triangulation as sonic localizers, infrared light-emitting diode (LED) emitters with optical linear charge-coupled device (LCCD) camera triangulation arrays as optical localizers, passive optical motion detectors using shaped light patterns, magnetic field distortion sensors, and gravitometers and inertial movement sensors.

The use of a passive localization arm for neurosurgical guidance was first described by Watanabe.[25] The neuronavigator consisted of a personal computer programmed in C, an image display monitor, and an articulated arm with six joints, each of which was equipped with a 50 KΩ potentiometer. The arm end-point position was determined by digitizing the angles at each of the arm joints and inserting these into the forward kinematic equation. This elegant system had two major disadvantages. First, the potentiometers used for angle-position detectors in each of the arm joints were not finely incremented and allowed for only a coarse measurement of angular displacement. The linearity of potentiometers was also inconstant, introducing fluctuations into the measurement of the angles. The second disadvantage of the system was its limited computational abilities in supporting the video display of medical images.

The ISG Viewing Wand system (ISG Technologies, Toronto, Canada) has been employed by numerous surgeons. The interactive localization device for the ISG Viewing Wand system is a passive localization arm (FARO Medical Technologies, Miami, Fla.). The ergonomics of this arm are praiseworthy, although it has a tendency toward backlash and forward drag at times. This six-jointed arm employs electrogoniometers for angular detectors, thus limiting its accuracy and precision.

Guthrie and Adler[26] reported on an evolving series of passive localization arms for measuring angular joint displacement based on optical encoder technology. Earlier versions of localization arms from this group possessed five articulating joints with low-resolution optical encoders. To achieve higher levels of localization accuracy for more recent versions of the arm, higher resolution optical encoders have been encased in six articulated joints. Elegant counterbalancing of the joints of these arms has been the hallmark of the mechanical construction displayed by this group; the arms "float" much like a Calder mobile, with occasional backlash.

In 1986 Roberts et al.[27] first described microscope-based frameless stereotaxy. Spark-gap ultrasonic emitters were attached to an operating microscope in a known geometric configuration. Sound detectors for these ultrasonic noises were arrayed throughout the operating room. The combination of these ultrasonic emitters and their detectors created a three-dimensionally registered space through which the microscope moved. The focal length of the optics of the microscope was known, and accordingly, the microscope's focal point became a virtual end effector for the microscope/spark-gap emitter assembly. In this way, the microscope could be used as an optical interactive localization device for patient landmarks. A fundamental limitation of this system is the use of spark-gap emitters. Because the speed of sound in air is highly temperature dependent and the distances between ultrasonic emitters and their detectors are long, the temperature fluctuations commonly encountered in surgical suites cause variations in the speed of sound sufficient to produce potentially large errors in target position location. The pathways between detectors and emitters must be kept clear to prevent signal displacement by intervening structures or materials. Echoes from the multitude of surfaces in the operating suite produce significant interference with surgical localization. Considerable work has been carried out by this Dartmouth University group to correct for temperature fluctuations, echoes, and other sources of error in the system. The error in locating the focal point of the operating microscope in a recent clinical series of 17 patients was 6.33 ± 3.37 mm.

Interestingly, this system has been employed in a series of seven patients undergoing conventional neurosurgical procedures on the lumbosacral spine for herniated discs or spondylolisthesis. The mean accuracy of locating the operating microscope's focal point was 6.04 mm. At the level of the disc space, however, the combination of all sources of error coupled with mobility of the soft tissue resulted in an average error of 28.81 mm.

Recently, Barnett and colleagues[28-32] incorporated spark-gap ultrasonic emitter technology with a hand-held interactive localization device (Picker International, Highland Heights, Ohio). This pointing device carries the spark-gap emitters rather than coupling the emitters to the operating microscope. The repetitive (50 kHz) ultrasonic pulses produced by the interactive localization device are detected by three or more microphone/emitter units comprising a portable detector/calibration array that is mounted to the side rails of a standard operating table. The positioning of the detector/calibration array was believed to be superior to ceiling-mounted or wall-mounted placement; the shorter triangulation distances and optimal slant ranges measurably improved localization accuracy. This system demonstrates a fair degree of sensitivity to angulation of the interactive localization device with respect to the detector/calibration array. Careful positioning of the interactive localization device is necessary for proper intraoperative localization. Software algorithms for temperature and humidity fluctuation effects are critical to the functionality of the system.

Several groups have investigated the use of infrared LEDs as an alternative form of optical localization.[19,33,34] By having two or more infrared LEDs attached to a surgical instrument, the position in space of that instrument can be tracked over time by a triangulation technique employing three or more "cameras." These cameras are specialized 2000- to 4000-element LCCDs with cylindric lenses that focus light from the infrared LEDs onto the individual elements of the array. Three of these one-dimensional arrays are precisely oriented on an aluminum cross beam so that their overlapping visual fields define any point in three-dimensional space.

These optical triangulation techniques are highly accurate and precise, surprisingly robust within the noisy operating theater environment, and extremely flexible in their use. Line-of-sight considerations apply in this situation much as they do with sonic digitizer triangulation methods. Unlike sonic digitizers, infrared LED arrays are insensitive to temperature or humidity fluctuations. Interference from surgical light sources has not proved to be a problem. The infrared wavelength of their emissions is not disruptive to surgery.[35]

Bucholz and Smith[33] employed an array of two infrared LEDs attached to a surgical bipolar cautery forceps. Maciunas et al.[19] developed an alternative manifestation of this optical triangulation technique. The position of the interactive localization device is tracked by a precision-milled, three-camera LCCD array and embedded computer program with knowledge-based software using center-finding algorithms to better detect the infrared LEDs. The interactive localization device is studded with an array of multiple infrared LEDs to increase the robustness and accuracy of localization. In this way, "blind spots" are more easily avoided.

Heilbrun et al.[36] have proposed a technique of surgical guidance employing machine vision in which the three-dimensional position of an object in space is determined from its differential position on two-dimensional video images viewed from two different angles. Two video cameras situated approximately 1 m apart are aimed at the surgical work space. A "video localizer," consisting of eight fiducial objects set in a boxlike configuration of known dimensions, is placed within the field of view of the two video cameras. A "photogrammetric" projection algorithm defines the three-dimensional coordinates of the eight fiducial objects. Subsequently, the position and field of view of the video cameras remain unchanged. Thus the three-dimensional position of any object in the surgical work space of their field of view can be determined and tracked. Surgical instruments may be tracked within the surgical space of the video cameras by affixing fiducial markers to the surgical instruments in a known geometric configuration. The advantages of this method are its flexibility, its potential to track standard surgical instruments as stereotactic points with minimal modification, and its reliance on readily available video technology. It remains sensitive to line-of-sight considerations, the need for the video cameras to maintain their relationship with the preoperatively defined surgical space, limitations to the resolution of currently available video technology, and the computationally intensive nature of intraoperative registration.

Many investigators have employed a magnetic field guidance system manufactured by Polhemus Navigation Sciences (Colchester, Vt.) for directing endoscopic visualization and dissection. A magnetic field is established by a transmitter antenna near the patient's head, and its strength is measured by a receiving antenna mounted on the surgical instrument. Because magnetic field strength diminishes as a function of the distance between the transmitter and the receiving antenna, the tip of the receiving instrument is measured in x, y, and z planes of space in relation to the repetitive direct-current pulse magnetic field in x, y, and z hemispheres. This process is carried out at 100 Hz. Magnetic field guidance has the attraction of being mechanically simple and inexpensive. Unfortunately, it has proved to be less accurate than other technologies in clinical settings and is susceptible to both static and active field distortion in the surgical suite environment because of the presence of common metals as well as electromagnetic field interference. The Regulus navigation system (Stereotactic Medical Systems, Rochester, Minn.) employs software with algorithms that attempt to compensate for the static magnetic field inhomogeneities to minimize the drift and inaccuracies encountered in the clinical use of magnetic localization systems.

Regardless of the interactive localization system used, attention must be paid to the degradation of registration information through system drift, head movement, and other sources of noise. Other than optical encoder-based joint-position sensors in linked passive arms and active, infrared-emitting diode-based optical triangulation systems, all other technologies to date have demonstrated some degree of drift of positional information over time. Head movement in the pinion head-holder has been identified as a very real source of positional drift. Optical systems have incorporated a reference emitter to track head movement and readjust the registration accordingly; for this to function properly, the reference emitter must be attached to the head proper, something that is not always done. In spinal surgery, the movement of anatomic structures during surgical manipulation is so significant that it is virtually imperative to consider a reference emitter for each mobile element to achieve maximal accuracy.

Whenever any interactive localization device is used, some error with its use should be anticipated. As a result, there is inevitable error accumulating during fiducial localization and registration, which is compounded during target localization. The surgeon can therefore assume that the target localization accuracy of any system will always be worse than the displayed fiducial registration accuracy due to this "double sampling error" and can apply the requisite caution in relying on these systems.

INTEGRATION OF REAL-TIME DATA

It's like déjà vu all over again.
—Yogi Berra

Despite the registration of image to physical space, digital scan information remains historical data and is subject to becoming outdated during the course of the surgical manipulation of tissues. The feedback loop of navigation can be closed by incorporating real-time intraoperative imaging and monitoring; these data are used to refine and modify the patient-specific maps being used for surgical guidance. The use of historically obtained (preoperative) imaging sets is further augmented by intraoperative updating and reregistration with real-time microendoscopy, spatially resolved electrophysiology and cortical mapping techniques, ultrasonography, and interventional CT and MR imaging. By digitizing the video output from intraoperative visualization techniques (ultrasonography, endoscopy, tomography, and electrophysiologic recordings), these images may be treated as simply another source of spatially registered medical information.[5,37,38]

Preliminary steps are being taken to incorporate this information into surgical guidance databases. Microscopes pose a considerable challenge to engineers attempting to produce a surgically accurate and useful device. Despite claims to the contrary, every surgeon must realize that these devices involve a real learning curve if used properly. The depth of field of microscopes, misalignments of their optical axis, miscalibrations of image injection systems, and visually confusing or deceiving perspective distortions must be taken into consideration with every clinical use. Because visually augmented reality can be most compelling, even when it is misregistered or incorrect, interpretation of this information as it is presented dictates extreme caution. Individual surgeons have varying degrees of stereoscopic vision and three-dimensional visualization skills, and this may affect how much can be gained with the use of these systems. Some microscopes assume right-eye dominance in their displays, limiting their use to those of us who are left-eye dominant. Video microscopy has been widely discussed as a means of integrating digital tomographic information and real-time video. Nevertheless, this system awaits the introduction of higher resolution LCCD arrays before it can replace optical microscopy for surgery; at present, it represents nothing more than a technical curiosity.

In the meantime, spatially registered endoscopy is becoming incorporated into routine clinical practice. The use of angled eyepieces can be visually confusing at times, and no good solution for registering flexible endoscopes is currently available. Slippage of the infrared LED attachments or miscalibration of the device can lead to erroneous positional data.

Intraoperative tomography offers the promise of high-resolution digital volumetric imaging data for continuous real-time updating of the surgical field. Intraoperative CT has been employed extensively, and intraoperative MR image scanning has been introduced into neurosurgery. The potential benefits of these devices include reregistration of preoperative databases when structures shift during surgery, visual assessment of the adequacy of surgical resection, and minimally invasive heating of selected tissues under imaging control. To date, the restrictive physical environment of these scanners has somewhat impeded their surgical utility. The considerable expenditures for the hardware and facilities of such systems have raised concerns about their cost-effectiveness in any but high-volume clinical settings.[39]

TISSUE DISPLACEMENT

All current medical registration techniques involve rigid body assumptions. This allows the computational load to be manageable and leads to therapeutically appropriate interfaces. With any surgical intervention, however, some movement of soft tissue is inevitable. For some time this has been a recognized limitation in the indiscriminate reliance on these navigation systems. Recent quantitation of this effect during craniotomies has indicated superficial brain shifts approaching 1 cm intraoperatively.[40] Deeper structures, especially those along the cranial base, along the falx, or near the deep gray nuclei, in fact, shift less than do the superficial overlying structures. This improves the reliability of navigation the deeper one goes, permitting these systems to be used safely and effectively. Nonetheless, this remains an issue of concern not only academically but for every clinical application.

First and foremost, the presence of tissue distortions mandates that the highest level of accuracy and freedom from drift be maintained for any SNS. Otherwise, the accumulation of errors threatens to engulf any effort at localization in positional noise.

Second, certain precautions are necessary. It appears that the greatest shift is in the direction of gravity. Thus, in a given proposed surgical trajectory, the critical structures of interest may prove to shift deeper along the trajectory rather than away in an unpredictable manner. Minimizing osmotic diuretics does not, at present, seem to be of any significant benefit, and standard surgical considerations should not be jeopardized. The venting of ventricular cerebrospinal fluid can produce unpredictable shifts in superficial structures and should be avoided until after the primary approach has been accomplished. Debulking of tumors may be modified by minimizing the "inside to outside" approach to debulking, making an effort to define the outer margins of intrinsic tumors with subsequent debulking carried out at the earliest opportunity.[32,34,41,42]

Some authors have described "refreshing" the registration by reregistering to shifted cortical or subcortical anatomic fiducials to keep up with these shifts, but this has the potential for transmitting extremely confusing information to the surgeon. Until more systematic protocols and software for accomplishing this procedure in a safe manner have been developed, it remains of limited benefit. Research is under way to integrate intraoperative imaging studies such as ultrasonography, CT, and MR imaging to warp preoperative images to a new registration based on tissue displacement. Although highly promising for the future, no reliable method is yet available for clinical use.

ROBOTICS

Currently, there is considerable speculation as to the applicability of robotic control technologies and the employment of virtual reality computer interfaces to integrate the various imaging databases obtained for a given patient. This automation of the surgical process will likely increase rather than decrease the involvement of the neurosurgeon in ensuring oversight, calibration, and knowledge-based feedback.

JUDGMENT AND CLINICAL EXPERIENCE

First, do no harm.
—Hippocrates

As in all other aspects of neurosurgery, the clinician is called on to definitively assess the conflicting or confusing sets of information about a patient's status and diagnosis. Rather than uncritically accepting whatever spatial and diagnostic information is provided, the surgeon must continue to exercise surgical judgment based on training and clinical experience to achieve optimal clinical results. Although a computer can effectively handle vast quantities of quantitative imaging data, it does not at present have the knowledge-based intelligence to appropriately weigh the evidence as it is presented and to distinguish between disease and healthy tissue or between surgical danger and safe passage. This weighing of factual information will remain the greatest responsibility (and generate the greatest excitement) in the clinical decision-making process for the surgeon.

Numerous limitations and pitfalls become apparent in the use of surgical navigation devices. Nonetheless, these are exceedingly useful devices and benefit neurosurgery on a daily basis. Given their deficiencies, how can they be so useful? There are a number of ameliorating factors that mitigate the detrimental aspects of this technology. First and foremost, most of us have the pleasure of spending our lives practicing in the median range of the universal Gaussian distribution of error rather than at the 99th percentile limits of confidence. Accordingly, by definition, most of the time these systems will perform better than they do in the worst-case scenario. In any event, most of the lesions that we approach are larger than the limits of resolution for these systems, and the overconfigured safety cushion provided by tight tolerances for accuracy pays off in reliable performance in most clinical situations. When a primary brain tumor is resected, the tumor architecture and biology provide an indistinct border to the target lesion, causing most surgeons to bracket the lesion coordinates for safety's sake. During a craniotomy, direct visualization of the lesion provides real-time feedback to update the registration intraoperatively. During functional stereotactic procedures such as thalamotomies or pallidotomies, electrophysiologic feedback is ultimately the technique for reregistering the appropriate anatomy and successfully completing the operation. The neurosurgeon must bring to bear all the available tools for localization of cerebral function and lesional anatomy to accurately distinguish them.[2,7,32,34,40-43]

And, in spite of pride, in erring Reason's spite, one truth is clear, whatever is, is right.
—Pope, *Essay on Man, I*

References

1. Galloway RL, Maciunas RJ. Stereotactic neurosurgery. Crit Rev Biomed Eng 18:207-233, 1990.
2. Maciunas RJ, ed. Clinical Frontiers of Interactive Image-Guided Neurosurgery. Neurosurg Clin N Am 1996.
3. Maciunas RJ, ed. Interactive Image-Guided Neurosurgery. Park Ridge, Ill.: American Association of Neurological Surgeons, 1993.
4. Maciunas RJ, Galloway RL, Latimer JW. The application accuracy of stereotactic frames. Neurosurgery 35:682-695, 1994.
5. Galloway RL Jr, Berger MS, Bass WA, et al. Registered intraoperative information: Electrophysiology, ultrasound, and endoscopy. In Maciunas RJ, ed. Interactive Image-Guided Neurosurgery. Park Ridge, Ill.: American Association of Neurological Surgeons, 1993, pp 247-258.
6. Kelly PJ. Computer-assisted stereotaxis: New approaches for the management of intracranial intra-axial tumors. Neurology 36:535-541, 1986.
7. Kelly PJ, Daumas-Duport C, Scheithauer BW, et al. Stereotactic histologic correlation of computer tomography and magnetic resonance imaging–defined abnormalities in patients with glial neoplasms. Mayo Clin Proc 62:450-459, 1987.
8. Maciunas RJ, Fitzpatrick JM, Gadamsetty S, et al. A universal method for geometrical correction of magnetic resonance images for stereotactic neurosurgery. Stereotact Funct Neurosurg 66:137-140, 1996.
9. Plante E, Turkstra L. Sources of error in quantitative analysis of MRI scans. Magn Reson Imaging 9:589-595, 1991.
10. Chang H, Fitzpatrick JM. A technique for accurate magnetic resonance imaging in the presence of field inhomogeneities. IEEE Trans Med Imaging 11:319-320, 1992.
11. Dong S, Fitzpatrick JM, Maciunas RJ. Rectification of distortion in MRI for stereotaxy. In Proceedings of the Fifth Annual IEEE Symposium on Computer-Based Medical Systems, 1992, pp 181-189.
12. Maurer CM Jr, Aboutanos GB, Dawant BM, et al. Effect of geometrical distortion correction in MR on image registration accuracy. J Comput Assist Tomogr 20:666-679, 1996.
13. Sumanaweera TS, Glover GH, Binford TO, et al. MR susceptibility misregistration correction. IEEE Trans Med Imaging 12:251-259, 1993.
14. Maurer CM, Fitzpatrick JM. A review of medical image registration. In Maciunas RJ, ed. Interactive Image-Guided Neurosurgery. Park Ridge, Ill.: American Association of Neurological Surgeons, 1993, pp 17-44.
15. Pelizzari CA, Chen GTY, Spelbring DR, et al. Accurate three-dimensional registration of CT, PET, and/or MR images of the brain. J Comput Assist Tomogr 13:20-26, 1989.
16. West J, Fitzpatrick JM, Wang MY, et al. Comparison and evaluation of retrospective intermodality image registration techniques. J Comput Assist Tomogr 21:554-566, 1997.
17. Adler JR Jr. Image-based frameless stereotactic radiosurgery. In Maciunas RJ, ed. Interactive Image-Guided Neurosurgery. Park Ridge, Ill.: American Association of Neurological Surgeons, 1993, pp 81-89.
18. Ge Y, Fitzpatrick JM, Votaw JR, Gadamsetty S, et al. Retrospective registration of PET and MR brain images: An algorithm and its stereotactic validation. J Comput Assist Tomogr 18:800-810, 1994.
19. Maciunas RJ, Fitzpatrick JM, Galloway RL, et al. Beyond stereotaxy: Extreme levels of application accuracy are provided by implantable fiducial markers for interactive image-guided neurosurgery. In Maciunas RJ, ed. Interactive Image-Guided Neurosurgery. Park Ridge, Ill.: American Association of Neurological Surgeons, 1993, pp 259-270.
20. Mandava VR, Fitzpatrick JM Jr, Maurer CR, et al. Registration of multimodal volume head images via attached markers. In Proceedings of the SPIE Medical Imaging Conference, 1992, pp 271-282.
21. Wang MY, Maurer CR, Fitzpatrick JM, et al. A knowledge-based technique for localizing externally attached markers in MR and CT volume images of the head. In Proc Ann Int Conference IEEE Eng Med Biol Soc 15:120-121, 1993.
22. Shelden C, McGann G, Jacques S, et al. Development of a computerized microstereotaxic method for localization and removal of minute CHS lesions under direct 3-D vision [Technical report]. J Neurosurg 52:21-27, 1980.

23. Drake JM, Joy M, Goldenberg A, et al. Computer- and robot-assisted resection of thalamic astrocytomas in children. Neurosurgery 29:27-33, 1991.
24. Maciunas RJ, Galloway RL, Fitzpatrick JM, et al. A universal system for interactive image-directed neurosurgery. Stereotact Funct Neurosurg 58:108-113, 1992.
25. Watanabe E. The neuronavigator: A potentiometer-based localization arm system. In Maciunas RJ, ed. Interactive Image-Guided Neurosurgery. Park Ridge, Ill.: American Association of Neurological Surgeons, 1993, pp 135-148.
26. Guthrie BL, Adler JR Jr. Computer-assisted preoperative planning, interactive surgery, and frameless stereotaxy. Clin Neurosurg 38:112-131, 1992.
27. Roberts DW, Strohbehn JW, Hatch JF, et al. A frameless stereotaxic integration of computerized tomographic imaging and the operating microscope. J Neurosurg 65:545-549, 1986.
28. Barnett GH. Surgical management of convexity and falcine meningiomas using interactive image-guided surgery systems. Neurosurg Clin N Am 7:274-284, 1996.
29. Barnett GH, Kormos DW, Steiner CP, et al. Frameless stereotaxy using a sonic digitizing wand: Development and adaptation to the Picker Vistar medical imaging system. In Maciunas RJ, ed. Interactive Image-Guided Neurosurgery. Park Ridge, Ill.: American Association of Neurological Surgeons, 1993, pp 113-120.
30. Barnett GH, Kormos DW, Steiner CP, et al. Intraoperative localization using an armless, frameless stereotactic wand. J Neurosurg 78:510-514, 1993.
31. Barnett GH, Kormos DW, Steiner CP, et al. Use of a frameless, armless wand for brain tumor localization with two-dimensional and three-dimensional neuroimaging. Neurosurgery 33:674-678, 1993.
32. Gomez H, Barnett GH, Palmer J. Contemporary stereotactic neurosurgery at the Cleveland Clinic. Review of 501 consecutive cases. Cleve Clin Med 60:399-410, 1993.
33. Bucholz RD, Smith KR. A comparison of sonic digitizers versus light-emitting diode-based localization. In Maciunas RJ, ed. Interactive Image-Guided Neurosurgery. Park Ridge, Ill.: American Association of Neurological Surgeons, 1993, pp 179-200.
34. Maciunas RJ, Berger MS, Copeland B, et al. A technique for interactive image-guided neurosurgical intervention in primary brain tumors. Neurosurg Clin N Am 7:245-266, 1997.
35. Horstmann GA, Reinhardt HF. Micro-stereometry: A frameless computerized navigating system for open microsurgery. Comput Med Imaging Graph 18:229-233, 1994.
36. Heilbrun MP, McDonald P, Wiker C, et al. Stereotactic localization and guidance using a machine vision technique. Stereotact Funct Neurosurg 58:94-98, 1992.
37. Berger MS. Ultrasound-guided stereotaxic biopsy using a new apparatus. J Neurosurg 65:550-554, 1986.
38. Berger MS, Kinkaid J, Ojemann GA, et al. Brain mapping techniques to maximize resection, safety, and seizure control in children with brain tumors. Neurosurgery 25:786-792, 1989.
39. Moriarty TM, Kikinis R, Jolesz FA, et al. Magnetic resonance imaging therapy: Intraoperative MR imaging. Neurosurg Clin N Am 7:323-331, 1996.
40. Hill DLG, Maurer CL Jr, Wang MY, et al. Estimation of intraoperative brain surface movement. In Troccaz J, Grimson E, Mosges R, eds. CVR Med-MRCAS '97. Berlin: Springer-Verlag, 1997, pp 449-458.
41. Berger MS, Deliganis AV, Dobbins J, et al. The effect of extent of resection on recurrence in patients with low-grade cerebral hemisphere gliomas. Cancer 74:1784-1791, 1994.
42. Galloway RL, Maciunas RJ, Failinger AL. Factors affecting perceived tumor volumes in magnetic resonance imaging. Ann Biomed Eng 21:367-375, 1993.
43. Olivier A, Germano I, Cukiert A, et al. Frameless stereotaxy for surgery of the epilepsies: Preliminary experience. J Neurosurg 81:629-633, 1994.

PART II

Clinical Applications

5

Minimal Access Craniotomy

Gene H. Barnett, M.D.

The primary application of surgical navigation systems (SNSs) for intracranial use by most practitioners is likely to be fashioning minimal access craniotomies.[1-13] Knowing the precise location of an intracranial lesion as well as vascular and cortical relationships may permit very small cranial openings and minimize the need for intracranial exploration. Computer-assisted minimally invasive craniotomies appear to be associated with reduced neurologic and wound complications, operative time, and patient discomfort compared with traditional techniques.[1,2,6,7,14]

Proper use of SNSs to select a surgical trajectory[15] requires the ability to interpret SNS displays and strategies to manage brain movement after opening the dura. This chapter reviews these issues as well as techniques I have used in several hundred minimal access craniotomies.

SURGICAL TECHNIQUE

Display Interpretation

A surgical trajectory that avoids functionally eloquent cortex and tracts is defined. Although the ultimate target is generally the center of the tumor or lesion, the best approach may not always be via the shortest distance. Simple triplanar (i.e., axial, sagittal, and coronal) displays are inadequate for optimal planning of a surgical trajectory for several reasons: (1) They may be misleading, particularly with respect to the margins of a tumor that project to the scalp surface (Fig. 5-1). For instance, novice users of SNSs will often move the pointing device (wand) on the scalp surface to where the tumor margin disappears on a given plane and mark that spot as the projected tumor boundary. To do so is *only* valid if the final surgical trajectory is truly parallel to the line of projection. This situation only exists at the vertex, immediately above the ears, and above the inion and nasion. Elsewhere, physical constraints usually demand that the scalp and bony openings will be perpendicular to the surface of the skull in that region, and this may depart as much as 45 degrees from the line of projection when the above technique is used. (2) It is difficult to interpret the surgical trajectory with respect to vascular structures, especially major cortical and parasagittal veins, since these struc-

A

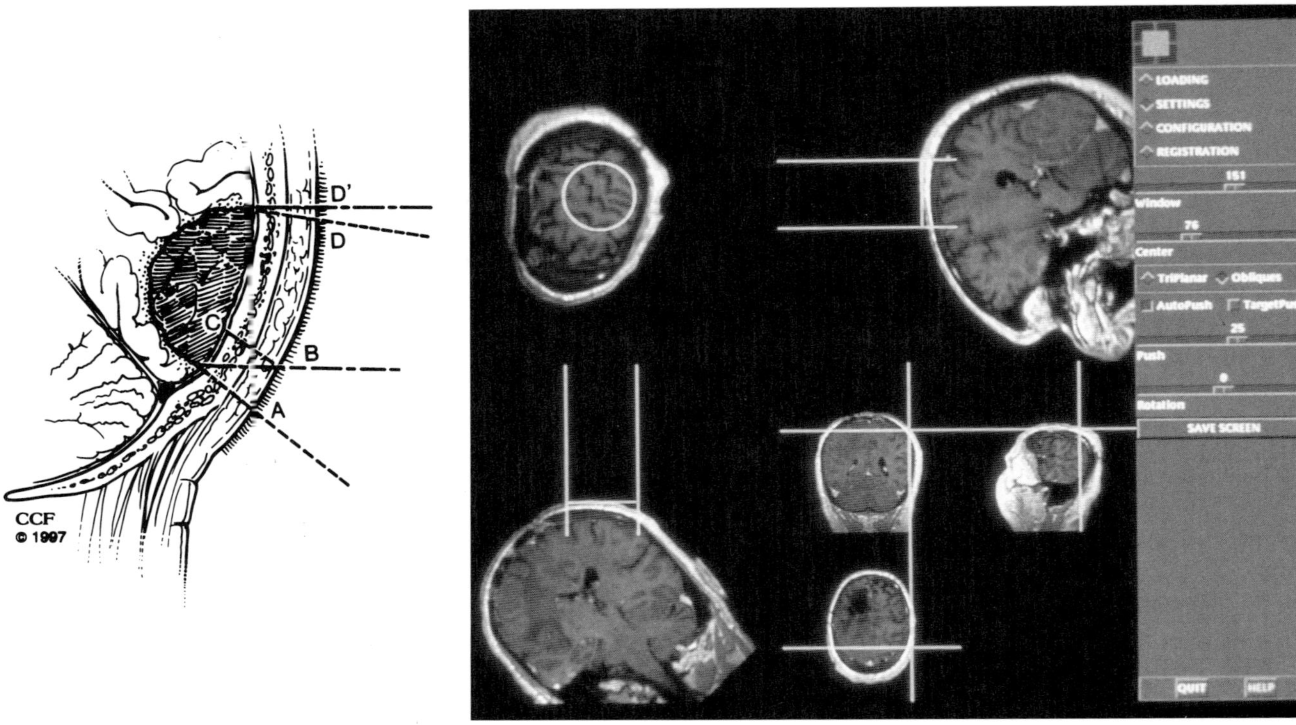

B

Figure 5-1. A, Proper placement of a minimal access craniotomy requires proper use of SNS displays. Approaches must account for the curvature of the skull. If a standard triplanar display is used (i.e., sagittal, coronal, or transverse), the craniotomy margin must be placed on a line perpendicular to the skull at the most extreme portion of the tumor *(A)* and not on a line either horizontal *(B)* or vertical on the display; otherwise the actual inner margin of the cut will be misdirected *(C)*. This effect is minimized at the 12, 3, 6, and 9 o'clock positions of each display (*D* and *D'*). **B,** Oblique displays are perhaps better suited to defining placement of the bony opening as long as the axis is perpendicular to the skull.

tures typically appear as nondescript spots of high intensity on most triplanar displays. (3) Often the relationship of the surgical trajectory to cortical anatomy and its inferred function (see Chapter 17) is obscure.

For these reasons, we believe that presentations that are directed or "steered" by the pointing device are quite valuable. Using a pair of perpendicular views that both *contain* the wand axis can be used to ensure that the surgical trajectory is truly perpendicular to the skull, and a view that is *perpendicular* to the wand axis at a user-selectable depth provides accurate projection of the lesion margins as well as visualization of vascular and cortical anatomy that may suggest redirection of the planned surgical trajectory (Fig. 5-2).

Patient Positioning, Preparation, and Opening

Ideally, the patient should be positioned so that this surgical trajectory is nearly vertical to minimize problems with intraoperative movements of the brain and tumor ("brain shift").[1,6,7] The minimal access craniotomy is located directly

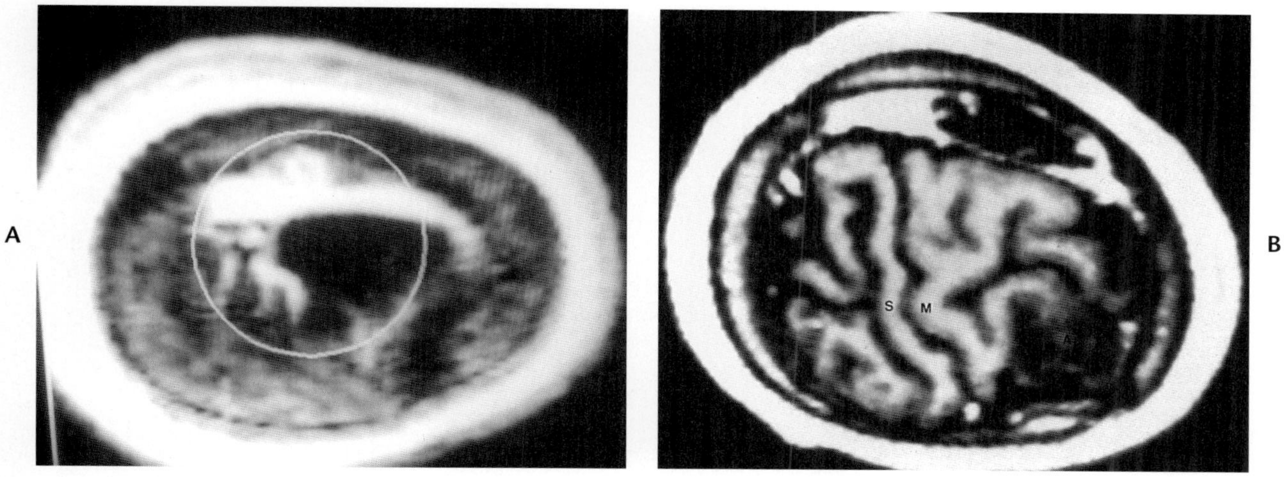

Figure 5-2. A, Oblique display showing superior sagittal sinus and draining vein. **B,** Oblique display showing motor strip *(M)*, sensory strip *(S)*, and astrocytoma *(A)*.

over a superficial lesion using the method described above to project the tumor boundary. Placement of the minimal access craniotomy for subcortical lesions is generally directed so as to avoid functionally eloquent cortex and major veins, and often the brain is entered through a sulcus to minimize parenchymal dissection.[1,6,7] Lesions requiring frontal or temporal lobectomy are best accessed through minimal access craniotomies located at the posterior boundary of the lesion, typically at the coronal suture or a few centimeters posterior to the temporal tip, respectively.

The head is secured in a fixation device so as to avoid displacement of reference fiducials (if used), to allow line-of-sight between the SNS wand, head tracker, and detector (as required by the SNS), and to allow a near vertical surgical trajectory. The hair is shaved about 1 cm on either side of the prospective incision and the region prepared with an antiseptic solution such as povidone-iodine[16] (Fig. 5-3). Draping is tacked in place with skin staples to cover the remaining hair, and a lazy S-shaped incision centered on the surgical trajectory is then fashioned (Fig. 5-4). Skin clips are usually not required if hemostasis is secured early. The periosteum is elevated, and self-retaining retractors are placed (Fig. 5-5) in lieu of fish hooks or other retractors that may move the head in the positioning device and risk spatial misregistration unless the head tracker mounts to the C-arm of the Mayfield device. A small bone flap is elevated using either a trephine or craniotome (Fig. 5-6). Although use of a trephine may provide a spatial reference when used with some SNSs,[6,7] it is more likely to result in cortical laceration than a craniotome in some hands. Dural tacking sutures are then placed through a small hole drilled around the periphery of the craniotomy. For most lesions, the dura is opened in a cruciate fashion with attention directed to underlying venous structures viewed on the SNS (Fig. 5-7). It is advantageous to tent the dural flaps with sutures placed at the base of the leaflets rather than the apices. Dural-based lesions are approached by opening the dura peripherally (Fig. 5-8).

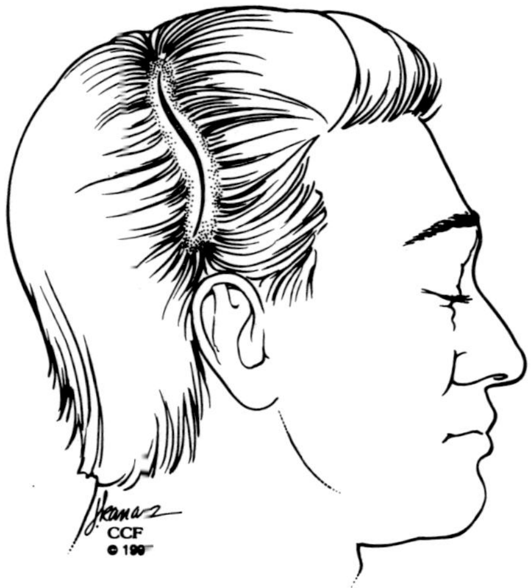

Figure 5-3. Minimal access craniotomy for malignant glioma begins with clipping the hair 0.5 cm on either side of the proposed incision, which is centered on the SNS-defined surgical trajectory.

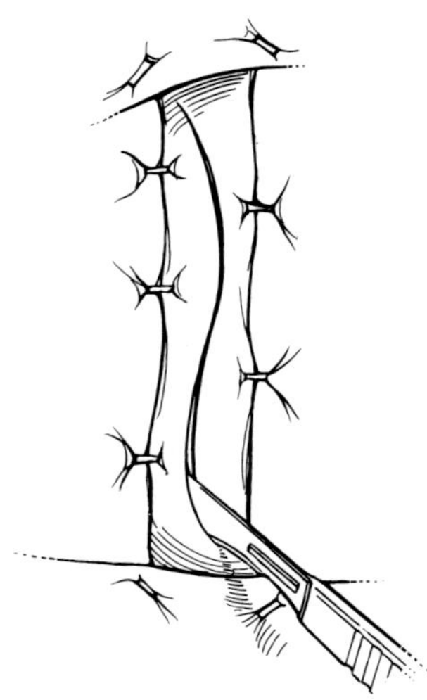

Figure 5-4. Drapes are stapled over the remaining hair and a lazy S-shaped incision made. Hemostasis can usually be obtained by cautery without the need for clips.

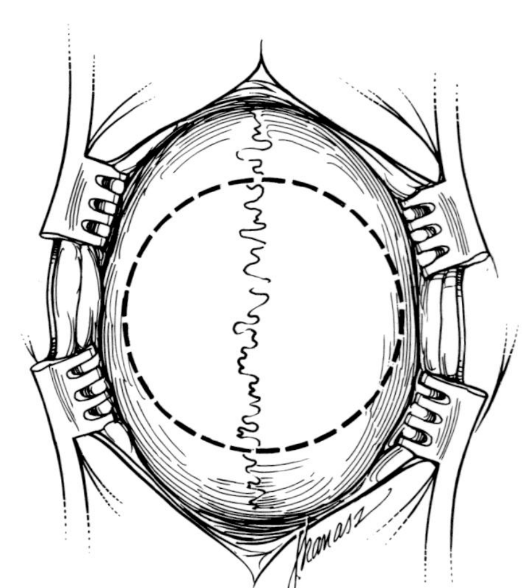

Figure 5-5. The periosteum is elevated and self-retaining retractors placed to provide an adequate opening for craniotomy.

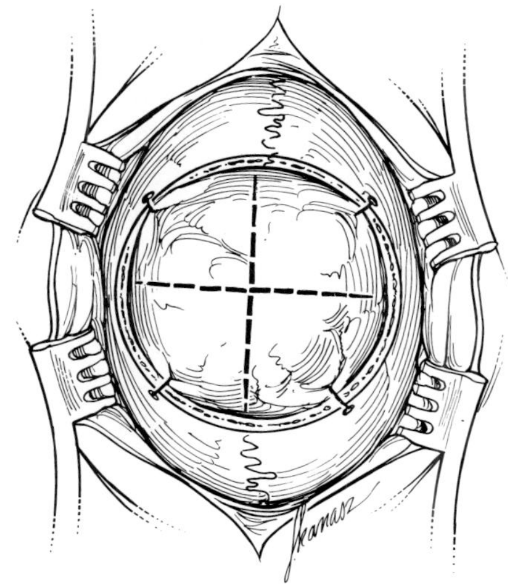

Figure 5-6. A small bone flap (1 to 2 inch) is then fashioned using a trephine or craniotome.

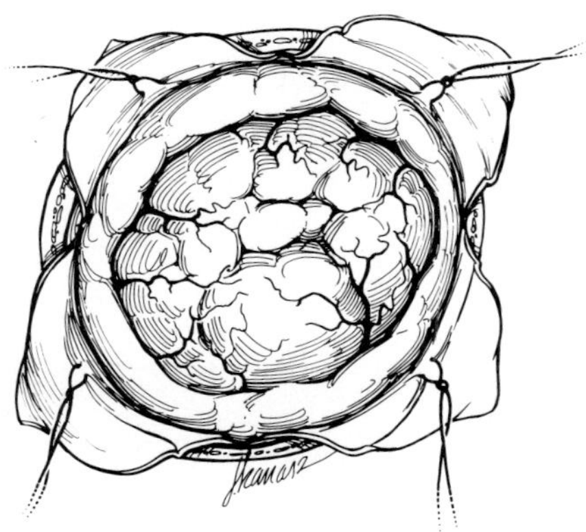

Figure 5-7. The dura is opened in four or more leaflets. It is best to retract the leaflets with sutures at their bases. This provides better exposure than when the apices are used. The superficial tumor is situated in the center of the minimal access craniotomy and is bounded by sulci laterally. The accuracy of the SNS can be confirmed by localizing in one of the sulci.

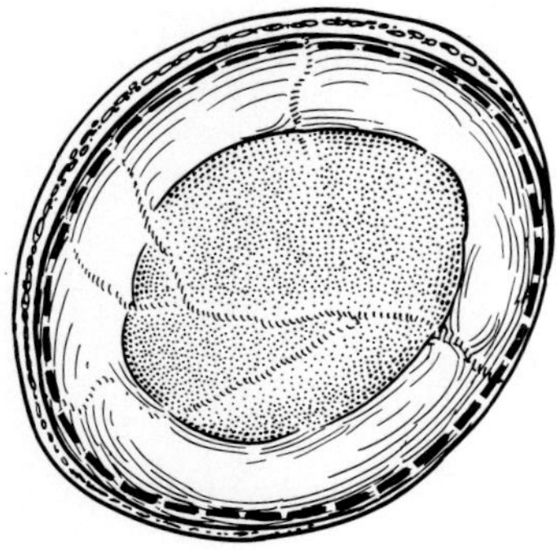

Figure 5-8. Dural-based lesions require opening the dura peripherally (dotted line).

The exposed cortical anatomy and veins provide an ideal opportunity to confirm the accuracy of the SNS prior to cerebrotomy. The view perpendicular to the wand should clearly show the veins, gyri, and sulci, especially when MRI is used for guidance, and correlate to what the surgeon sees. It is important to bear in mind that at this point the brain is often displaced a few millimeters through the dural plane so that there is often a predictable discrepancy of depth when using this technique. Triplanar displays can also be used to track visible sulci to ensure there is concordance.

Superficial lesions, particularly gliomas, often conform to sulci, and when visually different from the surrounding brain (see Fig. 5-7) provide a reference to confirm the accuracy of the SNS.

Lesion Resection and Brain Shift

The localization function of an SNS can provide valuable information as to the boundary between solid tumor and brain, particularly when contrast-enhanced MRI is used for navigation (Fig. 5-9). Optimal use of these devices, however, requires some modification of traditional microsurgical technique. Traditional gutting of the tumor followed by centripetal resection to surrounding brain[14] often renders preoperative imaging inaccurate as a navigational guide. As the tumor shrinks, the SNS is still referenced to the original tumor size, thereby

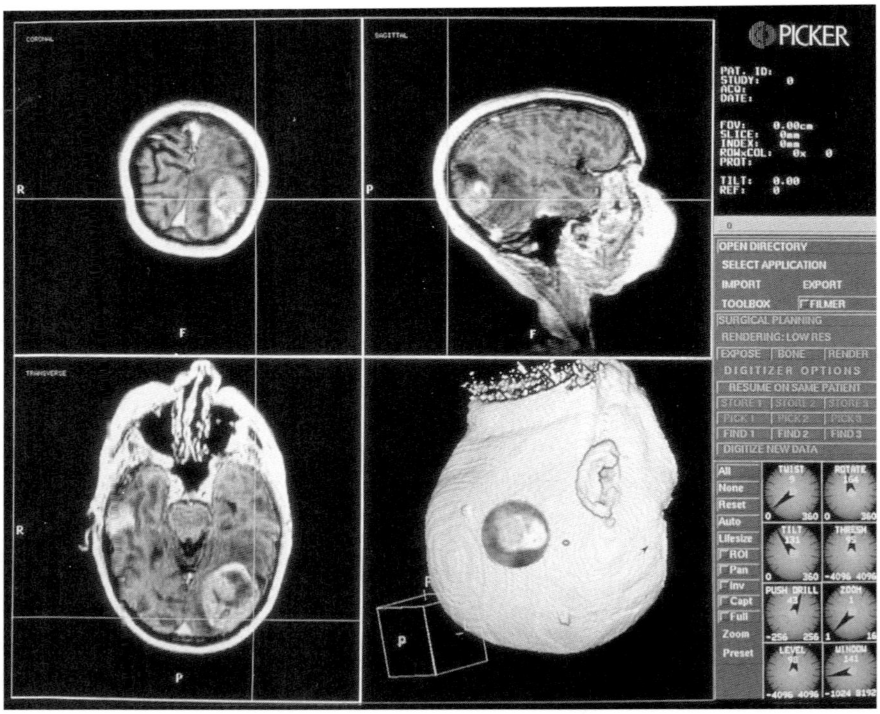

Figure 5-9. A triplanar display showing the location at the edge of the brain-tumor interface (crosshairs).

suggesting that more tumor remains than actually does. Similarly, it is unwise to decompress cystic portions of the tumor early in the resection because this may unpredictably displace the entire region of interest. For these reasons, when the SNS is used to assist in tumor-brain boundary definition, tumor resection is best accomplished by an en bloc resection.[1,2,6,7] The tumor-brain interface, defined using visual, tactile, and SNS information, is developed (Fig. 5-10), working first around the superficial portion of the tumor and then proceeding to its base (Fig. 5-11). If the resection is complete as documented by radiography, primary hemostasis is usually obtained easily without the need for lining the cavity with hemostatic agents (Fig. 5-12). Not all tumors can be removed in one piece without sacrificing safety. In such cases attention is first directed to regions where SNS information would be most useful, such as the portion nearest eloquent brain or deep nuclei. When brain distortion or shift is suspected, it is better to leave some tumor behind than risk intrusion into sensitive areas. Updated image data sets with ultrasound[17] or intraoperative MRI (see Chapter 18) may permit better and safer resection than is feasible with preoperative imaging alone.

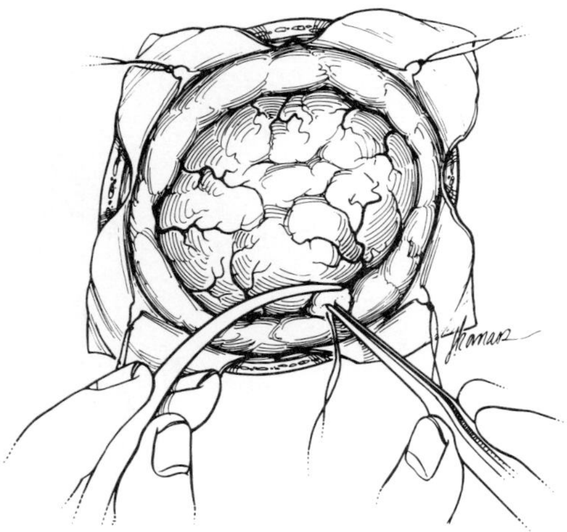

Figure 5-10. The sulcus is opened and the plane of dissection carried into the gyrus.

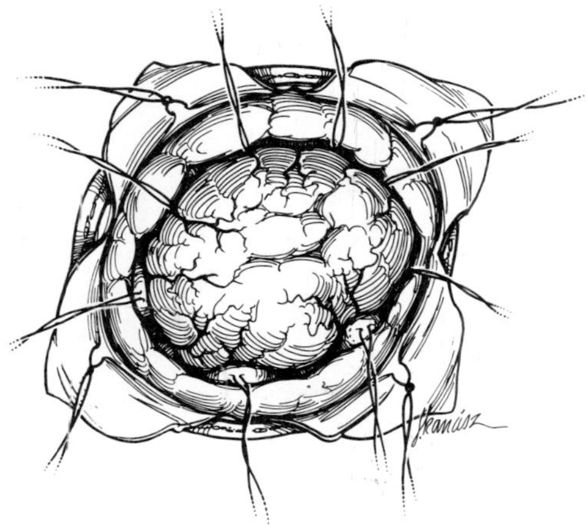

Figure 5-11. The localization function is used to assist in defining the plane around the entire solid portion of the tumor. If the lesion is not located in functionally eloquent brain, resection can be extended in an effort to obtain better margins.

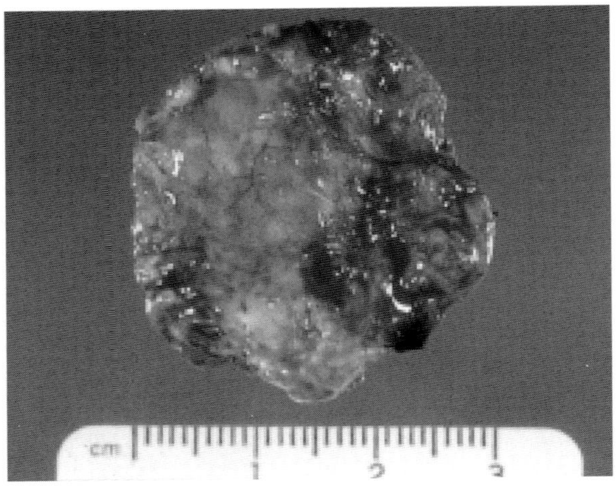

Figure 5-12. The tumor is then removed in essentially one piece and hemostasis obtained, usually without the need for topical agents.

Figure 5-13. Dural approximation is usually sufficient unless the ventricles or cisterns have been entered.

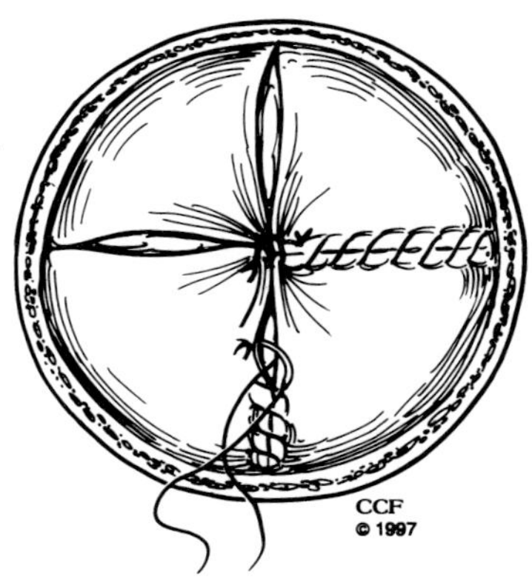

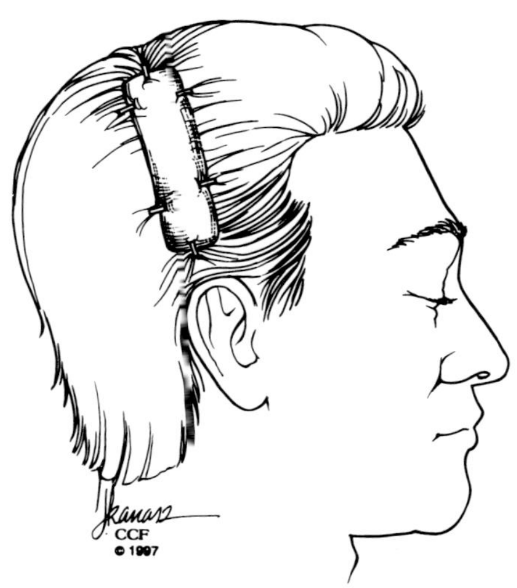

Figure 5-14. Antibiotic ointment is applied and a mini dressing stapled to the scalp.

Closure

Wound closure is accomplished by reapproximation of dural leaflets (Fig. 5-13). If the ventricles or large subarachnoid spaces are encountered, a watertight closure is desirable. The bone may be secured with suture, wire, or bone plates. A subgaleal drain may be placed if desired, followed by conventional closure of the galea and scalp. Antibiotic ointment is placed on the incision and a small dressing is stapled to the skin (Fig. 5-14).

SUMMARY

Minimal access craniotomy may be facilitated by use of SNSs, but optimal results require knowledge of the limitations of SNSs based on preoperative imaging and some modifications of traditional neurosurgical techniques.

References

1. Barnett GH. Stereotactic techniques in the management of brain tumors. Contemp Neurosurg 19:1-9, 1997.
2. Barnett GH, Kormos DW, Steiner CP, Weisenberger J. Use of a frameless, armless stereotactic wand for brain tumor localization with two-dimensional and three-dimensional neuroimaging. Neurosurgery 33:674-678, 1993.
3. Doshi PK, Lemieux L, Fish DR, Shorvon SD, Harkness WH, Thomas DG. Frameless stereotaxy and interactive neurosurgery with the ISG viewing wand. Acta Neurochir Suppl 64:49-53, 1995.
4. Golfinos JG, Fitzpatrick BC, Smith LR, Spetzler RF. Clinical use of a frameless stereotactic arm: Results in 325 cases. J Neurosurg 83:197-205, 1995.
5. Guthrie BL, Adler JR Jr. Computer-assisted preoperative planning, interactive surgery, and frameless stereotaxy. Clin Neurosurg 38:112-131, 1992.
6. Kelly PJ. Volumetric stereotactic surgical resection of intra-axial brain mass lesions. Mayo Clin Proc 63: 1186-1198, 1988.
7. Kelly PJ, Kall BA, Goerss S, Earnest F IV. Computer-assisted stereotaxic laser resection of intra-axial brain neoplasms. J Neurosurg 64:427-439, 1986.
8. Maciunas RJ, Galloway RL Jr, Fitzpatrick JM, Mandava VR. Edwards CA, Allen GS. A universal system for interactive image-directed neurosurgery. Stereotact Funct Neurosurg 58:108-113, 1992.
9. Manwaring KH. Magnetic field guided endoscopic dissection through a burr hole may avoid more invasive craniotomies. A preliminary report. Acta Neurochir Suppl 61:34-39, 1994.
10. Murphy MA, Barnett GH, Kormos DW, Weisenberger J. Astrocytoma resection using an interactive frameless stereotactic wand. An early experience. J Clin Neurosci 1:33-37, 1994.
11. Rhoten RP, Luciano M, Barnett GH. Computer-assisted neuro-endoscopy (CANE). Neurosurgery 40: 635-638, 1996.
12. Roberts DW, Strohbehn JW, Friets EM, Kettenberger J, Hartov A. The stereotactic operating microscope: Accuracy refinement and clinical experience. Acta Neurochir Suppl 46:112-114, 1989.
13. Smith KR, Frank KJ, Bucholz RD. The NeuroStation—A highly accurate, minimally invasive solution to frameless stereotactic neurosurgery. Comput Med Imaging Graph 18:247-256, 1994.
14. Walters CL, Schmidek HH. Surgical management of intracranial gliomas. In Schmidek HH, Sweet WH, eds. Operative Neurosurgical Techniques: Indications, Methods and Results. Philadelphia: WB Saunders, 1988, pp 431-450.
15. Barnett GH, Steiner CP, Weisenberger J. Target and trajectory guidance for interactive surgical navigation systems. Stereotact Funct Neurosurg 66:91-95, 1996.
16. Winston KR. Hair and neurosurgery. Neurosurgery 31:320-329, 1992.
17. Trobaugh JW, Richard WD, Smith KR, Bucholz RD. Frameless stereotactic ultrasonography: Method and applications. Comput Med Imaging Graph 18:235-246, 1994.

6

Cerebral Metastatic Disease

Barton L. Guthrie, M.D.

Resection of cerebral metastases is one of the most rewarding applications of cranial surgical navigation systems. This technology permits a minimally invasive operation that is associated with a short convalescence for patients who may have little quality life remaining. Cranial graphic-interactive navigation systems allow virtual planning of the least destructive surgical routes and are particularly helpful if craniotomies for more than one metastasis are planned. This chapter describes our experience in treating cranial metastasis at the University of Alabama at Birmingham, with emphasis on the application of a mechanically linked localization system called the Operating Arm system (Radionics, Brookline, Mass.).

Radiosurgery using the medical linear accelerator and Gamma Knife is our preference for management of cerebral metastases of less than 3 cm in diameter. Craniotomy is reserved for tumors larger than 3 to 4 cm since the complications of radiosurgery, especially symptomatic radionecrosis, are unacceptably high.

PATIENT POPULATION

Computer-assisted localization was used to treat 206 cerebral metastatic tumors in 100 patients from November 1, 1992, through March 31, 1996. Eighty-one patients were treated with radiosurgery and 19 with craniotomy. Six patients underwent both craniotomy and radiosurgery. Fifteen of the craniotomies were

Table 6-1. Patient Population

Procedure	No. of Patients
Craniotomy	13
Radiosurgery	
Medical linear accelerator (LINAC)	60
Gamma Knife	27
Radiosurgery and craniotomy	
Tumor >3 cm	2
Radionecrosis	4

performed to resect tumors larger than 3 cm in diameter. Four craniotomies were performed to debulk intractable radionecroses 12 to 30 months after radiosurgery; each of these four patients had tumors 2.5 cm or larger.

CRANIOTOMY

Preoperative Preparation

Patients were thoroughly informed about the use of computer-assisted guidance, which may range from craniotomy to navigation through the brain to the lesion.

Six surgical wound staples are affixed to the scalp to serve as localization fiducials for the preoperative CT scan. Preinjection of lidocaine is not necessary. To improve fiducial effectiveness, the scalp staples are positioned as far apart as possible in the following configuration: one in the midline at the hairline, one at the inion, one under each parietal boss, and one just below each superior temporal line a centimeter forward of the pinna. This positioning may be modified so that skeletal pinions do not shift the staple location.

In most cases 5 mm scan slices are adequate. If greater accuracy is required, 3 mm slices are obtained. The patient must remain immobile in the scanner to prevent increased error. A strip of tape across the forehead is usually sufficient to stabilize the head if the patient is cooperative.

The patient is positioned for the craniotomy in the operating room. A major advantage of frameless guidance is that any head position can be accommodated. After the patient is positioned for the craniotomy and before the skin is prepared, the localization device is fixed to the head-holder and registration is accomplished by touching four of the six staples in a defined sequence. The other two staples are used for accuracy testing.

Operative Planning

The surgeon and operating room personnel must be familiar with the image-interactive Operating Arm system to maximize its efficiency. The device is used to mark the general location of the craniotomy before shaving the patient's hair. If the lesion is close to the cortical surface, the skin incision line can be drawn over it with confidence that the craniotomy is accurate. If the tumor is more than several millimeters from the cortex, it is not adequate to pick a point on the head "just above the tumor" because head tilt during image acquisition may cause an erroneous estimate of trajectory. The *trajectory* feature, available on all surgical navigation systems, must be used for planning. I localize the craniotomy by drawing the margins of the tumor on the scalp as projected along the surgical trajectory, thereby ensuring optimal placement of the craniotomy to avoid operating at an angle under the bone edge. The tumor margin is marked so as to accommodate reported system error. For example, if the system reports a 4 mm error, the diameter is marked as roughly 4 mm larger than the actual tumor and centered on the tumor epicenter. This is an example of how the surgeon can use the feature of calculated error provided by these systems.

A straight incision is centered over the drawn tumor margins (or the projected margins if the tumor is deep). A curved incision may be required for cosmetic reasons, such as if a tumor lies within the frontal lobes below the hairline. Just enough hair is shaved to accommodate the incision, and the region is prepped and draped. The Operating Arm system is draped and the sterilized tip is attached in a sterile fashion through the drape. Anatomic correlation is used to confirm that the system has retained calibration.

Mechanical devices such as the Operating Arm system must not be draped too tightly since this limits the motion of the digitizer joints and may cause unmeasured "sagging" of the connection clamp, which will introduce error. I have found that an ultrasound drape works well. The digitizer (the Arm) itself is positioned on the side where the anesthetist is located so that it is away from the surgeon-nurse instrument path.

Surgical Technique

In about half of these cases the tumor was located very near the surface so that the Operating Arm system was used primarily to plan a minimal skin incision and craniotomy. In the other half the trajectory feature was used for optimal placement of the craniotomy and planning the surgical trajectory. The following observations and technical considerations were noted:

- Deep and periventricular lesions require constant "trajectory siting" for dissection. In these cases the Operating Arm system is used to pass a ventricular catheter to the tumor. The surgical dissection can then be quickly carried out along the catheter without constant reference to the graphics. This simple maneuver can substantially expedite the approach to deep tumors.
- It is important to navigate to cystic lesions prior to drainage. Cyst drainage and brain sagging can invalidate system registration to the preoperative image.
- Metastases usually have a margin that is visible intraoperatively. Therefore image-interactive technology may best be used to simply "get there." Good microneurosurgical technique is essential for complete resection.
- Intraoperative use of image-interactive surgery becomes more valuable if the metastasis is located deep. Brain shift is less likely along the deep margins of the tumor, allowing reliable localization throughout the procedure. This is most valuable in preventing inadvertent entry into the ventricles.
- Occasionally metastatic tumors will have lobular projections or irregular cysts. Image-interactive systems are invaluable in "tracking down" these eccentric components of the tumor, especially if the lesion is in or near eloquent brain. The surgeon is advised to approach these areas relatively early in the procedure to avoid the problem of brain shift.

SUMMARY

The most useful applications of the Operating Arm system in this series of 13 craniotomies for metastatic tumors were in designing a small incision and craniotomy that permits minimally invasive craniotomies and short hospital stays; for approaching deep tumors, either through its navigation features or by passing a catheter to the lesion; and for locating and assisting with resection of tumors with irregular and difficult margins, especially near eloquent brain structures.

7

Intracranial Gliomas

Michael W. McDermott, M.D., F.R.C.S.(C)

Primary glial neoplasms, especially astrocytomas in adults, behave clinically in a malignant fashion because of their infiltrating nature, making them microscopically truly "unresectable" by nature of their brain location. However, local recurrence is still the major cause of failure in patients even after intensive local therapies. The recurrence is within 2 cm of the original site in 80% to 90% of cases.[1] Recurrence distally within the central nervous system or systemically is uncommon. Local therapies, in which open operation for tumor resection plays a major role, have been shown to improve patient survival. Although there is some controversy surrounding the role of debulking surgery for elderly patients with malignant gliomas, a number of retrospective and prospective randomized trials conducted by the Radiation Therapy Oncology Group have documented the benefit of surgical resection in improving survival for patients with supratentorial malignant gliomas.[2-5] Our experience at UCSF tends to confirm the value of open operation for these patients, both at the time of diagnosis and in selected cases at the time of recurrence.[6] For malignant gliomas in the pediatric population, previous studies have shown that surgical resection has been an important factor in determining outcome.[7] Some authors have pointed out the distinction between assessing the residual volume of disease rather than the percentage resection as the variable to be analyzed.[4,8] Regardless of the measure of resection, appropriately selected patients with gliomas live "better, if not longer" after debulking surgery.

Given that surgical resection is an important component in the management of patients with intracranial gliomas, any technique that can improve orientation within brain tissue at the time of surgery and assist in determining the margins of solid tumor tissue with surrounding infiltrated brain should improve the safety and efficacy of these procedures. In the past we have relied on a conceptualized three-dimensional volume of an intra-axial tumor based on our knowledge of neuroanatomy, imaging studies, intraoperative two-dimensional imaging information from ultrasound studies, and visual and tactile feedback to orient ourselves with respect to margins of solid tumor tissue and surrounding brain. During a surgical procedure involving a confined operative and visual field, once surface sulcal and gyral landmarks have been excluded and we proceed using the operating room microscope in a subcortical dissection, orientation becomes a problem. Surgical navigation systems (SNSs) help maintain orientation and provide additional information from preoperative imaging sets. These systems are not designed to replace the standard surgical techniques or the surgeon's judgment in determining the completeness or safety of surgical resection. The problems associated with these systems are that the preoperative registration accuracy is affected by intraoperative brain shift, distortion, and removal of cerebrospinal fluid. Despite such problems, these systems represent a significant advancement in the performance of more efficient, safe, and complete surgical resection as compared with technologies available in the past. At our institution it has become the standard approach for surgical resection of primary intracranial gliomas.

PREOPERATIVE PREPARATION

We prefer the Elekta ISG Viewing Wand that uses skin-based fiducials as part of the registration process. Because intracranial anatomic detail is better defined by MRI, we use this as the imaging study of choice for intra-axial tumors. The standard approach is to use a volume acquisition with 124 slices, 1.5 mm thick in the axial plane, that has no skip and has a field of view of 26 using an SPGR sequence with intravenous contrast. Radiology technicians are careful to avoid compression of the tragus, straps over the forehead, or sponges in the headrest that would distort the skin surface, which is used for part of the registration process.

For discrete, nonenhancing, presumed low-grade intra-axial neoplasms, standard T1 imaging may not define the boundaries clearly. If we need a T2 volume for surgery, we use a fast spin echo (FSE) image without fat suppression, which allows the skin surface to be seen for reconstruction and registration and allows better definition of the margins of the nonenhancing lesion. In these cases cod liver oil capsules are used as opposed to vitamin E since the latter are not seen on the FSE images. In the future, revisions to the image sequence coding and software for the system should allow a variety of image sequences to be presented for interactive display during surgery.

Because the system relies on skin-based fiducials for registration of imaging to physical space, a potential source of error is skin movement over the skull because of patient positioning or the effects of scalp movement with pin fixation. We now define our skin fiducial placements as either anterior, lateral (half and half), or posterior (Table 7-1). Anterior fiducials are placed over the junction over the frontozygomatic process with the body of the zygoma bilaterally, and supraorbital margin anterior to the superior temporal line bilaterally; two are placed in the midline in the region of the glabella. The total number of fiducials used for this anterior setup is six, five of which are used for the registration process and one of which is reserved for an accuracy test of the registration process. For the lateral setup, fiducials are placed ipsilateral to the lesion, over the frontozygomatic process, and at the supraorbital margin; two are placed in the region of the glabella. In addition, fiducials are placed over the mastoid, one in the region of the parietal eminence and two in the region of the posterior midline vertex, as well as one below the inion. For the posterior setup, fiducials are placed on the mastoid processes bilaterally and parietal eminences bilaterally; two are placed in the pos-

Table 7-1. Fiducial Sets for Different Brain Locations

Fiducial Set	Fiducial Location	No.
Anterior	Junction over frontozygomatic process/body	2
	Superior orbital margin	2
	Glabella	2
Lateral (half and half)	Ipsilateral frontozygomatic process/body	1
	Ipsilateral superior orbital margin	1
	Glabella	2
	Ipsilateral mastoid tip	1
	Ipsilateral parietal eminence	1
	Posterior midline vertex	1
	Inion	1
Posterior	Mastoid tips bilaterally	2
	Parietal eminence bilaterally	2
	Posterior midline vertex	2
	Inion	1

terior midline vertex; and one is placed just below the inion. Even with these fiducial placements appropriate for the tumor's anatomic location in the brain, problems with image registration can be improved by using a combination of skin-based surface fiducials and random surface points.

In the operating room we use pin fixation for all patients, including those who require local anesthesia for intraoperative speech mapping. Ultra-short-acting intravenous anesthetic agents in combination with local anesthetic field blocks permit use of the Mayfield pin apparatus in patients who require speech/language assessment. We have had no problems with this technique.

Once the registration process has been completed and the accuracy of the registration confirmed, the surgeon can use the device in manual mode to review the anatomy of the tumor in three planes and "scroll" through the tumor volume. When the operative approach and plan are confirmed, the device is switched to the active mode to localize the tumor under the scalp and skull and help plan skin incisions. After the scalp flap has been turned back, the wand can be brought back into the field to confirm the margins for the craniotomy/craniectomy.

SURGICAL TECHNIQUE

Supratentorial Region

Frontal Lobe Tumors

For intra-axial tumors of the frontal lobe, use of SNSs is straightforward. Fiducials are placed in an anterior position, and the patient's head is usually straight up or rotated 20 degrees to the opposite side (Table 7-2). When a frontal lobectomy is planned, one of the issues that the surgeon should be aware of is the inaccuracy of the registration of position for brain structures as brain shift occurs with drainage of cerebrospinal fluid or coagulation and cutting of parasagittal draining veins, both of which allow the frontal lobe to move posteriorly and inferiorly. To allow the surgeon to assess this degree of shift, we place small black dot tickets on the surface of the brain at the start of the procedure similar to the

Table 7-2. Head Rotation for Patient Positioning and Fiducial Set Selection

Head Rotation* (degrees)	Fiducial Set	Anatomic Location
0-60	Anterior	Frontal Temporal Parietal
60-120	Lateral (half and half)	Medial temporal Posterior temporal, occipital Posterior parietal, occipital Cerebellopontine angle
120-180	Posterior	Posterior medial temporal Occipital Posterior fossa

*0 degrees = supine, brow up, no rotation; 180 degrees = prone, Concorde, face down.

numbers or letters used during functional mapping. A second registration is required at the beginning of the procedure if the surgeon plans to use these "brain landmarks." With this second registration set, these black dot tickets on the surface of the brain can be used as landmarks so the surgeon can check the minimum tip-to-landmark distance to assess the degree of shift at the brain surface.

Temporal Lobe Tumors

Tumors of the anterior temporal lobe are approached in a similar fashion to those of the frontal pole. For midtemporal and posttemporal tumors where the head will be rotated beyond 60 degrees from the upright position, a lateral or half-and-half fiducial placement technique will be used. This avoids artifact created by using fiducials on the dependent portions of the skin surface that sag away from the bone with extremes of positioning. Lesions that are in the medial portion of the temporal lobe are also subject to lack of anatomic correlation with registration when retraction is required for elevation of the temporal lobe to gain access to the medial structures. The surgeon can become reoriented relative to the dura of the middle cranial fossa, the lateral wall of the cavernous sinus, and the free edge of the tentorium to estimate the degree of shift of temporal lobe structures caused by retraction. Tumors in a posterior medial temporal lobe location can be exposed also via a supratentorial medial suboccipital route to minimize temporal lobe elevation for access.

Parietal Lobe Tumors

For tumors in the nondominant parietal lobe, the main concern is the effect that patient positioning will have on fiducial placement. Again, the surgeon should consider this prior to the operation so that the appropriate fiducial set can be placed before imaging studies. In the dominant hemisphere we have been able to use the ISG system with the patient awake for speech and motor mapping in pin fixation.

Occipital Lobe Tumors

For tumors in this location, a posterior fiducial set should be placed. For these fiducials, the scalp will have to be shaved prior to the imaging study so that the fiducials can be reliably secured to the skin. Again, the mastoid process bilaterally, the parietal eminences bilaterally, the midline vertex, and the inion are used for fiducial placement.

Other Brain Locations

SNSs are particularly helpful using a trajectory view for accessing tumors within the ventricular cavity. This trajectory view can be used to guide the surgeon transcortically to the ventricle and also allow determination of where to begin an incision along the corpus callosum. Although the intraventricular landmarks assist with orientation during the procedure, surgical navigation devices are particularly helpful in determining the posterior margin of large tumors. All too often in the past we assumed a greater extent of surgical resection was needed for intraventricular lesions based on postoperative imaging studies than was actually the case. This seems to have become less of a problem since using this device.

This device has also proved particularly helpful to pediatric surgeons for the surgical debulking of optic chiasm hypothalamic gliomas. Significant resections have been accomplished safely, and anecdotal evidence suggests that the extent of resection of these tumors may also influence outcome, although this remains to be analyzed. Orientation with respect to the lateral, posterior, and superior margins of these lesions is of course crucial and is assisted by the SNS.

Focal low-grade contrast-enhancing neoplasms within the brainstem are now being approached surgically by our pediatric colleagues, and there is again some evidence that this may improve tumor control. Lesions of the midbrain, diencephalon, pons, and medulla can be approached accurately and selective incisions made in the pial surface. Because these lesions are located in the brainstem, errors in registration related to brain shift are minimized the closer one is to the central axis of the brain. Surgeons should be mindful of the focal length objective of the microscope and the length of the probe to be used. The shorter the focal length for the microscope lens, the more difficulty the surgeon will have in placing the probe deep into the wound toward the brainstem at the time of surgery. Lenses of 350 to 400 mm are most appropriate, and the long probe should be used for deep transsylvian approaches or subtemporal transtentorial approaches to the brainstem.

Infratentorial Region

Cerebellar Tumors

A posterior fiducial set is of course necessary for accurate registration in patients with cerebellar tumors, whether the patient is positioned prone or in the Concorde position. Tumors within the cerebellar hemisphere or vermis can be more accurately localized, and again, the deeper location of lesion in the hemisphere, the less important are issues related to brain shift. However, supracerebellar infratentorial approaches to anterior vermian lesions require consideration of the effects of inferior displacement of the cerebellum during tumor exposure.

Fourth Ventricular Tumors

Exophytic brainstem tumors or tumors filling the fourth ventricle are ideally imaged in the sagittal plane to maintain the surgeon's orientation with respect to the floor of the fourth ventricle. When the rostral or caudal portion of the normal ventricular floor cannot be seen because of the tumor mass, these SNSs assist with maintaining orientation of position relative to the position of the floor of the fourth ventricle above and below the margin of tumor. Patients with tumors that do not arise from the floor of the fourth ventricle primarily, such as medulloblastomas, can also benefit from the use of the device by allowing the surgeon to become reoriented as the resection proceeds and presumably increasing the efficiency and safety of tumor resection.

Posterior Fossa Biopsies

In the past, frame-based stereotaxy has been used for biopsy in selected cases prior to instituting therapy, and the options are either a transcerebellar route through the middle cerebellar peduncle, a precoronal transventricular intra-axial trajectory, or less commonly, a transtentorial route. Limited craniectomies can be performed using the image-guided system, and a small corridor down to the lesion can be safely developed using the in-line trajectory view. Lesions down to the junction of the dorsal pons and middle cerebellar peduncle have been approached in this fashion.

CLINICAL EXPERIENCE

During a prospective clinical trial of the ISG wand at UCSF between 1993 and 1994, the device was used for operation on an intra-axial primary brain neoplasm in 61% of cases. In this group of 51, 66% of the patients had high-grade gliomas, and 25% were being operated for recurrent disease. The average time for registration was 13 minutes during this study, and the additional time for setup of the equipment in the operating room was approximately 18 minutes. The majority of the surgeons (85%) believed the device was easy to use, and most (76%) thought the device was helpful in assisting them with tumor resection. There were no breaks in the sterile field or adverse patient events. Table 7-3 lists the pathologic diagnoses for these 51 patients.

The experience with the device now includes over 400 cases and the system is considered standard equipment, at least for supratentorial neoplasms and for first-time operations and reoperations for intra-axial neoplasms. Because of time constraints and use of the device twice in one day, patients scheduled for surgery starting in the morning are scanned the afternoon before surgery, and patients scheduled for operations later in the day are scanned the morning of surgery. Operating room technicians and the surgeon work together to perform the registration process, and fiducial locations for registration can be selected ahead of time

Table 7-3. Pathologic Diagnoses for Intra-Axial Neoplasms

Newly Diagnosed		Recurrent	
Glioblastoma multiforme	16	Recurrent glioblastoma multiforme	8
Anaplastic astrocytoma	7	Recurrent anaplastic astrocytoma	3
Oligodendroglioma	7	Recurrent oligodendroglioma	3
Astrocytoma	2	Recurrent astrocytoma	1
Juvenile pilocytic astrocytoma	2		
Ependymoma	2		
Mixed oligoastrocytoma	1		
Ganglioglioma	1		

on the computer, which speeds up the process. Intraoperatively, particularly when working under the microscope, the surgeon requires the assistance of operating room personnel to freeze the image position so that he or she can safely turn away from the microscope to look at the computer screen. In an attempt to overcome this problem, we have adapted a small 4.5-inch diagonal active liquid crystal display flat video monitor to the operating room microscope and hard-wired the monitor back to the ISG computer.

TECHNICAL CONSIDERATIONS

The choice of the operative approach to a primary intra-axial neoplasm may influence how accurately preoperative imaging reflects intraoperative localization during the resection. Generally there are two approaches for removing malignant gliomas in the supratentorial compartment in a noneloquent location. The first is by limited corticectomy and internal debulking; the second is a larger area of corticectomy immediately superficial to the area of underlying brain abnormality. In the first approach considerable retraction along the corticectomy is required to expose peripheral margins of the tumor, and this retraction may add to the displacement of brain tissue, thus affecting the accuracy of the intraoperative location of the probe tip. With a more generous superficial corticectomy, such retraction is usually not required, and one would suppose that artifacts from retraction in this situation would be minimized. We have avoided the "fence-posting" technique employed by surgeons using frame-based systems in which catheters are placed stereotactically at the margins of the tumor and then the operation carried out following these catheters. Instead, once we have outlined the area for corticectomy, we proceed initially with a resection in a narrow trough at the margins of lesion down to the inferior extent of the tumor as visualized through the microscope and as represented on the ISG system. Once troughs around the margin of the tumor have been created, presumably the margins have been more accurately defined, as opposed to proceeding first to internal debulking where brain shift may interfere with accurate localization based on preoperative images.

We have also noted that there is a significant difference between first and second operations on a patient with a glioma, and this relates to the effect of prior therapies on the relative elasticity of brain. For initial operations, the brain is relatively more elastic, and tumor removal allows normal tissue to move into the

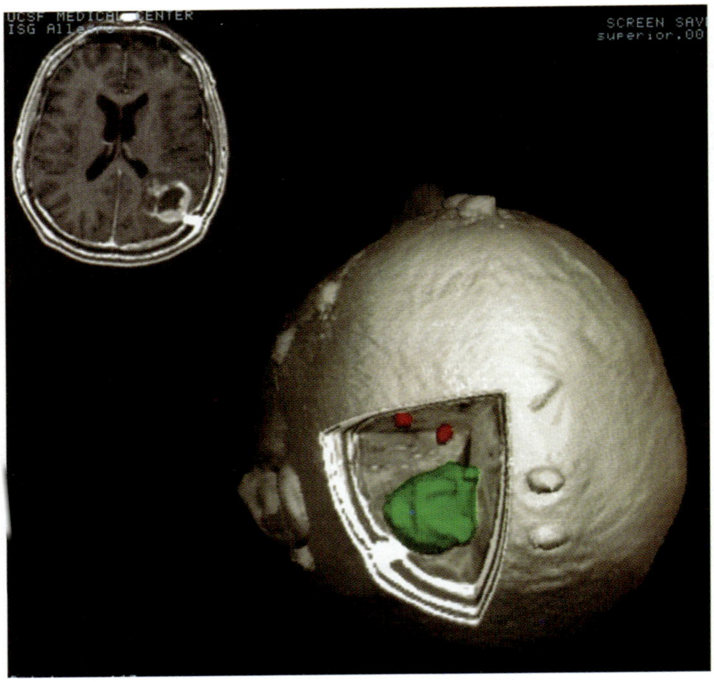

Figure 7-1. Three-dimensional image of patient with recurrent glioma showing reconstructed tumor volume (green) and position of somatosensory dipoles (red) from magnetic source imaging study.

space created by the resection cavity. This movement may make subsequent localization inaccurate and information related to visual and tactile clues as to the margins of solid tumor tissue with surrounding more normal edematous or infiltrated brain is thus more important. With recurrent tumors, the brain is less elastic and does not rebound back into the resection cavity after removal of tissue. On the other hand, with recurrent tumors the visual and tactile clues as to the junction between solid tumor tissue and surrounding brain is less well defined. Despite these limitations, we have found SNSs to be particularly helpful with achieving a more complete resection in these recurrent cases.

The surgeon should also be mindful of the fact that these SNSs are adjuncts to standard surgical techniques; they do not replace them. Anatomic localization does not guarantee functional localization, and in areas of eloquent tissue, intraoperative electrophysiologic monitoring and mapping are essential to reduce the likelihood of postoperative deficits. The combination of SNSs and electrophysiologic monitoring has allowed for more complete resection of lesions previously thought to be unapproachable or amenable only to "subtotal" removal of solid tumor tissue. Recently we have been successful in superimposing magnetic source imaging–derived somatosensory dipoles on two-dimensional and three-dimensional ISG images (Figs. 7-1 and 7-2). This has been helpful in localizing the primary sensory cortex during surgery.

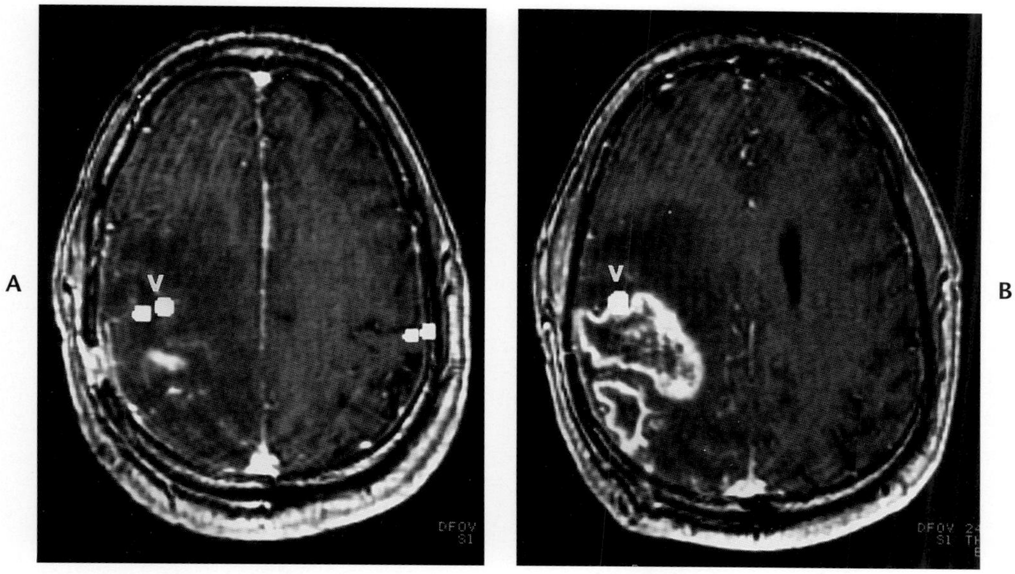

Figure 7-2. Two-dimensional axial images from different vertical slices in the same patient as in Fig. 7-1 showing representation of somatosensory dipoles *(v)* anterior to tumor for digits **(A)** and lip **(B)**.

SUMMARY

Our experience with one SNS has been gratifying. Surgeons have found the device easy to use, reliable, and informative. At our institution it has become standard equipment for resection of supratentorial intra-axial neoplasms and will likely become a specialty standard within the next 5 years. Future applications of the technology include combining functional MR or magnetic source imaging data with the SNSs, possibly reducing the need for intraoperative functional localization, at least at the cortical surface. Since intraoperative volumetric localization is possible for multiple sites within a tumor, there are basic science research questions comparing pathology, proliferative indices, special stains, and molecular biologic analyses with the results of diffusion-weighted, cerebral blood volume and spectroscopy MR-based imaging.

References

1. Sneed PK, Gutin PH, Larson DA, et al. Patterns of recurrence of glioblastoma multiforme after external irradiation followed by implant boost. Int J Radiat Oncol Biol Phys 29:719-727, 1994.
2. Curran WJ, Scott CB, Horton J, et al. Recursive partitioning analysis of prognostic factors in three Radiation Therapy Oncology Group malignant glioma trials. J Natl Cancer Inst 85:704-710, 1993.
3. Devaux BC, O'Fallon JR, Kelly PJ. Resection, biopsy and survival in malignant glial neoplasms. A retrospective study of clinical parameters, therapy and outcome. J Neurosurg 78:767-775, 1993.
4. Rostomily RC, Spence AM, Duong D, et al. Multimodality management of recurrent adult malignant gliomas: Results of a phase II multiagent chemotherapy study and analysis of cytoreductive surgery. Neurosurgery 35:378-388, 1994.
5. Simpson JR, Horton J, Scott C, et al. Influence of extent of surgical resection on survival in patients with glioblastoma multiforme: Results of three consecutive Radiation Therapy Oncology Group (RTOG) clinical trials. Int J Radiat Oncol Biol Phys 26:239-244, 1993.

6. Barker FG II, Prados MD, Chang SM, et al. Radiation response and survival time in patients with glioblastoma multiforme. J Neurosurg 84:442-448, 1996.
7. Duffner PK, Horowitz ME, Krischer JP, et al. Postoperative chemotherapy and delayed radiation in children less than three years of age with malignant brain tumors. N Engl J Med 328:1725-1731, 1993.
8. Berger MS, Deliganis AV, Dobbins J, et al. The effect of extent of resection on recurrence in patients with low-grade cerebral hemisphere gliomas. Cancer 74:1784-1791, 1994.

8

Intracranial Meningiomas

Gene H. Barnett, M.D. • *Wayel Kaakaji, M.D.*

The surgical approach to resection of intracranial meningiomas presents several challenges that are rarely encountered with primary or metastatic intraparenchymal tumors.[1,2] Not only must the bony opening be centered over the tumor, but its margins must more than encompass the dural attachment of convexity and parasagittal lesions to reduce the risk of recurrence.[3] Also, resection of lesions of the falx may be facilitated if the relationship of the tumor to veins draining into the superior sagittal sinus is known. Finally, tumors of the skull base often eclipse the view of the major cerebral arteries, potentially leading to catastrophic consequences.[4,5] Many of these problems unique to meningioma surgery and others common to all intracranial tumors may be mitigated with the use of real-time navigational information.[6]

Although image-guided frame stereotaxy (IGFS) gained some acceptance as a technique to guide resection of primary and metastatic brain tumors,[6-12] its role as an adjunct to meningioma surgery proved far more limited, being used almost solely to position minimal access craniotomies over small convexity lesions.[8] In theory, IGFS could be used to locate multiple targets[13] as would be required to design the size and shape of a bone flap; however, the logistics of using a frame to access a *single* target for craniotomy proved to be more than most neurosurgeons were willing to suffer.

The guidance, orientation, and localization information provided by contemporary surgical navigation systems (SNSs) provides far more useful stereotactic information than even the most sophisticated frame systems.[14-20] Our insights and opinions on how to best use SNSs during surgery for intracranial meningiomas are presented.

METHODS

The SNS has been previously described.[14,15] Early on the SNS used ultrasonic pulses produced by emitters affixed to a probe or other surgical instrument. These were then detected by an array of three or more microphones situated in an array affixed to or near the surgical field. The time delays between pulse production and detection for each possible emitter/microphone pair were determined electronically and their respective distances calculated after correction for the local speed of sound. Guidance, localization, and orientation information is presented on one of several multiplanar displays generated by a portable computer workstation and presented on computer monitors or a head-mounted display.[5] This work has subsequently been extended using an active light-emitting diode system using a trackable head reference and dual two-dimensional charge-coupled device cameras.

PATIENT POPULATION

The perioperative course of 48 patients undergoing 49 craniotomies for meningioma (Table 8-1) with the assistance of an SNS was reviewed. The patient data were prospectively entered into a computer database and charts retrospectively reviewed. Clinical outcome was evaluated 6 to 8 weeks after surgery. Five additional patients undergoing implantation of I-125 seeds for intracranial meningioma were also assessed. Substantial changes in performance (Karnofsky Performance Scale) of 20 or more points, steroid dose of 30% or more, or neurologic examination (e.g., loss or return of vision) were considered noteworthy. Minor nonneurologic complications such as urinary tract infections and deep vein thromboses are not included.

CLINICAL EXPERIENCE

Resection

Eighteen patients had resection of convexity meningiomas (5 falcine, 4 parasagittal, 1 tentorial, and 20 of the skull base). Of these, six were of the anterior and 12 of the middle cranial fossae. The mean age of patients was 55.8 years (median 53, range 23 to 81). Thirty-five of the patients were women (73%).

Morbidity data by anatomic site are presented in Table 8-2. One patient had transient aphasia after resection of a left frontal tumor. Serious sustained neurologic morbidity occurred in four patients: Cranial nerve palsies occurred in three patients with tumors invading the cavernous sinus (one also had a hemiparesis due to injury of perforator vessels) and a giant petroclival meningioma. One patient had persistent hemiparesis after intracranial hemorrhage due to anticoagulation in an effort to preserve patency of a vascularized myocutaneous flap that had repeatedly thrombosed. There was one death due to systemic complication of pneumonia and subsequent multiorgan failure and one death from other causes. There were three wound complications. Vision was not harmed in any patient.

Implants

Five patients underwent permanent implantation of I-125 seeds. All were poor surgical risks with stable or no symptomatology. Two lesions were falcine or parasagittal and three skull base in origin. There were no early or late complications from the procedure. All patients were discharged on the day of surgery. The

Table 8-1. Patient Characteristics

Sex/Age (yr)	Location	Type	2-Month Outcome	Complications
F/46	R. frontal convexity	Trephine	Same	
M/40	R. frontal convexity	Trephine	Improved	
M/78	R. frontoparietal convexity	OCC	Improved	
M/60	L. frontal convexity	OCC	Died	MOF
F/44	L. petroclival	Craniectomy	Same	
F/53	L. frontal parasagittal	Trephine	Same	
F/46	L. frontal convexity	OCC	Same	Transient aphasia
F/67	L. frontal convexity	Trephine	Same	
F/75	R. falcine	OCC	Improved	
F/32	Falcine	Trephine	Same	
F/44	R. cavernous sinus	CC	Same	CNI
M/53	R. sphenoid wing	OCC	Improved	
F/37	Falcine	OCC	Improved	
F/47	Planum sphenoidale	OCC	Same	
M/71	R. frontal convexity	OCC	Improved	
F/74	L. petroclival	Craniectomy	Worse	CNI
M/23	R. sphenoid	CC	Improved	
F/30	L. parietal convexity	OCC	Improved	Wound infection
F/59	L. sphenoid	CC	Improved	
F/42	R. cavernous sinus	CC	Worse	CNI
F/41	R. parietal convexity	OCC	Improved	
M/23	R. sphenoid	CC	Worse	ICH
M/60	R. frontal convexity	OCC	Improved	
F/68	R. anterior clinoid	CC	Same	
M/78	R. parietal convexity	Trephine	Same	
M/25	R. medial sphenoid wing	CC	Worse	CNI, hemiparesis
F/56	L. frontal convexity	Trephine	Same	
M/27	L. falcine	Trephine	Same	
F/72	R. central convexity	Trephine	Same	
F/74	R. parietal convexity	OCC	Same	
F/52	L. sphenoid wing	CC	Same	
F/46	L. parietal convexity	Trephine	Improved	
F/77	L. sphenoid wing	CC	Dead from other causes	
F/41	L. sphenoid wing	CC	Same	
F/81	R. sphenoid wing	CC	Improved	
F/66	L. central convexity	Trephine	Same	
F/53	L. occipital convexity	Trephine	Improved	
M/66	Olfactory groove	MAC	Same	
F/38	Tuberculum sella	CC	Improved	
F/71	R. tuberculum sella	CC	Same	
M/45	L. parasellar	CC	Improved	
F/46	R. central convexity	Trephine	Improved	
F/50	L. parasagittal	OCC	Same	
M/69	Olfactory groove	MAC	Improved	Transient CSF rhinorrhea
F/70	R. parasagittal	OCC	Improved	
F/76	R. sphenoid wing	CC	Same	
F/63	R. falcine	CC	Improved	
F/76	L. parasagittal	OCC	Same	
M/52	Tentorial	CC	Improved	Meningitis

OCC = optimize conventional craniotomy; CNI = cranial nerve injury; ICH = intracranial hemorrhage; MAC = minimal access craniotomy; MOF = multiorgan failure; NA = not applicable due to insufficient follow-up.

Table 8-2. Morbidity Associated with Meningioma Location

Site	Morbidity	Quantity
Convexity	Multiorgan failure	1/18
	Wound infection	1/18
	Transient aphasia	1/18
Falcine		0/5
Parasagittal region		0/4
Tentorial region	Meningitis	1/1
Skull base		
Anterior	CSF rhinorrhea	1/6
Middle	Cranial nerve palsies	3/12
	Hemiparesis	2/12
	Intracranial hemorrhage	1/12
Posterior	Cranial nerve palsies	1/2

number of seeds ranged from one to five. The initial tumor volume ranged from 21.1 to 208.2 cm^3 (mean 64.7 cm^3). Four tumors were reduced 25% to 40% in volume. Total dose delivered ranged from 7000 to 15,000 cGy (mean 10,800). One patient had a measured increase in volume of 16% (within the range of error) and no additional symptoms. The Karnofsky Performance Scale score improved in three patients and remained unchanged in two.

SURGICAL TECHNIQUE

Resection

Preoperative Planning

Most SNSs provide some mechanism to rehearse or plan operations using their sophisticated orientation and display facilities. This feature can provide important information on surgical risk and may influence decisions on surgical approach. For instance, the relationship of deep anterior or middle skull base meningiomas to the carotid artery can substantially affect resectability and risk. Visualization of underlying cortical or venous anatomy, either directly on oblique displays (see Chapters 5 and 17) or by fusion with physiologic data (e.g., PET or functional MRI) or vascular imaging (e.g., MR venography and angiography) may allow better prediction of risk of a motor or speech deficit. In our experience the need for these rehearsals, however, is the exception rather than the rule. Extensive preoperative planning is required and useful in a minority of cases, but it is comforting to know that it is available when indicated.

Convexity Lesions

Minimal Access Craniotomies. Small convexity lesions (i.e., 5 cm or less) are amenable to resection using trephinations or conventional craniotomies. In general MRI is preferred for use with the SNS. However, if preoperative MRI shows the absence of a dural tail and the lesion is far from parasagittal draining veins, CT may suffice.

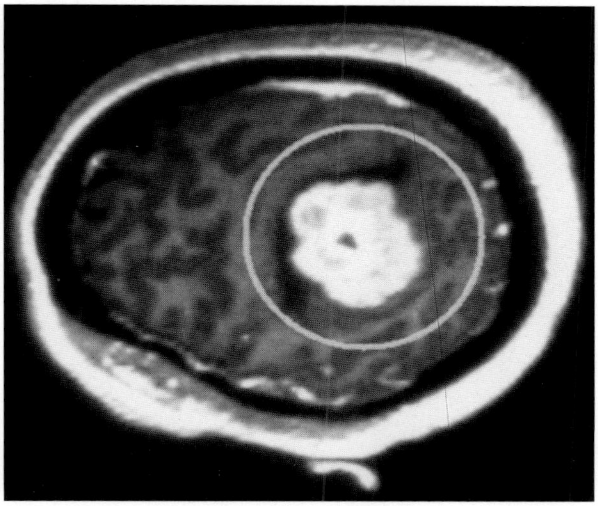

Figure 8-1. SNS oblique display that precisely defines the relationship between the center of the proposed craniotomy and the lesion.

After the patient's head is securely positioned and the SNS registered, a surgical trajectory may be defined. Early experience demonstrated that using simple triplanar displays (i.e., coronal, sagittal, and transverse planes) could be misleading when determining location of the craniotomy because of the curvature of the skull (see Chapter 5). Displays that contain the axis of the pointing device and one or more images normal to it (so-called oblique displays) provide far more accurate localization (Fig. 8-1). A craniotomy that is at least ½ inch larger than the maximum diameter of the tumor's dural base is prescribed.

A lazy S-shaped incision twice as long as the diameter of the intended trephination is planned centered on the surgical trajectory. The patient's hair is clipped rather than shaved, and this area is restricted to 0.5 cm to either side of the intended incision. Although shaving is probably unnecessary,[21] this limited clip facilitates suture placement and removal and yet is a cosmetic improvement for patients. The area and surrounding hair is scrubbed for 10 minutes or more prior to draping along the shaved areas using skin staples to secure the towels.

After incision, angled self-retaining retractors are used to provide exposure. Reorientation with the SNS then confirms proper centering of the craniotomy. Although a craniotome may be used, a pneumatically driven trephination may be faster in experienced hands. If the bone shows any evidence of tumor invasion, it is either terminally irradiated for use at closure or discarded and replaced by cranioplasty. Correct orientation is once again confirmed with the SNS. If MRI is used for navigation, the relationship of cortical veins to the craniotomy can be inspected and this information used to plan dural opening. Tacking sutures are placed at the perimeter of the dural exposure.

The dura is then incised peripherally (Fig. 8-2) and the lesion delivered using conventional techniques. Dural closure is typically unnecessary. A sheet of collagen foam or film is placed over the brain, the bone replaced, and the scalp closed followed by application of a sterile dressing.

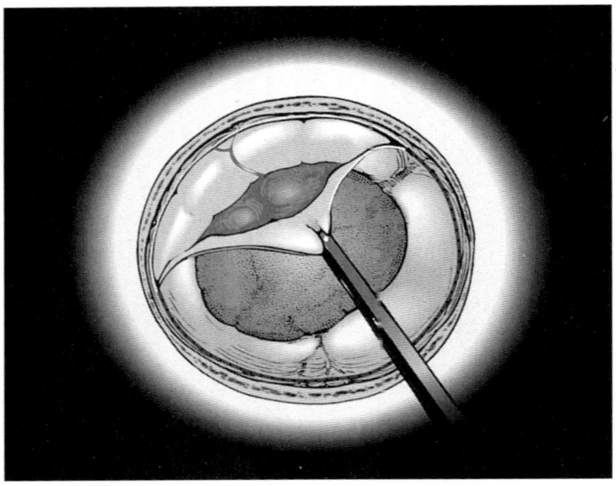

Figure 8-2. A typical peripheral dural opening for resection of a convexity lesion.

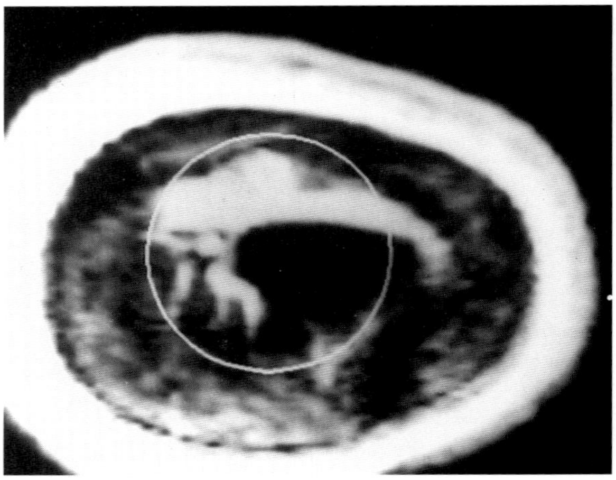

Figure 8-3. Surface veins may be readily visualized using the SNS prior to dural opening and tumor resection.

Large Convexity Lesions (Optimal Access Craniotomies). The general principles of tackling larger convexity meningiomas are much the same as for their smaller counterparts. The extent of the bony opening is once again determined using oblique displays, moving the pointing device to map the outline of the dural attachment. We favor larger S-shaped incisions over more conventional horseshoe or question-mark–shaped flaps since the former facilitates management of hair during draping, incision length is typically smaller and therefore opening and closure are expedited, and vascular compromise of the scalp (both arterial and venous) is minimized. Large self-retaining retractors provide exposure.

The craniotomy is fashioned using a craniotome after the tumor perimeter is once again confirmed using the SNS with oblique displays. Since large tumors are more likely to involve cortical veins, the venous anatomy should once again be studied using the SNS (Fig. 8-3). If large veins underlie the tumor, preservation of these vessels is probably best accomplished by exposing and resecting the tumor from the proximal portion of the vein distally.

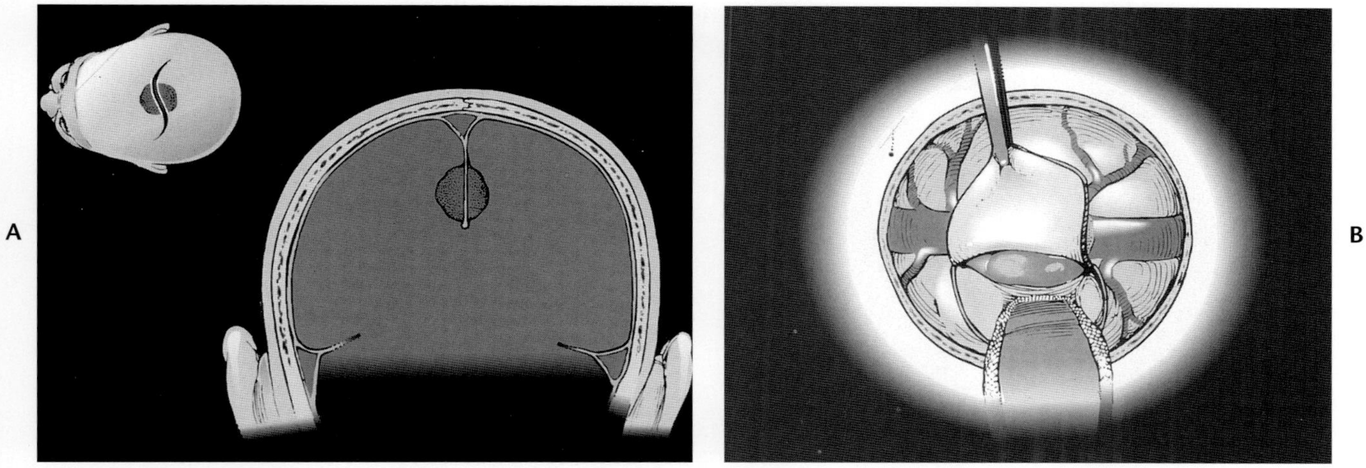

Figure 8-4. A, Coronal orientation of incision to access a falcine meningioma. This allows for venous control and reconstruction of the superior sagittal sinus should it be violated. **B,** The SNS allows visualization of multiple veins draining into the superior sagittal sinus to plan a surgical corridor between these vessels.

The SNS may help define the tumor-brain interface in the case of gliomas[15-17,19]; however, the boundary of meningiomas are readily apparent. Also, since they are extra-axial, they are tethered in place by their attachments to dura and skull. For both reasons, tissue movements (so-called brain shift) from use of diuretics, cerebrospinal fluid (CSF) drainage, or tumor resection are minimal when compared with SNSs to assist in resection of intra-axial tumors.

Tumor resection and closure are performed using conventional techniques.

Parasagittal and Falcine Lesions

Small Lesions. Parasagittal lesions less than 5 cm in size and even some larger falcine lesions can be successfully resected using minimal access craniotomies. It is important to plan the incision and bone opening to allow for control and reconstruction of the superior sagittal sinus in the event of laceration. Therefore the long axis of the S-shaped incision is positioned in a coronal plane, allowing access to the contralateral dura, and the incision is lengthened accordingly. If a trephine is used, a craniotome should be on hand in case contralateral bony removal is required and to minimize the risk to the sinus itself. The final opening of the inner table over the sinus may be performed using small chisels.

Once again, it is advantageous to exploit the ability of an SNS (using MRI) to display underlying venous anatomy when operating on tumors in these areas. The craniotomy may be situated to maximize the surgical corridor between draining veins when accessing falcine lesions (Fig. 8-4), even when this may not necessarily be the shortest approach. In contrast, when parasagittal lesions dictate the location of craniotomy, the dural opening can be planned to avoid underlying veins until they can be directly visualized.

A

B

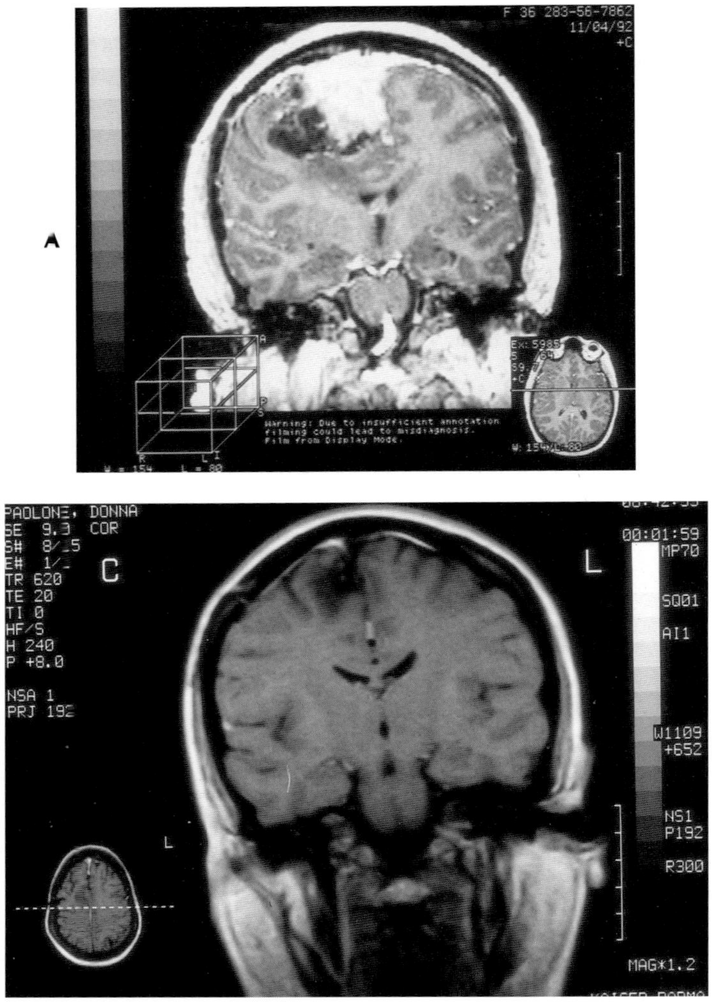

Figure 8-5. Large parasagittal lesion before **(A)** and after **(B)** resection guided by an SNS. Information on the lesion's boundaries and venous anatomy provided by the SNS was particularly helpful.

Large Lesions. Even enormous lesions can benefit from the ability of SNSs to determine underlying tumor boundaries and venous structures (Fig. 8-5). The surgical techniques are a combination of those for large convexity lesions and those for small tumors of the falx. Large, coronally oriented S-shaped incisions are favored and the bony opening tailored to encompass all dural attachments and tails of the tumor. Conventional bone flaps are elevated, exposing the superior sagittal sinus as required. Dural opening is begun in areas shown to be free of large draining veins. The opening is then extended under direct vision to areas shown to be suspect. When the SNS shows that cortical veins have been displaced to either side of the tumor and there is little risk of harming an underlying vein, the tumor may be resected from lateral to medial. Conversely, should the lesion appear to be obscuring one or more veins, the dural resection should be carefully extended along the sinus to expose the proximal aspect of the vein and attempt to resect the lesion from medial to lateral. Tumor debulking should be performed as required.

Tentorial Lesions

The benefits of SNSs when approaching meningiomas of the tentorium are somewhat limited. It is unusual for an experienced surgeon to need such a device to find these lesions, and large arteries are usually not lurking behind these tumors. Those vessels that may be nearby (e.g., posterior cerebral and superior cerebellar) are usually too small to be reliably identified on the SNS display; however, deep venous structures may be visualized. As such, the greatest benefit of navigational information in this setting relates to the venous anatomy.

In addition to deep veins, approaches to these lesions (both supra- and infratentorial) typically require craniotomies near the transverse sinus, and the SNS can readily be used to locate and avoid this structure. More important, the location of the vein of Labbé can be precisely identified and avoided during dural opening for supratentorial lesions. Similarly, draining veins of the occipital lobe may be identified when an interhemispheric approach is planned.

Skull Base Lesions

Anterior Fossae. The principal advantages of SNS for anterior skull base lesions are as follows:

1. Define relationship of the tumor to the optic nerves
2. Define relationship of the tumor to internal carotid arteries and proximal anterior and middle cerebral vessels
3. Locate frontal air sinuses
4. Determine one's position in the tumor when approaching more posterior structures.

Olfactory groove lesions may be approached using minimal access techniques through the eyebrows with excellent exposure and surprisingly good cosmetic results (Fig. 8-6). Brow hair should not be shaved since it may not regrow. The pericranium is reflected inferiorly, and the skull is opened using a craniotome. Prior to this the extent of the frontal air sinuses can be determined with the SNS to facilitate skull opening; the sinuses are then obliterated. Variants on pterional or subfrontal craniotomies may also be used for meningiomas of the anterior fossa. In these cases the SNS may be used to avoid the frontal air sinus on the operative side.

An SNS is rarely required to locate a tumor of the anterior skull base; however, it can be quite helpful during lesion debulking to determine one's position in the tumor, particularly if the posterior portion abuts or involves the optic nerves or major arteries. Inadvertent puncture of the posterior tumor wall can lead to disabling or fatal consequences.

Middle and Posterior Fossae. Meningiomas arising along the sphenoid wing are accessed easily using variants of a pterional approach without the need for

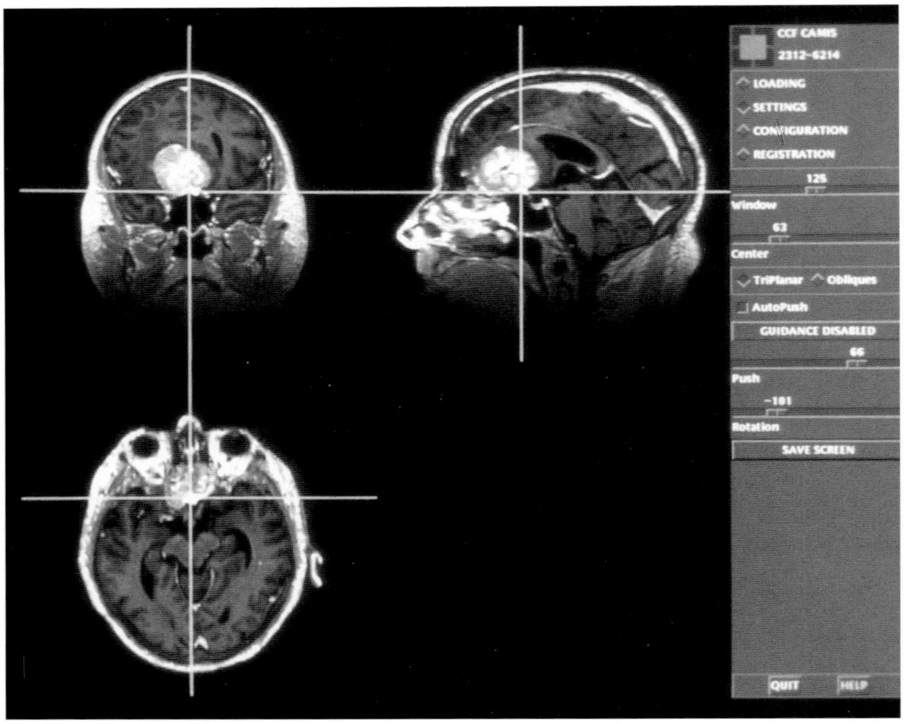

Figure 8-6. This large anterior fossa meningioma can be approached through a minimal access craniotomy located in the eyebrows.

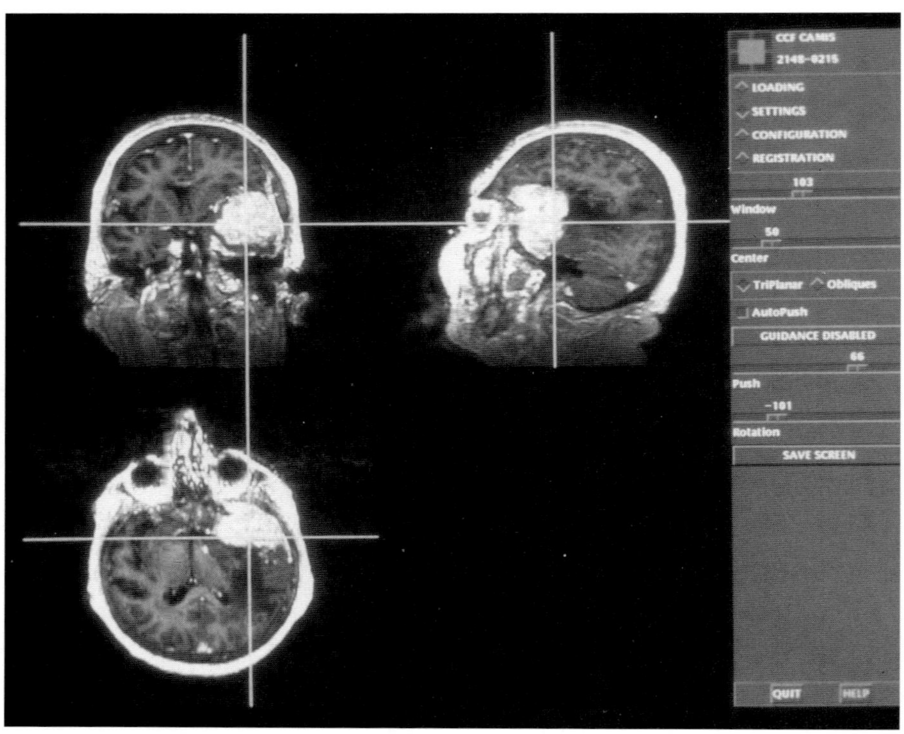

Figure 8-7. The SNS may be helpful when resecting skull base tumors such as this sphenoid wing meningioma by defining the surgeon's location in the tumor and position relative to arterial anatomy. This knowledge may prevent catastrophic vascular injury.

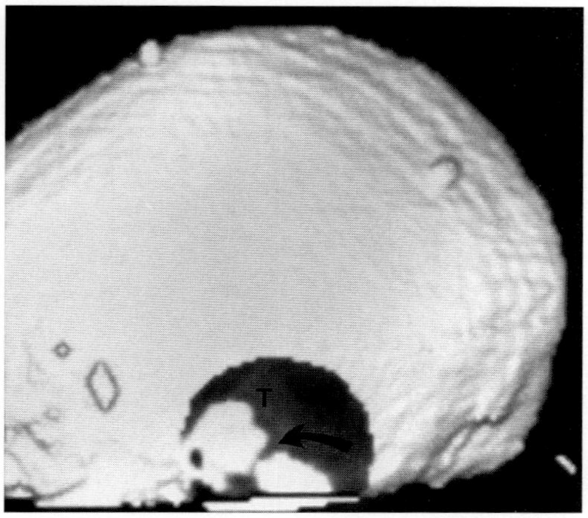

Figure 8-8. Navigational images of petroclival meningioma *(T)* using CT guidance showing internal auditory meatus (arrow). Such information may help prevent injury to cranial nerves, which are generally not visible on CT or MR navigational images.

SNSs. For large or mesial tumors, including those of the cavernous sinus, SNSs can provide valuable intraoperative information on the surgeon's location in the tumor as well as the location of major vascular structures such as the internal carotid and middle cerebral arteries (Fig. 8-7). Even with significant tumor removal, SNSs provide useful information on the relationships of mesial structures, which remain relatively unchanged until most of the tumor attachments to the skull base are severed. SNSs are also useful for guidance during extradural approaches.

As yet, SNSs seem to offer little additional protection for most cranial nerves during surgery. Unfortunately, small cranial nerves are not typically visualized on conventional CT and MRI, and SNSs give no hint of their position except where they pass through visualizable structures such as the superior orbital fissure. Even the location of portions of the optic nerve may be obscured when thinly stretched over the surface of an adjacent mass. Meticulous microsurgical technique and appropriate neurophysiologic monitoring minimize the risk to these friable structures more so than the SNS itself.

The situation is much the same for petroclival tumors; in this case the best use for SNSs is in determining one's location in the tumor and avoiding inadvertent entry into an obscured basilar artery. As for tentorial lesions, SNSs can assist in optimal positioning of the bone and dural opening with respect to nearby venous sinuses. Since most of the cranial nerves in the posterior fossa are not easily identified on MRI, particularly when draped over tumor, SNSs are of little benefit in nerve preservation. An exception is determining the location of the internal auditory meatus when it is obscured by a petroclival meningioma (Fig. 8-8).

Permanent I-125 Implants

Patient selection is critical. Candidates should have minimal symptoms (e.g., seizures controlled with anticonvulsants) or should be considered a poor surgical risk[22-24] (Fig. 8-9). The number and location of I-125 seeds are determined by the radiation oncologist. The patient's head is secured in a Mayfield three-point fixation device. Although the operation may be done with the patient awake, we prefer to use a general anesthetic.

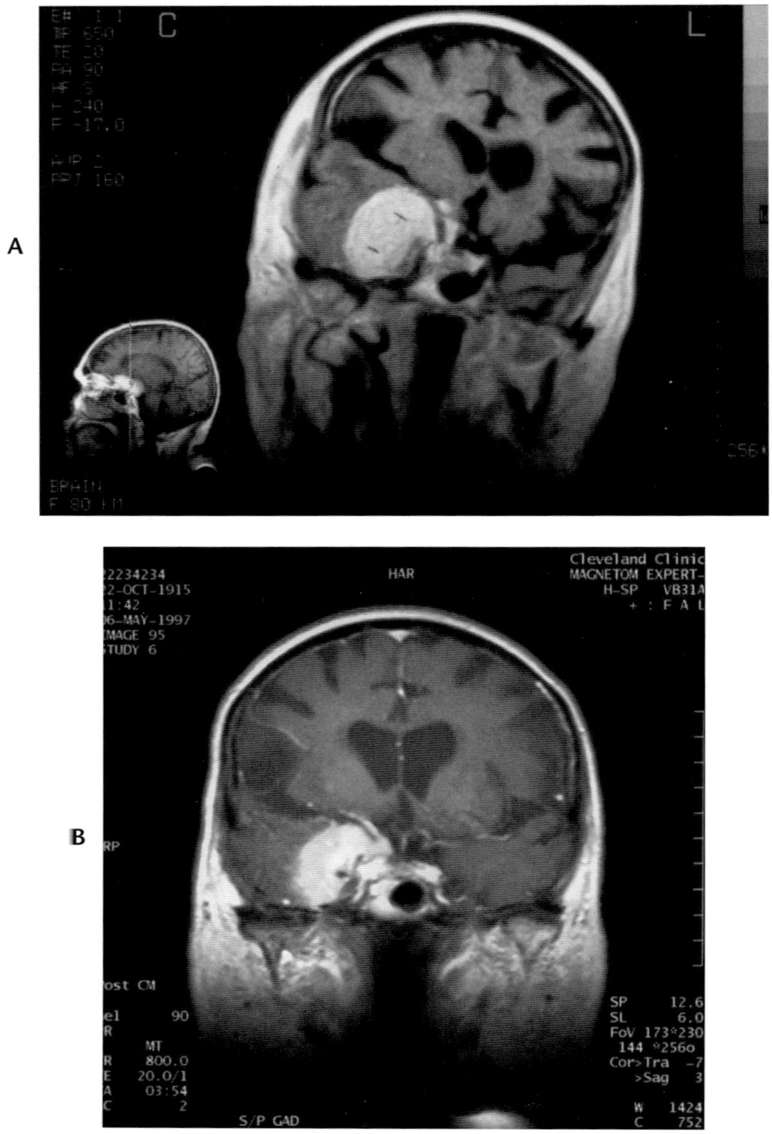

Figure 8-9. Patient with cavernous sinus/sphenoid wing meningioma before **(A)** and 18 months after **(B)** treatment with permanent I-125 implant (black dot). Note reduction in brain edema and mass effect.

The placement targets of the seeds are defined on the SNS. A small area of hair is clipped around the prospective entry point and the skin widely prepared with povidone-iodine scrub and solution. The scalp is punctured, a twist drill hole fashioned, and a cannula advanced just short of the target (to account for the length of the seed). A modified obturator is then used to drive the seed to the target site (Fig. 8-10). The scalp is closed with a single simple suture, a Band-Aid applied, and the patient awakened. Seed placement is confirmed with radiographs, and a CT scan of the head is obtained prior to discharge to exclude bleeding.

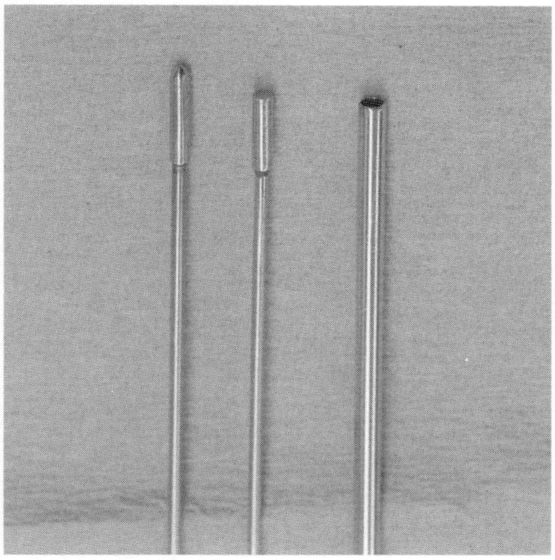

Figure 8-10. Instruments used to deliver I-125 seeds for permanent implantation into meningiomas. Left: Cannula. Right: Obturator used to pass cannula to target. Middle: Obturator shortened to be flush with end of cannula, thereby allowing seed to be pushed to end of cannula.

SUMMARY

It is not surprising that there are no large published series using IGFS as an adjunct to craniotomy for meningioma. With the exception of small convexity lesions, finding the tumor is not the navigational problem. Rather, optimizing the bone and dural opening, avoiding arterial and venous structures, defining the frontal air sinuses, and determining one's location within a large tumor devoid of landmarks are the pertinent issues. An SNS can provide the instantaneous localizing and orientation information that is required to address these problems and is an effective means of doing so. Permanent implantation of radioactive seeds into meningiomas that are either unresectable or when surgery poses unacceptable risk appears to be another promising area for SNSs in the management of some of these tumors.

We wish to thank Ms. Sharon Preztak for her assistance with the preparation of this manuscript and Picker International for material and software support.

References

1. Kelly PJ, Kall BA, Goerss SJ. Results of computed tomography-based computer-assisted stereotactic resection of metastatic intracranial tumors. Neurosurgery 22:7-17, 1988.
2. Kumar PP, Good RR, Leibrock LG, Mawk JR, Yonkers AJ, Ogren FP. High activity iodine 125 endocurietherapy for recurrent skull base tumors. Cancer 61:1518-1527, 1988.
3. Chen TC, Rabb C, Apuzzo ML. Complex technical methodologies and their applications in the surgery of intracranial meningiomas. Neurosurg Clin N Am 5:261-281, 1994.
4. Barnett GH, Steiner CP, Kormos DW, Weisenberger J. Intracranial meningioma resection using interactive frameless stereotaxy-assistance. J Image Guided Surg 1:46-52, 1995.
5. Barnett GH, Steiner CP, Weisenberger J. Adaptation of personal projection television to a helmet-mounted display for intraoperative viewing of neuroimaging. J Image Guided Surg 1:109-112, 1995.
6. Barnett GH, Kormos DW, Steiner CP, Weisenberger J. Intraoperative localization using an armless, frameless stereotactic wand. J Neurosurg 78:510-514 1993.
7. Ebeling U, Hasdemir MG. Stereotactic-guided microsurgery of cerebral lesions. Minim Invasive Neurosurg 38:10-15, 1995.
8. Gomez H, Barnett GH, Palmer J. Contemporary stereotactic neurosurgery at the Cleveland Clinic. Review of 501 consecutive cases. Cleve Clinic J Med 60:399-410, 1993.

9. Kumar PP, Patil AA, Syh HW, Chu WK, Reeves MA. Role of brachytherapy in the management of the skull base meningioma. Treatment of skull base meningiomas. Cancer 71:3726-3731, 1993.
10. Kelly PJ. Volumetric stereotactic surgical resection of intra-axial brain mass lesions. Mayo Clin Proc 63:1186-1193, 1988.
11. Moore MR, Black PM, Ellenbogen R, Gall CM, Eldredge E. Stereotactic craniotomy: Methods and results using the Brown-Roberts-Wells stereotactic frame. Neurosurgery 25:572-577, 1989.
12. Guthrie BL, Adler JR. Frameless stereotaxy: Computer interactive neurosurgery. Perspect Neurol Surg 2(1):1-19, 1991.
13. Hassenbusch SJ, Anderson JS, Pillay PK. Brain tumor resection aided with markers placed using stereotaxis guided by magnetic resonance imaging and computed tomography. Neurosurgery 28:801-806, 1991.
14. Horstmann GA, Reinhardt HF. Micro-stereometry: A frameless computerized navigating system for open microsurgery. Comput Med Imaging Graph 18:229-233, 1994.
15. Vuorinen V, Heikkonen J, Brander A, Setala K, Sane T, Randell T, Paetau A, Pohjola J, Mantyla M, Jaaskelainen J. Interstitial radiotherapy of 25 parasellar/clival meningiomas and 19 meningiomas in the elderly. Analysis of short-term tolerance and responses. Acta Neurochir 138:495-508, 1996.
16. Watanabe E, Watanabe T, Manaka S, Mayanagi Y, Takakura K. Three-dimensional digitizer (neuronavigator): New equipment of CT-guided stereotaxic surgery. Surg Neurol 27:543-547, 1987.
17. Kelly PJ. Computer-assisted stereotaxis: New approaches for the management of intracranial intra-axial tumors. Neurology 36:535-541, 1986.
18. Roberts DW, Strohbehn JW, Hatch JF, Murray W, Kettenberger H. A frameless stereotaxic integration of computerized tomographic imaging and the operating microscope. J Neurosurg 65:545-549, 1986.
19. Barnett GH, McKenzie RL, Ramos L, Palmer J. Nonvolumetric stereotaxy-assisted craniotomy: Results in 50 cases. Stereotact Funct Neurosurg 61:80-95, 1993.
20. Simpson D. The recurrence of intracranial meningiomas after surgical treatment. J Neurol Psychiatry Neurosurg 20:22-39, 1957.
21. Barnett GH, Kormos DW, Steiner CP, Weisenberger J. Use of a frameless, armless wand for brain tumor localization with two-dimensional and three-dimensional neuroimaging. Neurosurgery 33:674-678, 1993.
22. Winston KR. Hair and neurosurgery. Neurosurgery 31:320-329, 1992.
23. Roberts DW, Nakajima T, Brodwater B, Pavlidis J, Friets E, Fagan E, Hartov A, Strohbehn J. Further development and clinical application of the stereotactic operating microscope. Stereotact Funct Neurosurg 58:114-117, 1992
24. Sekhar LN, Babu RP, Wright DC. Surgical resection of cranial base meningiomas. Neurosurg Clin N Am 5:299-330, 1994.

9

Transsphenoidal Hypophysectomy

Gene H. Barnett, M.D.

The renewed interest in the transsphenoidal approach to tumors of the pituitary gland has proved a major advance in the management of these disorders.[1,2] Both micro- and macroadenomas may be approached using the sulabial or transeptal variations with minimal risk. Complications, however, include lateral entry into the carotid artery or cavernous sinus as well as misdirection superiorly into the ethmoid sinus or brain. Although fluoroscopy with lateral imaging aids orientation, this real-time imaging modality is somewhat cumbersome and does little to assist with left-right orientation in the sphenoid sinus. The introduction of endoscopy makes accurate localization of instruments and the surgical approach even more critical.

Surgical navigation systems (SNSs)[3-6] have the potential to augment or even replace fluoroscopy as a means of localization and guidance in transsphenoidal surgery. My opinions using SNS in this setting are presented.

SURGICAL TECHNIQUE

Imaging

SNSs are primarily used for guidance to the sella and orientation in the sphenoid sinus. These structures are best characterized by CT. With CT-compatible fiducials, a three-dimensional data set can be obtained that encompasses these markers as well as the nasal air passages, sphenoid sinus, and sella. The additional cost incurred is minimal since surgeons typically require a CT scan of the sinus to better define bony anatomy in this region and the price of a three-dimensional study without contrast is infinitesimal compared to the potential expense of a single serious complication due to misdirection.

Patient Positioning, Preparation, and Opening

The patient is placed in a mild reverse Trendelenburg position with the head tilted laterally away and rotated slightly toward the surgeon. If the lesion is a macroadenoma, a lumbar subarachnoid drain is placed after induction of general anesthesia to allow injection of intracranial air to cap the tumor using lateral fluoroscopy and facilitate delivery of the tumor into the sella. A lumbar tap is not necessary for microadenomas. Surgery proceeds with skin and mucosal preparation of the nasolabial area as well as an abdominal site in the event a fat graft must be harvested.

The septum, turbinates, and ala are mobilized as required for the transeptal approach using either microsurgery or endoscopy, but mobilization is generally much more limited for the latter. After nasal passages are entered, the vomer is commonly used as a landmark to locate the midline anterior wall of the sphenoid sinus. At this time the SNS can be used in lieu of fluoroscopy to confirm both the lateral and rostrocaudal location of instruments prior to osteotomy and to provide guidance to the sella turcica (Fig. 9-1).

Septal anatomy in the sphenoid sinus can be complex and misleading. Failure to adequately remove septae within the sphenoid sinus reduces the working area and may result in less than optimal placement of the sellar osteotomy. In contrast, excessive lateral bony exploration can have disastrous consequences, including cranial nerve palsies, temporal lobe injury, false aneurysms of the internal carotid artery, and stroke or exsanguination from overt injury to the internal carotid artery. SNSs can provide rapid, accurate orientation in the sphenoid sinus when operating on either micro- or macroadenomas (Fig. 9-2).

After localization within the sphenoid sinus is confirmed, the sella is opened with chisels and the circular sinus managed with a cautery and/or Avitene. The SNS may be used at this time to help locate a microadenoma; however, its benefit in treating macroadenomas is more limited. The intracranial capsule of the tumor may descend as tumor is removed. Since most SNSs rely exclusively on preoperative image data sets, they may produce spurious information on the location of instruments in the tumor, suggesting that its tip is well within the lesion whereas it is actually poised to perforate the capsule with possible dire consequences. Visualization of suprasellar air on lateral fluoroscopy is far more revealing in this situation.

Closure and postoperative management are routine. The sellar wall is reconstructed according to the surgeon's preference, and the sphenoid sinus is packed if cerebrospinal fluid is seen.

DISCUSSION

The resurgence of the transsphenoidal approach to the sella required tools that provided better early diagnosis and intraoperative visualization.[1,2,7] Although bony landmarks are usually reliable, major complications from the procedure sometimes involve straying off course into the cranial vault, carotid artery, or cavernous sinus. Because the patient's head is typically fixated for such procedures, SNSs represent a straightforward means of reducing these risks with the added bonus, in cases of microadenomas, of obviating the need for fluoroscopy and its attendant radiation effects on operating room personnel. The technique should be equally applicable for a transsphenoidal approach to craniopharyngiomas and other suitable sellar lesions.[8]

In addition to microsurgical transsphenoidal hypophysectomy, SNSs may prove useful for directing traditional stereotactic pituitary ablation using cryohypophysectomy[9] or radiation implant techniques[10,11] as well as serving as an ad-

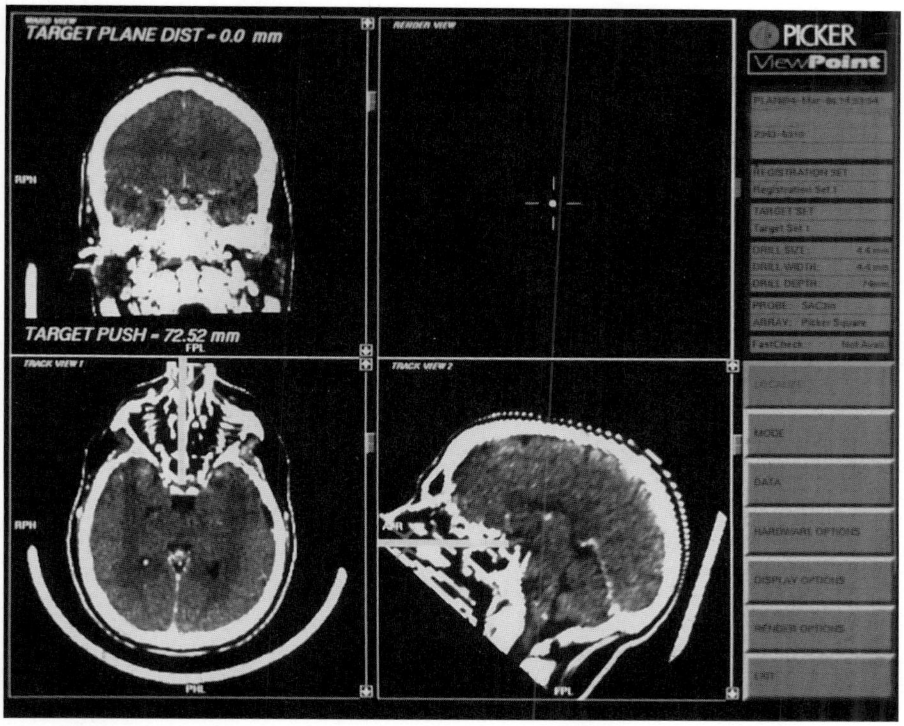

Figure 9-1. SNS guidance showing trajectory of surgical approach toward the sella. This can prevent misdirection superiorly into the cranial vault.

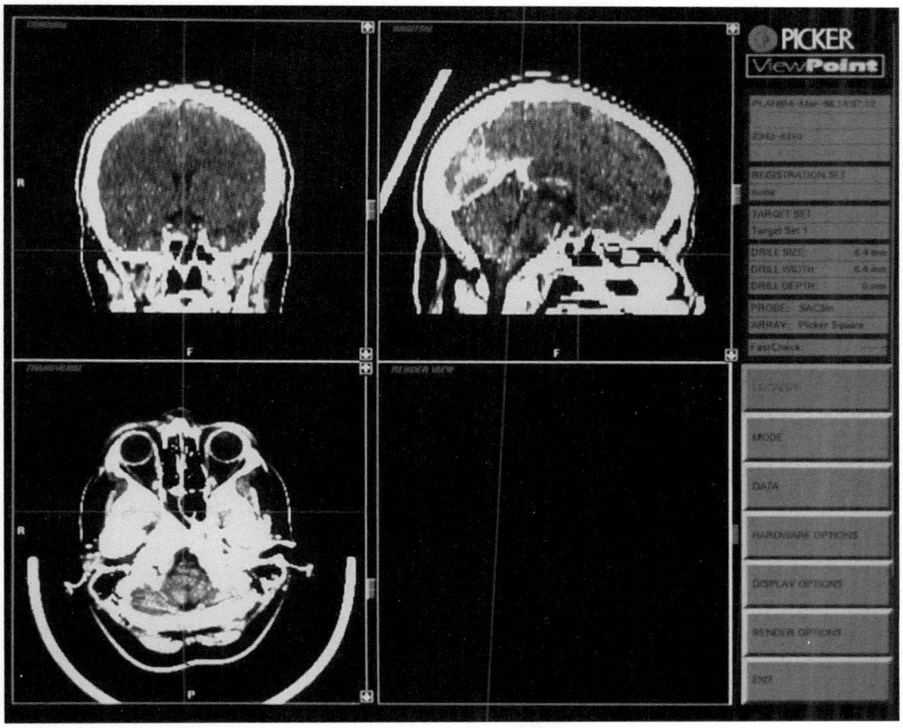

Figure 9-2. Localization of pointer tip on the septum in the sphenoid sinus. SNSs can define the lateral location in the sinus and help optimize resection of septal structures while minimizing the risk of entering the carotid artery or cavernous sinus.

junct to newer endoscopic techniques for treating these lesions. Stereotactic surgical microscopes continue to proliferate and may also prove to be beneficial in transsphenoidal sellar surgery.[12]

SUMMARY

SNSs may replace fluoroscopy in transsphenoidal surgery for pituitary microadenomas, providing guidance to the sellae and localization in the nasopharynx and sphenoid sinus. The best application may be as an adjunct to fluoroscopy in patients undergoing surgery for macroadenomas until real-time intraoperative imaging is practical since only dynamic imaging can show movements in the tumor capsule and the relationship of instruments to the tumor wall.

References

1. Hardy J. Transsphenoidal microsurgery of the normal and pathological pituitary. Clin Neurosurg 16:185-217, 1969.
2. Hardy J. Transsphenoidal hypophysectomy: Neurosurgical techniques. J Neurosurg 34:482-504, 1971.
3. Barnett GH, Kormos DW, Steiner CP, Weisenberger J. Intraoperative localization using an armless, frameless stereotactic wand. J Neurosurg 78:510-514, 1993.
4. Barnett GH, Kormos DW, Steiner CP, Weisenberger J. Use of a frameless, armless stereotactic wand for brain tumor localization with 2-D and 3-D neuroimaging. Neurosurgery 33:674-678, 1993.
5. Guthrie BL, Adler JR. Frameless stereotaxy: Computer interactive neurosurgery. Perspect Neurol Surg 2(1):1-19, 1991.
6. Maciunas RJ, Galloway RL Jr, Fitzpatrick JM, Mandava VR, Edwards CA, Allen GS. A universal system for interactive image-directed neurosurgery. Stereotact Funct Neurosurg 58:108-113, 1992.
7. Wilson CB, Dempsey LC. Transsphenoidal microsurgical removal of 250 pituitary adenomas. J Neurosurg 48:13-22, 1978.
8. Hardy J, Vezina JL. Transsphenoidal neurosurgery of intracranial neoplasm. Adv Neurol 15:261-274, 1976.
9. Rand RW. Stereotactic treatment of pituitary tumors. In Wilkins RH, Rengachary SS, eds. Neurosurgery. New York: McGraw-Hill, 1985, pp 899-901.
10. Hartog M, Doyle F, Fraser R, Joplin GF. Partial pituitary ablation with implants of gold-198 and yttrium-90 for acromegaly. Br Med J 2:396-398, 1965.
11. Molinatti GM, Camanni F, Massara F, Olivetti M, Pizzini A, Giuliani G. Implantation of yttrium 90 in the sella turcica in sixteen cases of acromegaly. J Clin Endocrinol Metab 22:599-611, 1962.
12. Roberts DW, Strohbehn JW, Hatch JF, Murray W, Kettenberger H. A frameless stereotaxic integration of computerized tomographic imaging and the operating microscope. J Neurosurg 65:545-549, 1986.

10

Vascular Malformations

Lucia Zamorano, M.D., Ph.D. • *Miguel Lis-Planells, M.D.* • *Zhaowei Jiang, Ph.D.*
Lutz Nolte, Ph.D. • *A. Majeed Kadi, M.S.* • *Fernando Diaz, M.D., Ph.D.*

Vascular malformations located in deep or eloquent areas of the brain represent a therapeutic challenge. Although surgical excision is the only method to prevent further neurologic deficit as a result of hemorrhage, poor accessibility to deeply seated malformations may carry a high risk of postoperative morbidity.[1,2] The same is true for vascular malformations located in or around eloquent brain regions such as speech and motor-sensory areas. Image guidance provides a three-dimensional view of the actual vascular malformation through computer simulation and an accurate means of determining its position in relation to adjacent brain structures (anatomic localization). It also allows the surgeon to plan a surgical strategy that takes into account the relationship of feeding, nidus, and draining vessels, thus ensuring the safest and most effective surgical approach to be selected.

In vascular malformations close to eloquent areas, digitized functional information is gathered into a specially developed software program (Neurological Surgery Planning System, Wayne State University, Detroit, Mich.) for localization of sensory, motor, and language functions derived from cortical and subcortical intraoperative mapping (functional localization). Finally, interactive image guidance permits a constant display of the position of surgical instruments during an operation and their relationship to the vascular malformation components, surrounding normal brain, and vascular structures, providing valuable guidance to the surgeon during the entire intraoperative period.

We will discuss our experience with 17 vascular malformations (13 patients) that were resected with interactive image localization using an infrared-based localization system developed at Wayne State University.

PATIENT POPULATION

The clinical presentation, age of the 13 patients, and location and type of lesion are summarized in Table 10-1. There were six arteriovenous malformations (AVM) and 11 cavernous malformations. Three patients had multiple cavernous

Table 10-1. Patient Data

Sex/Age (yr)	Location	Presentation	Type	Spetzler Martin Grade
F/16	Left temporal	Intracranial bleeding	AVM	Grade II
M/25	Right parietal	Intracranial bleeding	AVM	Grade III
F/52	Left parietal	Intracranial bleeding	AVM	Grade III
F/50	Right frontal	Headaches	AVM	Grade II
M/27	Right frontal	Intracranial bleeding	AVM	Grade I
M/50	Left frontal	Intracranial bleeding	AVM	Grade I
M/24	Left frontal × 2	Intracranial bleeding	CM	N/A
M/6	Thalamic (right, left), cerebellar	Seizures, intracranial bleeding	CM	N/A
F/43	Left parietal	Seizures	CM	N/A
F/35	Left temporal × 2	Seizures	CM	N/A
M/56	Pons	Intracranial bleeding	CM	N/A
M/15	Left caudate	Seizures, intracranial bleeding	CM	N/A
F/51	Right frontal	Intracranial bleeding	CM	N/A

CM = cavernous malformation.

malformations. All the patients with AVMs had intracranial hemorrhage except for one who had headaches. The patients with cavernous malformations were initially seen with either intracranial hemorrhage (n = 5) or seizures (n = 6). A partial embolization had been previously performed in one patient with an AVM. The clinical follow-up period ranged from 2 to 39 months.

SURGICAL TECHNIQUE

Image-guided resection of vascular malformation is a three-step process: image data acquisition, surgical planning, and interactive image localization. Interactive image localization comprises these three steps. We will only briefly describe the different steps since they have been extensively described elsewhere,[3,4] with special emphasis in their use related to vascular malformations.

Image Data Acquisition

Interactive image guidance requires one or multiple registered images derived from CT, MRI, MR angiography, PET, or digital angiography. Images from many sources must be registered to each other and to the patient's actual anatomy using a common point of reference such as points on a stereotaxy frame, markers, or anatomic surfaces. Although frameless methods of registration (markers or surfaces) have some advantages, notably that patients are more comfortable without a head frame and that images from different modalities do not have to be taken on the same day, in a patient with an AVM we consider it mandatory to obtain a registered angiogram, which is most easily accomplished using a stereotaxy frame. For tomographic images such as MRI, MR angiography, and PET, the frameless method can be used.

Gadolinium-enhanced MRI scans and contrast-enhanced CT scans were obtained in all patients in this study. In patients with AVMs the stereotaxy frame was placed using the Zamorano-Dujovny localizing unit for stereotactic digital angiography (MR angiography). In patients with cavernous malformations, MRI, MR angiography, and PET were not performed since these lesions cannot be visualized on angiograms. In patients with an AVM close to speech or functional areas, PET scans were obtained without a head frame and registered using either attached markers on the skin or surface matching algorithms.

Surgical Planning

The Neurological Surgery Planning System (NSPS 3.0) consists of multimodular software run on a computer workstation used for interactive surgical assistance in intracranial[3,4] and spine procedures[5,6] and for teaching purposes.[7,8] The first step of computer planning (and the only one necessary, if so desired) is multimodality image registration using point-based or surface algorithms.[3] For patients with AVMs, multimodality registration included images taken with a head frame (digital angiography) and images without the frame (MRI and MR angiography). From these, registered multiplanar two-dimensional and three-dimensional images are generated and displayed showing the lesion and related anatomic structures. At this stage the surgeon may plan the surgery using patient data and a computer-resident anatomic atlas. One goal of planning is to "optimize" the surgical approach, that is, find the best surgical corridor to the malformation. This process is referred to as optimization. Thus the optimal surgical corridor is selected and entry and target points defined to generate surgical trajectories. As we will show later, these trajectories can be simple linear approaches such as the classic stereotactic ones or can be quite complex nonlinear ones, corresponding to many of the standard neurosurgical approaches.

Specific localization of feeding arteries and draining veins can be achieved by digitizing the information extracted from the stereotactic angiogram. A two-dimensional display of the images perpendicular to the surgical trajectory can be generated corresponding to the surgeon's view of the operation.

Planning can be as simple as the image registration or include a more complex approach, depending on the neurosurgeon's choice. If a head frame is being used as a reference guide for one imaging modality (usually angiography), then stereotactic arc coordinates are generated during this stage.

Interactive Image Localization

Interactive image localization uses a digitizer or localizer to interactively display the location of a pointer or other instrument over the preregistered images. The system we use consists of an infrared-based system extensively described elsewhere.[3-8] In brief, the continuous localization is achieved by three infrared cameras continuously tracking the position of multiple light-emitting diodes (LEDs) mounted in a predefined relationship and referred to as a rigid body (Fig. 10-1). When these LEDs are mounted as a rigid body into different precalibrated surgi-

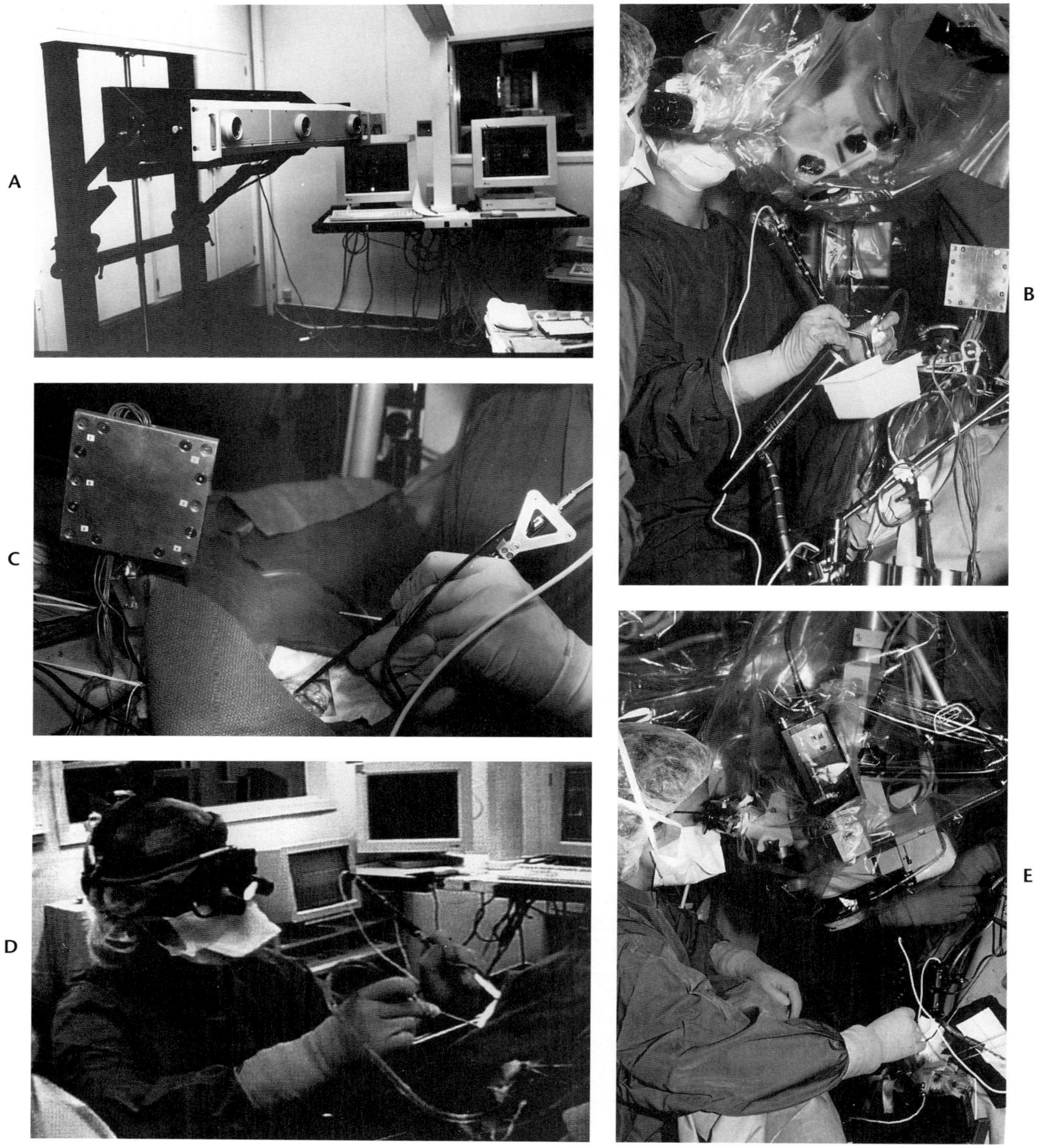

Figure 10-1. Infrared-based intraoperative localization. **A,** Three infrared cameras continuously detect the position of multiple LEDs mounted as a patient rigid body and as an instrument rigid body or pointer. **B,** Patient rigid body and pointer while defining the center of the craniotomy. **C,** During surgery close to the speech area the pointer is represented by the electrode with three LEDs mounted; this allows functional registered information. **D,** Intraoperative view of vascular malformations close to the surface or subcortical regions showing the infrared camera, the instrument rigid body, and the computer displaying the real-time location of the surgical instrument. **E,** Intraoperative view of vascular malformations located in deep regions; real-time localization can be obtained using the same instruments under the surgical microscope.

cal instruments such as the bipolar electrode or dissector, we refer to that as the surgical rigid body or pointer. Another rigid body is mounted into the head-holder or the stereotaxy frame and is used to continuously track the patient's head (patient rigid body). Lately we have added a third rigid body to our system called the surgeon rigid body that is placed on the surgeon's head and is used at the beginning of the procedure to indicate the spatial relationship of the surgeon's eye view and the patient's head. The objective of this third rigid body is ultimately to display the three-dimensional images corresponding to the exact surgeon's perspective on the operating room monitor.

The surgical procedure starts by registering or mapping the image studies with the intraoperative space (intraoperative registration). This is achieved by touching the pointer on at least three or four "real" points (i.e., points either on the patient or on a head frame) that can be easily located on the precaptured images. We have used known points on the stereotaxy frame, markers, and multiple points that generate a surface since intraoperative registration can be point- or surface-based. After this, any time the pointer is used, its tip position and trajectory are simultaneously displayed on the computer images, giving a real-time orientation.

In AVM surgery a centered incision is made, and craniotomy is performed according to the planned surgical approach. If the AVM is superficial, anatomic localization is easily achieved. Depending on the location of the AVM, language, motor, or sensory intraoperative mapping (functional localization) is performed using a bipolar stimulation electrode with an attached rigid body; thus the functional information obtained is also registered and saved and, from this point forward, continuously displayed on the precaptured images. The same is true when intraoperative electrocorticography is performed; any positive information can be spatially located using the pointer. If the AVM is deeply located, then a surgical corridor through noneloquent brain becomes necessary. This corridor corresponds to our preplanned trajectory. How can we transpose this computer-planned trajectory into the real operation? When the stereotaxy frame has been used, the stereotactic arc keeps the desired linear surgical trajectory. In frameless conditions the preplanned trajectory is reproduced, and the position of the pointer on the multiplanar, surgeon's perspective, and three-dimensional images is followed and compared with the ideal plotted trajectory. This "trial and error" procedure allows the surgeon to incrementally correct the position of the surgical instrument to stay on the trajectory while advancing toward the lesion. The trajectory is presented on all multiplanar two-dimensional and three-dimensional images on the operating room monitor as a projected line, and the tip of the instrument is shown as a cursor.

Some surgeons may prefer a more conventional approach and use the interactive display as an orientation tool and for constant feedback. Even in this instance variations in surgical approach can be easily accommodated, especially if registered intraoperative functional information shows it is necessary. The surgical corridor can be maintained by stereotactic or conventional brain retractors.

From here the procedure follows the conventional and ideal principles of AVM surgery. The feeding arteries are localized and disconnected followed by localization of the draining veins and microsurgical dissection of the nidus. The final step is disconnecting the draining veins to complete the excision of the lesion. Since vascular malformation surgery is primarily a microsurgical procedure, the most useful pointer in our experience has been the microsurgical dissector.

RESULTS

In our study all the AVM patients underwent postoperative angiography to confirm total excision of the lesion. The neurologic condition of all patients was unchanged. No instances of morbidity and mortality were reported for this group. Fig. 10-2 shows a small AVM within a hematoma that was resected under image guidance.

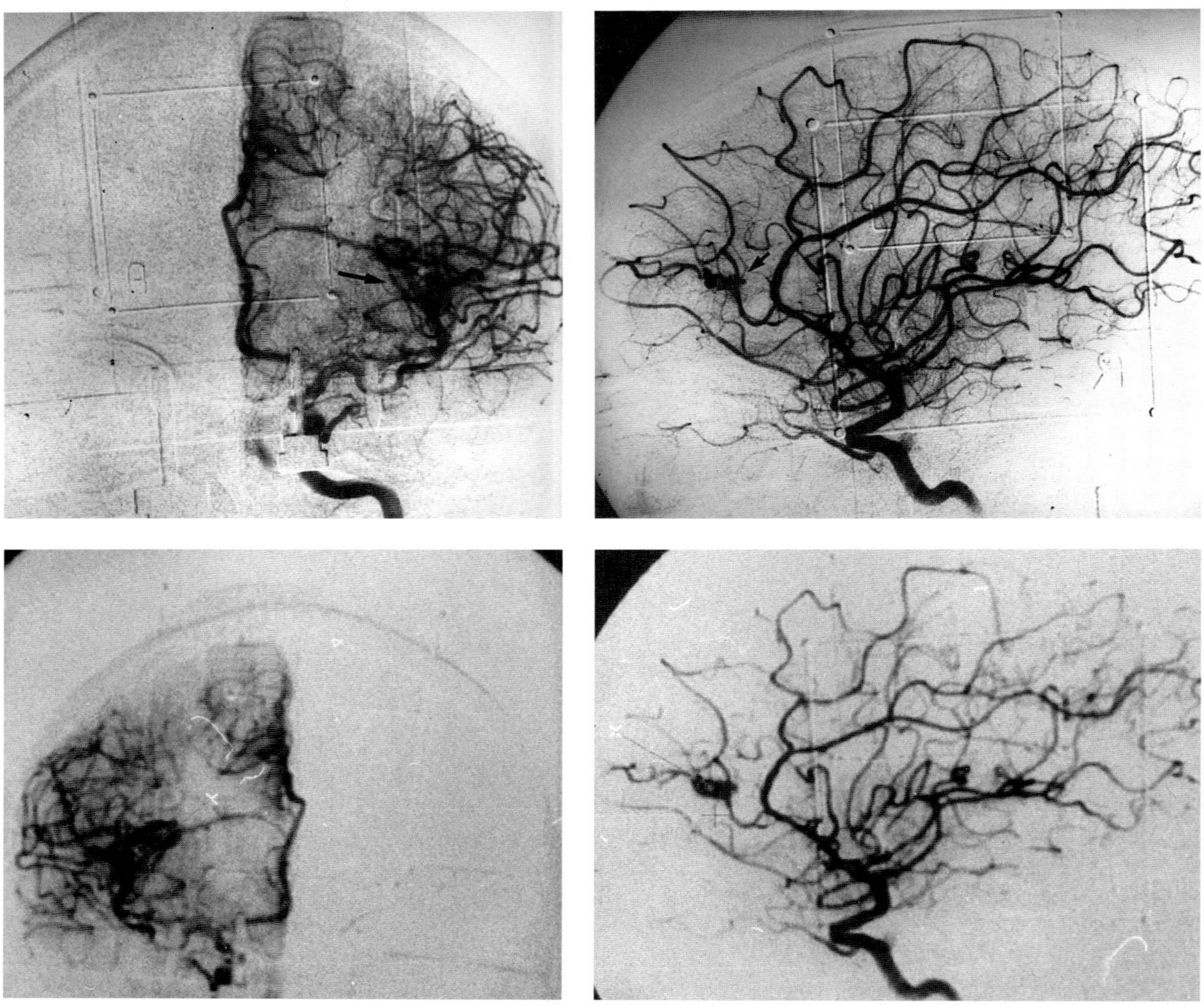

A B C D

Figure 10-2. Intracranial hemorrhage from ruptured AVM. This required finding and removing an AVM within a hematoma. Anteroposterior **(A)** and lateral **(B)** preoperative stereotactic angiogram showing the nidus, feeding artery, and draining vein. Note the location of the nidus in the lateral margin of the hematoma. The cursor shows the location of the surgical instrument during the operation on angiograms **(C and D)**.

Continued.

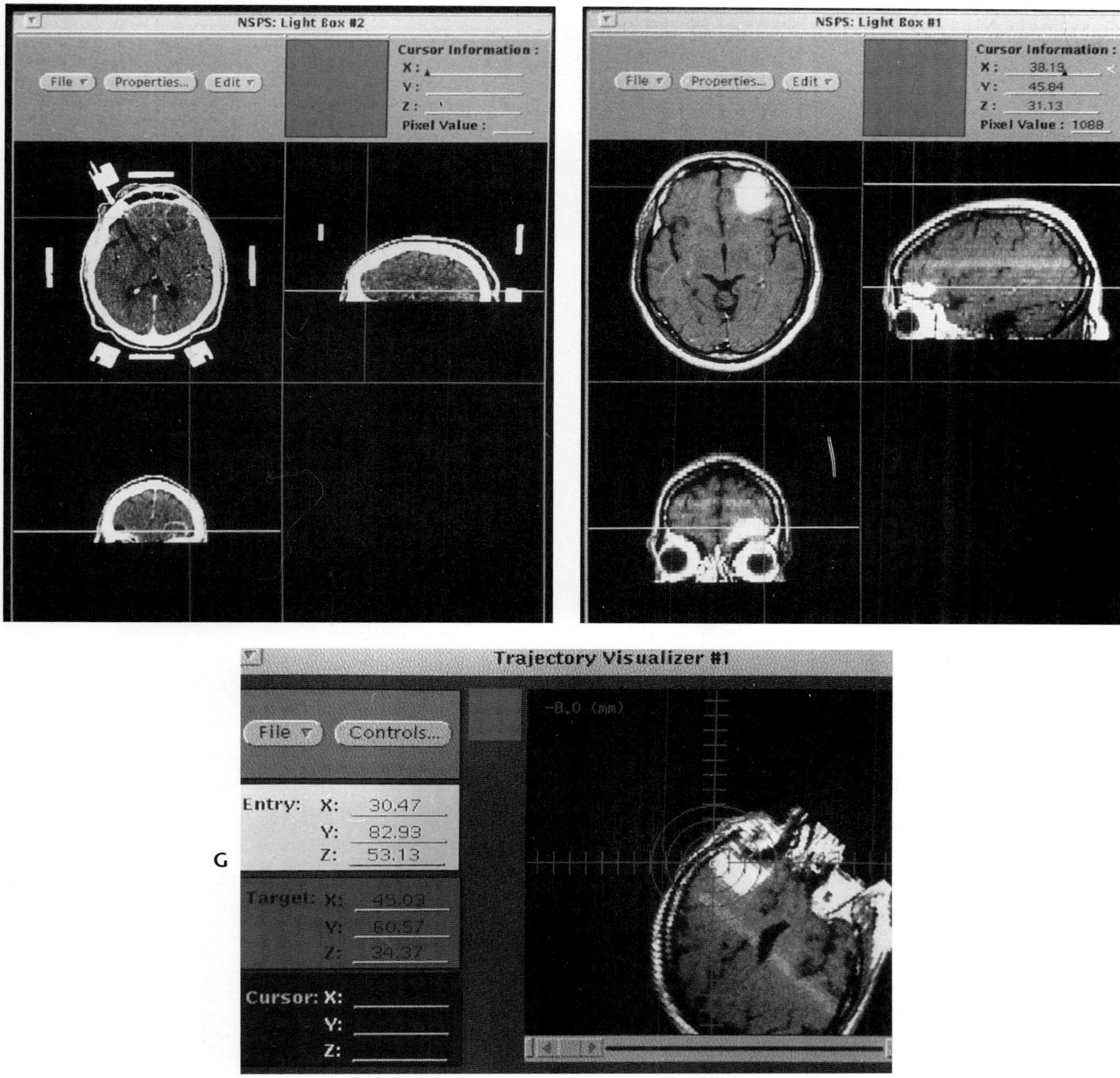

Figure 10-2, cont'd. CT scans **(E),** MR images **(F).** **G,** Localization seen from surgeon's perspective.

Continued.

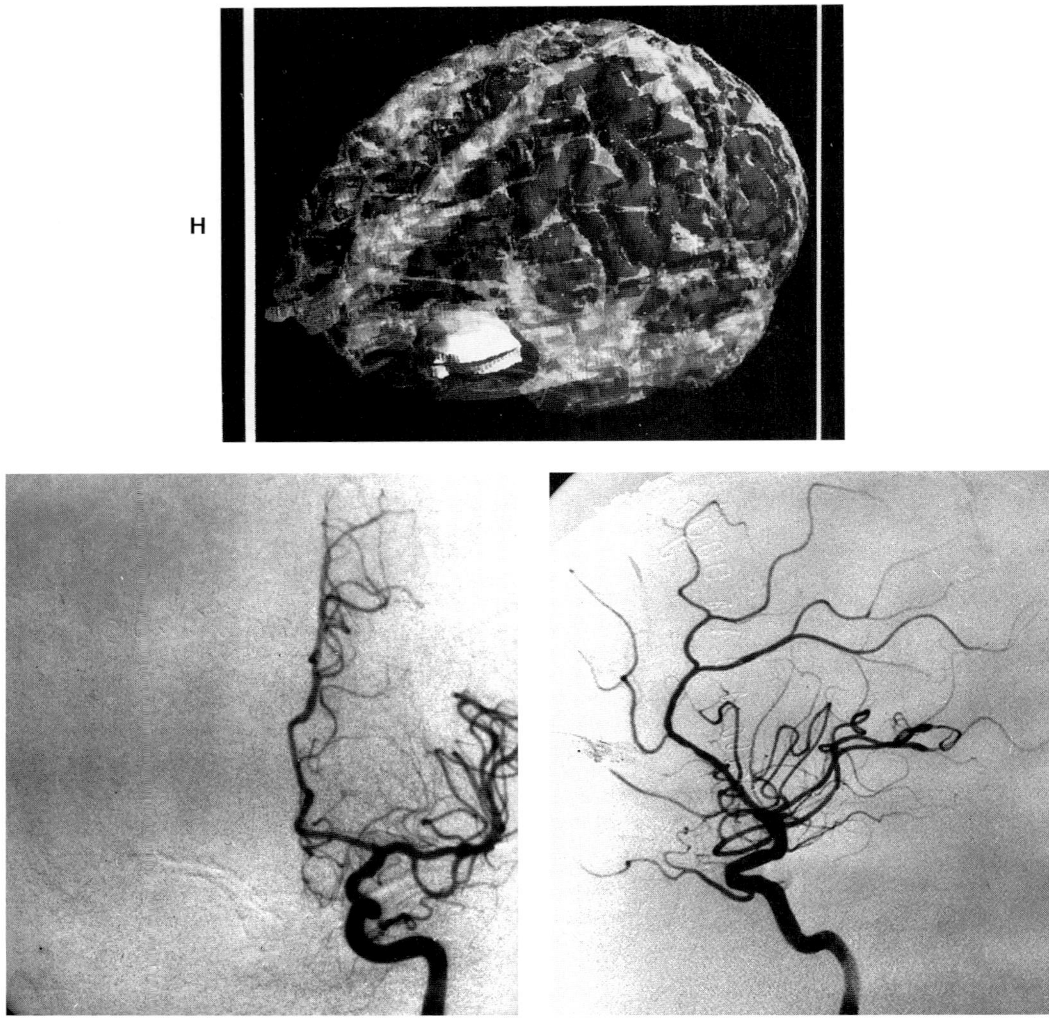

Figure 10-2, cont'd. Three-dimensional reconstruction of MRI **(H)** displaying the hematoma in relation to the brain surface. In all the views the line represents the surgical trajectory and the cursor shows the location of the surgical instrument. Postoperative angiograms showing excision of the AVM on anteroposterior **(I)** and lateral **(J)** view.

Follow-up MRI of the cavernous malformations confirmed total excision of the lesions in all patients. Fig. 10-3 shows two cavernous angiomas resected under image guidance. The most serious surgical complication was observed in a patient with a cavernous angioma located in the pons about 1.5 mm from the pial surface in the fourth ventricle. A total resection was performed. This patient had multiple cranial nerve deficits postoperatively that had gradually and continuously improved at 16-month follow-up.

Other complications reported in the patients with cavernous malformations included transient cerebellar ataxia in a 6-year-old boy with a cerebellar lesion and transient hemiparesis in a patient with a deep frontal cavernoma.

A

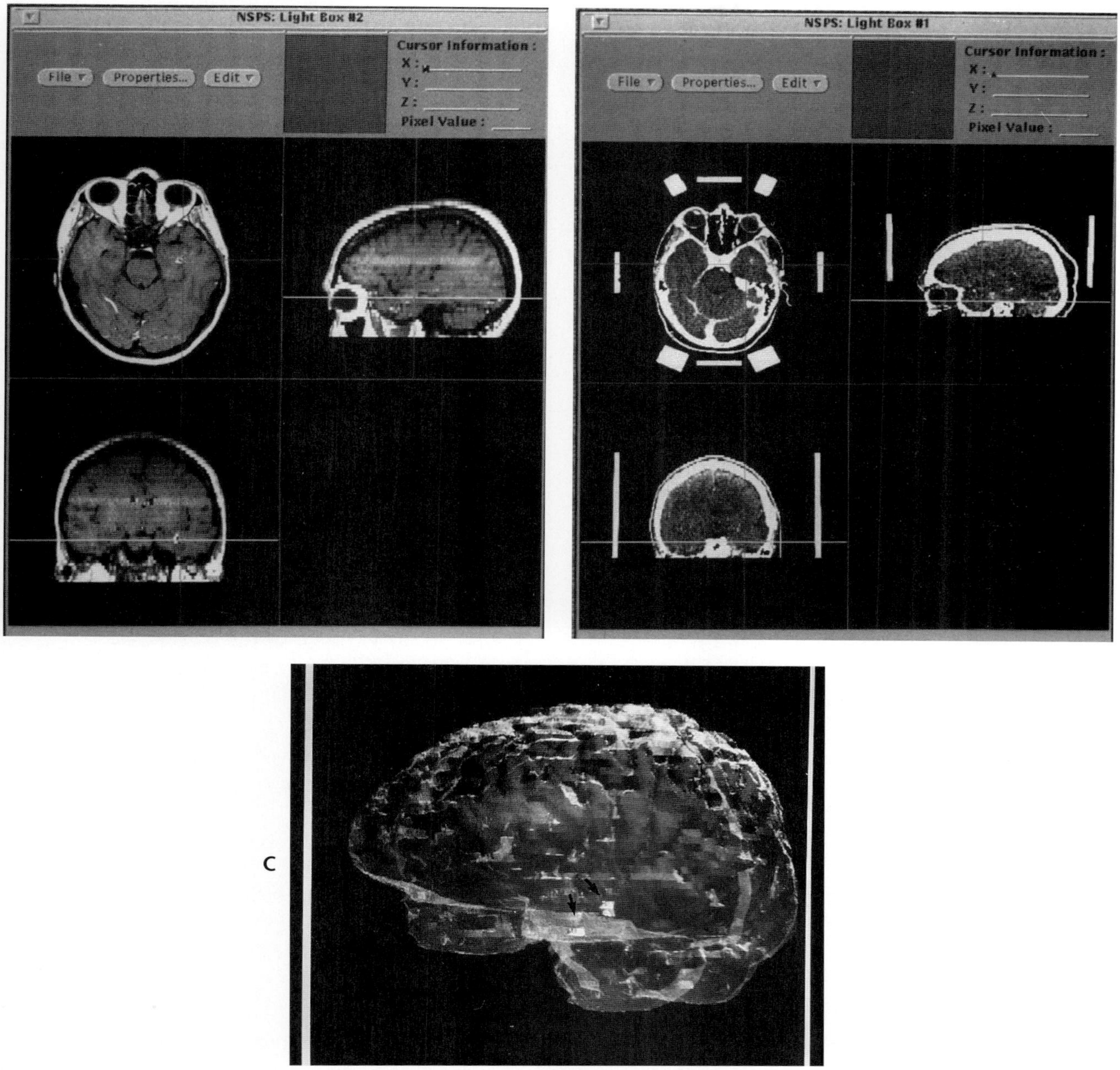

B

C

Figure 10-3. Multiple cavernous angiomas in the temporal lobe of a patient with seizures. The plan was to resect the two lesions with intraoperative electrocorticography without performing a complete temporal lobectomy if electrophysiologic data did not indicate it. CT and MR images were obtained and registered and intraoperative localization was done. MR **(A)** and CT **(B)** scans of the brain showing the surgical trajectories to the lesions. The cursor shows the position of the surgical instrument using the infrared system. **C,** Three-dimensional reconstruction of cavernous angiomas in relation to the brain surface.

Continued.

D

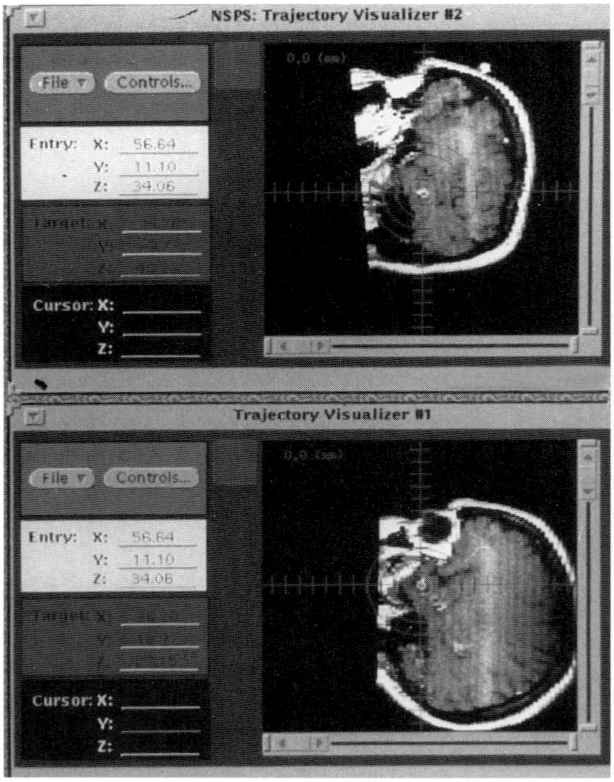

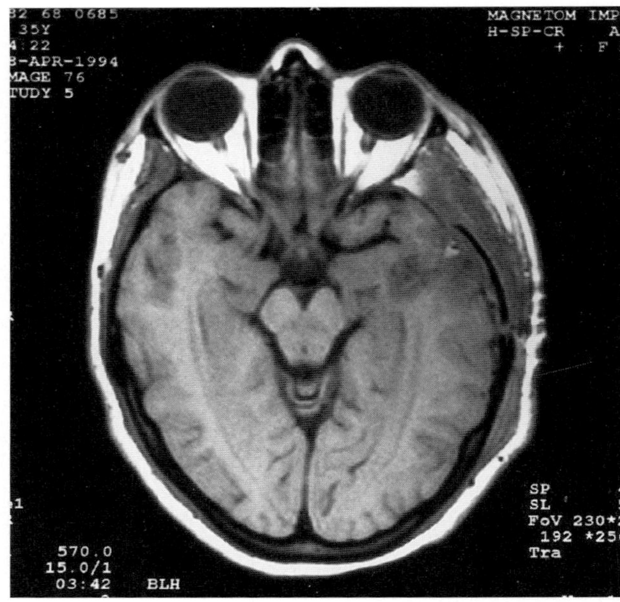

E

Figure 10-3, cont'd. D, Surgeon's perspective displaying the target of one of the trajectories. **E,** Postoperative MR scan showing resection of the lesions without performing a temporal lobectomy.

DISCUSSION

The various treatment modalities for AVMs include embolization, radiosurgery, and surgical resection. The decision to proceed with a surgical excision of an AVM is influenced by numerous factors such as the patient's age, size and location of the lesion, presence of hemorrhage that may facilitate the surgical approach, and neurologic status at the time of presentation.[9-13]

Small AVMs (nidus of less than 3 cm in diameter) are at a higher risk of bleeding.[14,15] Nevertheless, small AVMs are generally completely resected by microsurgical techniques if they are located in accessible areas. Small malformations seated in deep or eloquent areas of the brain represent a therapeutic dilemma: complete excision is the only option to prevent further hemorrhage, but the nidus, feeding arteries, and draining veins are difficult to localize, increasing the postoperative risk of neurologic deficit from injury to surrounding structures.[10,11,16-18]

Several reports in the literature have proposed stereotactic techniques for intraoperative localization of vascular lesions.[9,16-21] Stereotactic systems have been used primarily for centering the craniotomy and nidus localization. The nidus is generally reached by advancing a probe mounted on the stereotactic arc to the selected target. Our technique of image guidance is based on interactive multimodality imaging that allows surgical planning from a registered CT scan, MRI scan, and/or angiogram. The surgical plan includes not only a centered craniotomy and coordinates of a desired target, but also encompasses a two- and three-dimensional display of the surgical trajectory that includes localization of the nidus, feeding arteries, and draining veins. Multi-image planning provides the neurosurgeon with an important tool to optimize the surgical approach. The intraoperative interactive display gives constant feedback during surgery that is invaluable in keeping the surgeon oriented. Lesions can be resected completely and with minimal morbidity.

This is the first reported series using an infrared system for intraoperative localization of vascular malformations. This device enables the tracking of surgical instruments within the stereotactic field with an accuracy of 1 mm. The position of the tip of the instrument is displayed intraoperatively on the MRI scan and angiogram. This system is useful to determine the margins of the nidus, AVM, or cavernous malformation and provides fast localization of related brain and vascular structures. The infrared digitizer, as with any other intraoperative localizer, carries with it the risk of inaccuracy because of brain shifting. This is minimized by measures such as giving a low intraoperative dose of mannitol and using stereotactic retractors to maintain the surgical corridor without major brain displacement.

The natural history of cavernous malformations remains unclear. Recent reports indicate a risk of hemorrhage of 1.1% per lesion per year for familial cases[22] and 0.11% to 0.25% per lesion per year for sporadic cavernous malformations.[2,23] In general surgical excision of cavernous malformations should be considered for lesions that are symptomatic and present as hemorrhage, seizures difficult to control, and progressive neurologic deficit.[1,2,22,23] Cavernous malformations are safely approached with stereotactic image guidance. The 11 lesions in our series were completely resected.

Our postoperative superimposed deficit was absent for AVMs and transitory in two of the three cases reported for cavernous malformations. In these patients complications were related to the location of the lesions and not to intraoperative localization itself. Transient cerebellar ataxia was reported in a patient with a deep cerebellar cavernoma and transient hemiparesis occurred in a patient with a cavernoma involving the basal ganglia. One patient had multiple cranial nerve deficits after removal of a cavernous malformation located in the pons. There are two possible explanations for this complication. The lesion was not abutting the pial surface of the brainstem, which means that normal tissue was transected to reach the target, or manipulation of the brainstem itself during dissection may have caused the complication.

SUMMARY

Surgical navigation in the treatment of vascular malformations aids in the safe and complete removal of lesions that are small in size and located in deep or eloquent areas of the brain where accurate localization of the lesion is critical. Low postoperative morbidity is associated with smaller skin incisions, centered craniotomy, a planned surgical trajectory based on multimodality imaging, and fast, accurate localization of the nidus, feeding arteries, draining veins, and related neural structures. Accurate surgical navigation coupled in some cases with intraoperative functional mapping allows resection of these challenging lesions with the least possible morbidity. Image fusion capabilities, integration of imaging with physiologic monitoring, and interactive localization are expected to further improve the current management of vascular malformations in difficult locations.

References

1. Golfinos JG, Wascher TM, Zabramski JM, Spetzler RF. The management of unruptured intracranial vascular malformations. BNI Q 8:2-11, 1992.
2. Robinson JR, Award IA, Little JR. Natural history of the cavernous angioma. J Neurosurg 75:709-714, 1991.
3. Zamorano LJ, Nolte L, Jiang Z, Kadi AM. Image-guided neurosurgery: Frame-based and frameless approaches. Neurol Operative Atlas 3:403-422, 1993.
4. Zamorano L, Jiang Z, Kadi M. Computer-assisted neurosurgery system: Wayne State University hardware and software configuration. Comput Med Imaging Graph 18:257-271, 1994.
5. Nolte LP, Zamorano LJ, Jiang Z, Wang Q, Langlotz F, Berlemann U. Image guided insertion of transpedicular screws: A laboratory set-up. Spine 20:497-500, 1995.
6. Nolte LP, Zamorano L, Visarius H, Berlemann U, Langlotz F, Arm E, Schwarzenbach O. Clinical evaluation of a system for precision enhancement in spine surgery. Clin Biomech 10:293-303, 1996.
7. Zamorano L, Jiang Z, Nolte LP, Grosky W. Telepresence and virtual reality in computer assisted neurological surgery: Basic theory and a prototype. J Virtual Reality Med 1(Spring):54-59, 1995.
8. Jiang Z, Grosky W, Zamorano L, Nolte L, Kadi M. Immersive database system and virtual patient. J Virtual Reality Med 1(Fall/Winter):20-26, 1996.
9. Sisti MB, Solomon RA, Stein BM. Stereotactic craniotomy and resection of small arteriovenous malformations. J Neurosurg 75:40-44, 1991.
10. Wilson CB, Martin NA. Deep supratentorial arteriovenous malformations. In Wilson CB, Stein BM, eds. Intracranial Arteriovenous Malformations. Baltimore: Williams & Wilkins, 1984, pp 184-208.
11. Lee JP. Surgical management of thalamic arteriovenous malformations. Neurosurgery 32:498-504, 1993.
12. Tamaki N, Ehara K, Lin TK, Kuwamura K, Obora Y, Kanzawa Y, Yamashita H, Matsumoto S. Cerebral arteriovenous malformations: Factors influencing the surgical difficulty and outcome. Neurosurgery 29: 856-863, 1991.
13. Morgan MK, Johnston IH, Hallinan JM, Weber NC. Complications of surgery for arteriovenous malformations of the brain. J Neurosurg 78:176-182, 1993.
14. Spetzler RF, Hargraves RW, McCormick PW, Zabramski JM, Flom RA, Zimmerman RS. Relationship of perfusion pressure and size to risk of hemorrhage from arteriovenous malformations. J Neurosurg 76:913-923, 1992.
15. Piepgras DG, Sundt TM, Ragoowansi AT, Stevens L. Seizure outcome in patients with surgically treated cerebral arteriovenous malformations. J Neurosurg 78:5-11, 1993.
16. Davis DH, Kelly PJ. Stereotactic resection of occult vascular malformations. J Neurosurg 72:698-702, 1990.
17. Kelly PJ, Alker GJ, Zoll JG. A microstereotactic approach to deep-seated arteriovenous malformations. Surg Neurol 17(4):260-262, 1982.
18. Reinhardt HF, Herstmann GA, Gratzl O. Sonic stereometry in microsurgical procedures for deep-seated brain tumors and vascular malformations. Neurosurgery 32:51-57, 1993.
19. Cahan LD, Rand RW. Stereotactic coagulation of a paraventricular arteriovenous malformation. Case report. J Neurosurg 39:770-774, 1978.
20. Kandel EI, Peresedov VV. Stereotactic clipping of arterial aneurysms and arteriovenous malformations. J Neurosurg 46(1):12-23, 1977.
21. Dempsey PK, Kondziolka D, Lunsford LD. Stereotactic diagnosis and treatment of pineal region tumors and vascular malformations. Acta Neurochir 116:14-22, 1992.
22. Zabramski JM, Wascher TM, Spetzler RF, Johnson B. The natural history of familial cavernous malformations: Results of an ongoing study. J Neurosurg 80:422-432, 1994.
23. Del Curling OD Jr, Kelly DJ Jr, Elster AD, Craven TE. An analysis of the natural history of cavernous angiomas. J Neurosurg 75:702-708, 1991.

11

Spinal Surgery

Iain H. Kalfas, M.D.

Surgical navigation systems using surface reference marks rather than a stereotaxy frame provide an accurate and reliable means of *localizing* lesions within the brain and identifying underlying anatomic structures.[1-9] This can help minimize surgical morbidity and limit the length and expense of the procedure. For most spinal procedures, however, localization is not a significant problem. An intraoperative lateral radiograph is sufficient in most cases to localize the appropriate spinal level. Surgical navigation of the spine is not needed to identify a lumbar disc herniation, a vertebral body fracture, or an extramedullary spinal neoplasm. For those cases in which an intramedullary neoplasm or syrinx is difficult to precisely localize, intraoperative ultrasonography has proved useful.[10]

The purpose of applying stereotactic principles to spinal surgery is to improve the surgeon's orientation to the unexposed spinal anatomy. The three-dimensional anatomy of the spinal column can present difficulties for even the most experienced surgeon. Standard posterior surgical approaches expose only a portion of the spinal column at a given level. Although this limited exposure is not problematic for most laminectomy or discectomy procedures, it can be limiting in the setting of complex spinal column disorders such as fractures, neoplasms, or deformities.

The ability to conceptualize the three-dimensional anatomy of the spinal column from any particular approach varies among surgeons. It is highly dependent on the correct interpretation of both preoperative and intraoperative images. Image-guided spinal navigation facilitates this image interpretation process by providing optimal digitized images through multiple points and planes in the spinal column. This greatly enhances the surgeon's ability to "visualize" the unexposed spinal anatomy.

The evolution of spinal instrumentation devices as well as the development of more involved surgical approaches to the spine have expanded the options for managing complex spinal disorders. These procedures all require that the surgeon maintain his or her orientation to the unexposed spinal anatomy. In particular, the various screw fixation techniques that involve the placement of bone screws into the pedicles of the thoracic, lumbar, and sacral spine, into the lateral masses and across joints of the cervical spine, and across the vertebrae of the thoracic and lumbar spine require a thorough understanding of the spatial relationships of the unexposed spinal anatomy.

Although intraoperative fluoroscopy and serial radiography have proved useful intraoperative imaging tools, they can only provide a two-dimensional image of a complex three-dimensional structure. Consequently, the surgeon must estimate the position of unexposed spinal structures based on an interpretation of these images and a knowledge of the pertinent anatomy. Such inference can result in varying degrees of inaccuracy when placing screws in the spinal column.

For example, several studies have shown the unreliability of routine radiography in assessing pedicle screw placement in the lumbosacral spine. The rate of penetration of the pedicle cortex by an inserted screw ranges from 21% to 31% in these studies.[11-13] However, Steinmann et al.,[14] using an image-based technique for pedicle screw placement that combined CT axial images of cadaver spine specimens with fluoroscopy, was able to demonstrate a reduction of this screw insertion error rate to 5.5%.

The initial difficulty in adapting stereotactic principles to spinal surgery was identifying a frame of reference in which digitized images could be more directly applied to intraoperative anatomy. Unlike intracranial surgery, a frame system is not practical for spinal surgery. Furthermore, the use of surface landmarks or fiducials creates problems of spatial accuracy because of skin movement with respect to bony landmarks.[15,16] This poses less of a problem in intracranial applications because of the relatively fixed relationship of the overlying skin to selected bony landmarks.

The application of stereotactic technology to spinal surgery involves using the rigid spinal anatomy itself as a frame of reference. By selecting a series of corresponding points in a CT image set and in the exposed spinal anatomy, a point to point representation of the image data and the spinal anatomy can be established. The image data can then be reformatted and presented to the surgeon in multiple planes to optimally demonstrate the unexposed spinal column.[17]

However, unlike intraoperative ultrasonography or fluoroscopy, image-guided spinal navigation does not provide true real-time imaging. It does not show changes in the spinal anatomy as they occur. The images presented are all preoperative images. The system functions as a confirmatory tool to assist the surgeon in identifying unexposed anatomic structures and relating their position and orientation to the exposed spinal anatomy. It is not intended to function as a substitute for an understanding of the appropriate spinal anatomy and correct surgical indications and techniques. It is an alternative to the more conventional means of interpreting two-dimensional images of the spine, relating them to the surgeon's knowledge of the pertinent anatomy, and estimating the location of unexposed structures.

SURGICAL TECHNIQUE

Intraoperative localization for intracranial lesions using an armless, frameless stereotaxy wand system has been described previously.[1,2] The primary components of the system used for spinal navigation include an image processing computer workstation interfaced with a two-camera optical localizer (Fig. 11-1). The optical

A

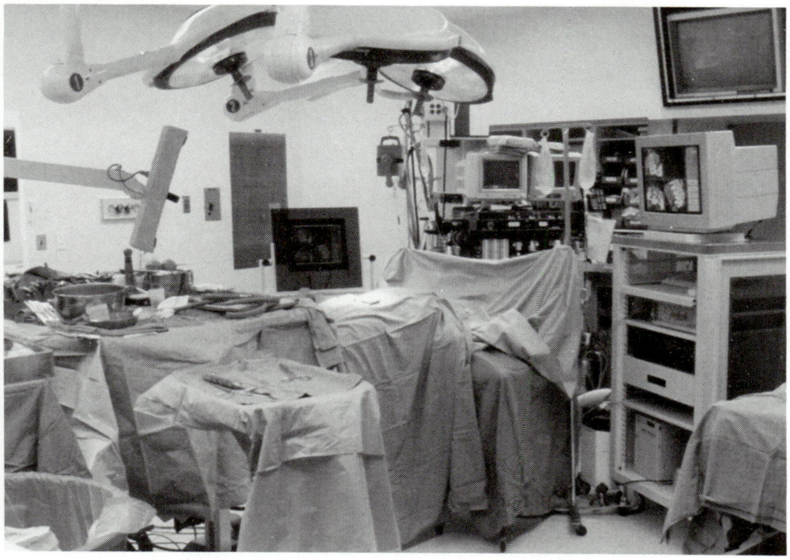

B

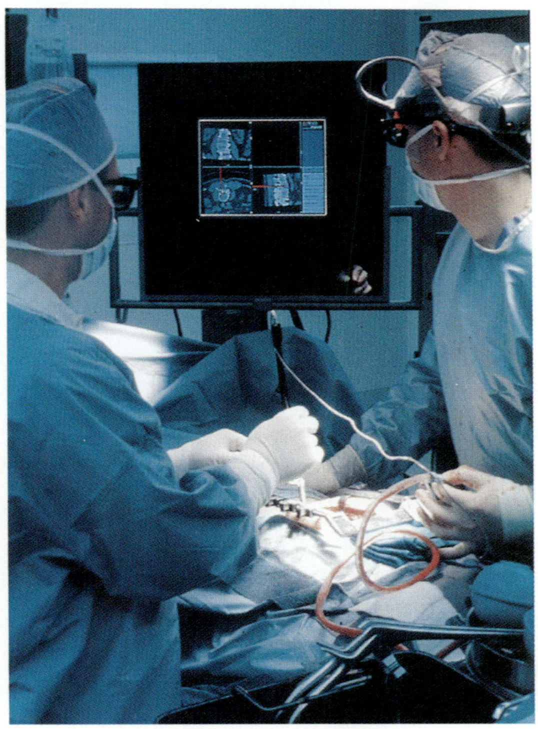

Figure 11-1. A, Operating room arrangement for image-guided spinal navigation. For lumbosacral procedures, the infrared camera detector is positioned near the foot of the table and aimed rostrally. For cervical procedures, it is positioned at the head of the table and aimed caudally. The image processing workstation is positioned across the table from the surgeon. A separate flat panel display screen connected to the workstation is positioned across the table from the assistant. **B,** Intraoperative use of image-guided spinal navigation.

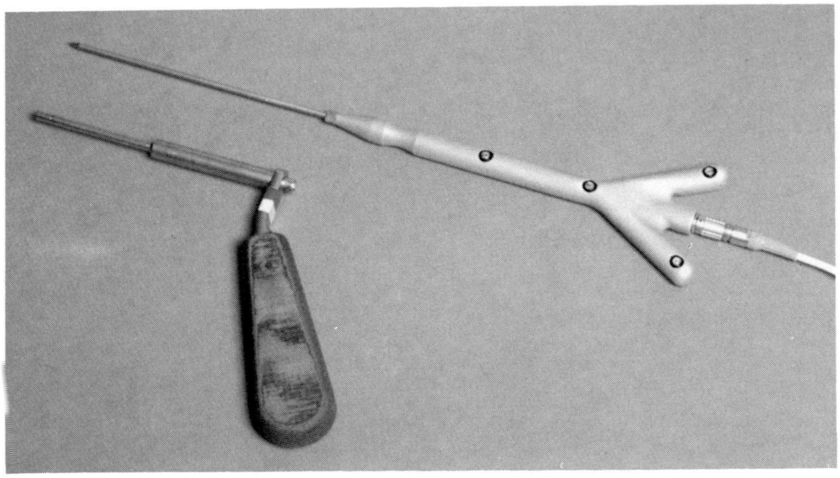

Figure 11-2. Hand-held wand and drill guide. The same wand can be used for both the registration and orientation process. The drill guide is used during the orientation process to mark the location of the entry point and the angle of trajectory. The wand can then be removed and a drill inserted through the drill guide.

localizer tracks infrared light emitted by a series of light-emitting diodes mounted on a customized hand-held wand or selected surgical instruments (Fig. 11-2). The position of the wand or selected surgical instruments can then be tracked in space using mathematical principles of localization by triangulation. These instruments serve as the interface between the surgeon and the computer workstation.

The surface anatomy of the exposed spinal column provides the frame of reference necessary for image-guided navigation. Specifically, any bony landmark that can be identified intraoperatively as well as in the preoperative image data set can be used as a reference point. The spatial position of each point selected can be defined by its specific x, y, and z Cartesian coordinates. The coordinates of a selected point in the image data set can be mapped onto its corresponding point in the surgical anatomy data set through a process termed registration.

Registration involves placing the computer cursor on a selected anatomic landmark in the CT or MRI data set while positioning the wand on the corresponding point in the surgical field (Fig. 11-3). The position of the wand tip is precisely tracked by the camera localizer system. When the wand is placed on a specific reference point, the spatial location of that point is relayed to the computer workstation. Three to five reference points at a single exposed spinal level (i.e., tips of a spinous process and the two transverse processes) are required for the registration process. Once the registration process is completed, reformatted multiplanar CT or MR images can be generated in near real time to precisely navigate through the unexposed spinal column and orient the surgeon to selected screw entry points and trajectories.

Selection of reference points for anterior spinal fixation procedures can be less precise because of the lack of prominent bony landmarks on the anterior surface of the spinal column. For anterior thoracic fixation procedures, the potential reference points available include the junction of the head of a rib with the adjacent

A

B

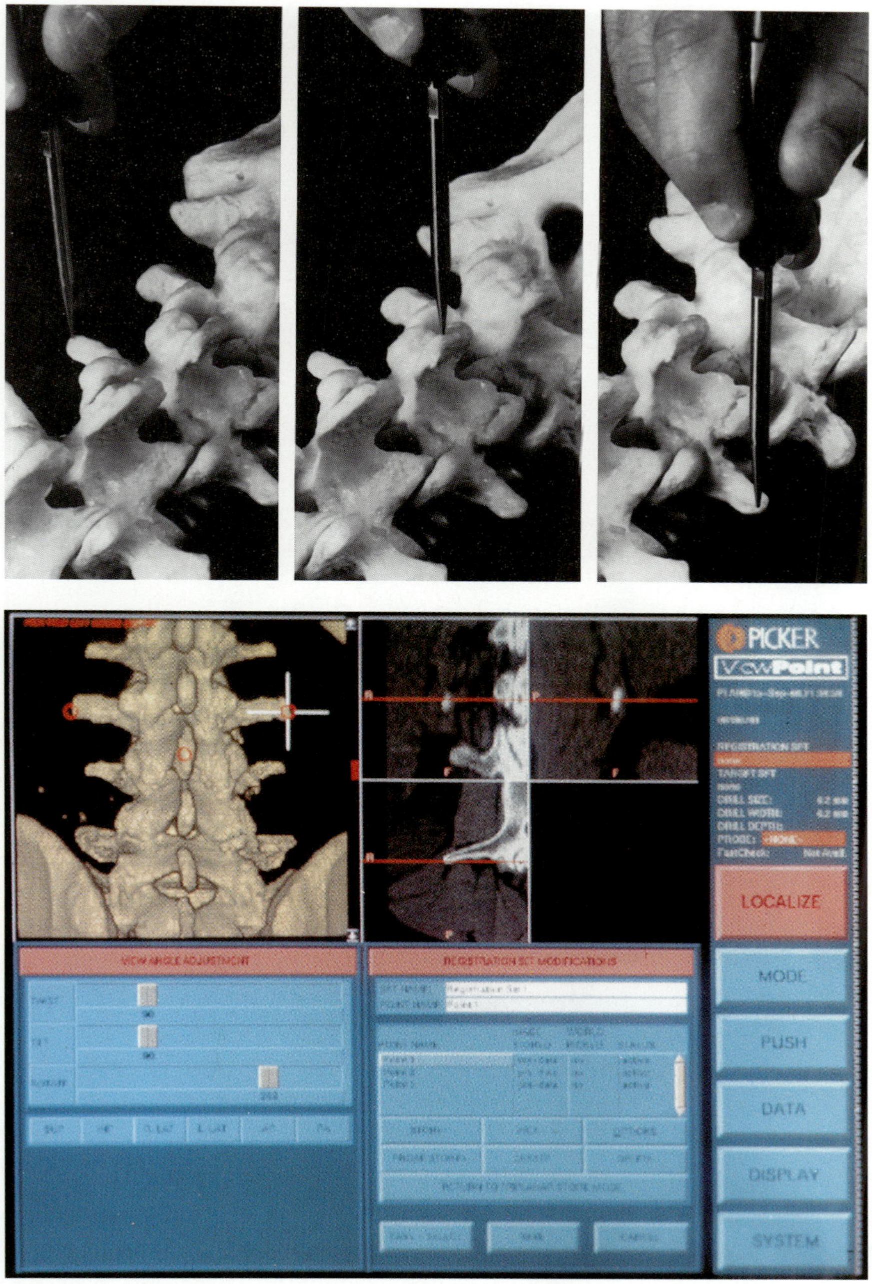

Figure 11-3. A, Demonstration of the registration process on a lumbar spine model. The wand is sequentially placed on three selected bony landmarks at the level to be instrumented. (In this demonstration these points are the L4 spinous process and the lateral tips of the two L4 transverse processes.) The computer workstation cursor is placed on those same points in the image data. The wand is activated on each point selected, effectively "linking" the spinal anatomy to the image data. This process can be repeated at any time during the procedure. **B,** Workstation screen demonstrating selection of registration points at the L3 level. The upper left screen quadrant represents a surface-rendered view of the imaged lumbar spine. The selected registration points (two transverse process tips and the spinous process tip) are identified by red circles placed on those points. When a specific registration point is highlighted (white crosshairs), the upper right screen quadrant will display the axial, sagittal, and coronal planes through that point. These triplanar views can be used to more precisely localize each registration point.

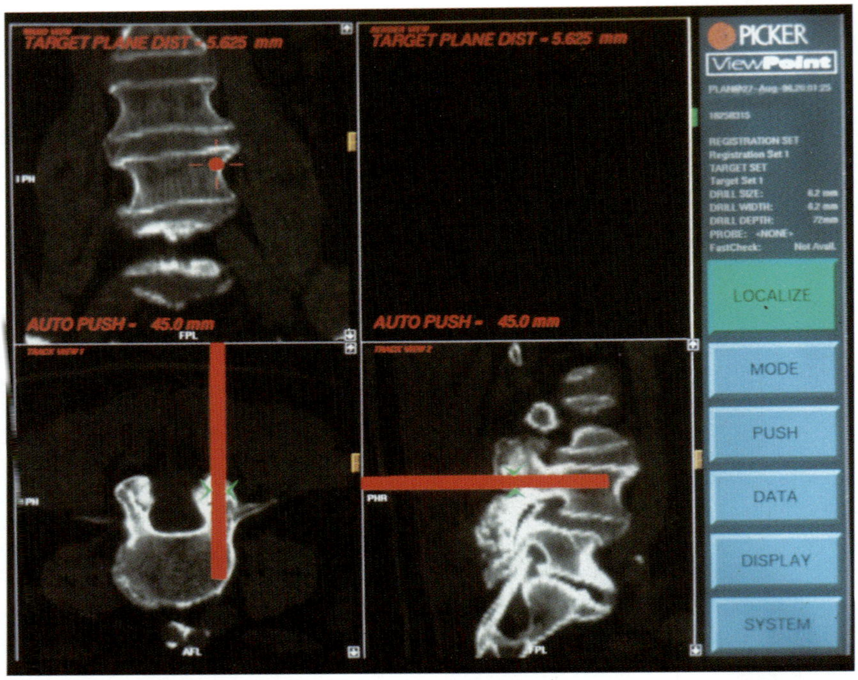

Figure 11-4 Workstation screen demonstrating a satisfactory trajectory through the L4 pedicle. The depth of the trajectory line is set at 45 mm. The cursor in the near-coronal view (left upper quadrant of the screen) indicates the distal end point of the trajectory line. The near-axial view and near-sagittal views are shown in the two lower quadrants.

disc or pedicle, the disc spaces themselves, and selected points on the lateral surface of the vertebral body. Although these reference points may not provide the same degree of millimetric accuracy as that provided by the selection of more distinct posterior bony landmarks, less precision is required for screw placement across a thoracic vertebra as opposed to insertion through a lumbar pedicle or across the C1-2 facet joint.

Once the registration process is completed, the image-guided system can be used to manipulate the image data set and correlate it with the exposed spinal anatomy. The images are reformatted and presented to the surgeon in multiple planes through any selected surface point. Typically, three different orthogonal planes oriented to the long axis of the wand are presented. As the axis of the wand changes with respect to the spinal column, the orientation of each plane will change. In most applications to spinal surgery the three planes commonly displayed will be a near-sagittal, a near-coronal, and a near-axial view. A cursor and a trajectory line with a diameter and width that can be adjusted according to the selected screw diameter are presented on the workstation screen. These indicate the proposed location and trajectory path through the selected point in the operative field. The length of the trajectory line relative to the imaged spine is displayed in millimeters, providing for accurate screw length selection (Fig. 11-4).

The images can be manipulated intraoperatively to show corresponding spinal anatomy in multiple planes and at a range of depths. By adjusting the length of

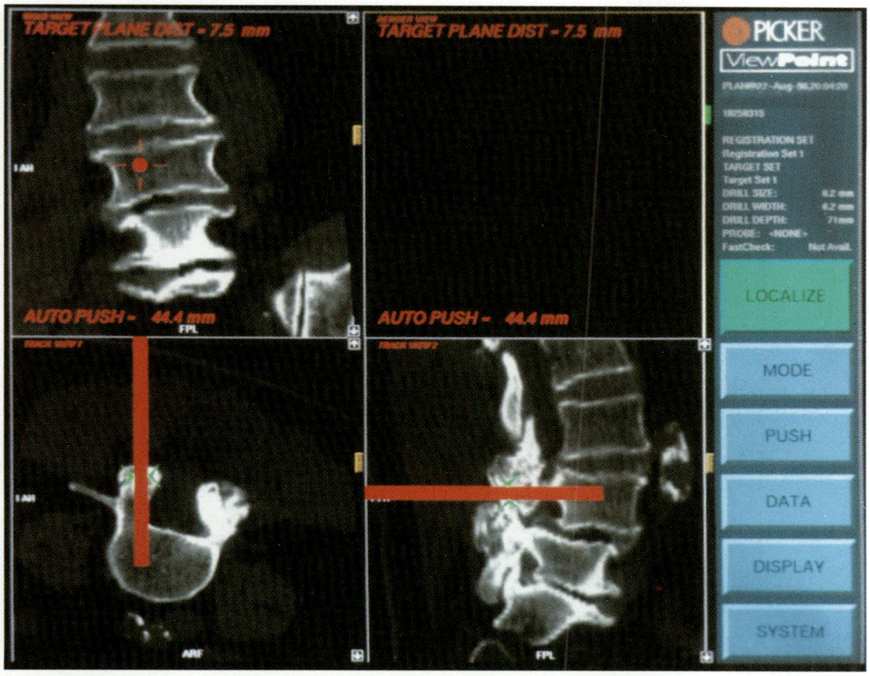

Figure 11-5. Workstation screen indicating an error in positioning of the hand-held wand. The near-axial view demonstrates that the trajectory selected through the L4 pedicle is too medial. A lateral fluoroscopic view would show only the sagittal trajectory seen in the lower screen quadrant and could result in incorrect screw placement. Movement of the wand medially would result in a redirection of the trajectory line in a corrected lateral position.

the trajectory line, a near-coronal reconstructed image corresponding to the end of the trajectory line can be generated. When the correct entry point and trajectory for a pedicle screw are selected, the near-coronal view will show a cursor lying within the boundaries of the pedicle on cross section. As the trajectory line is extended through the image set, the near-coronal plane will adjust accordingly to indicate the final position of a screw tip placed along that trajectory. Significant errors in sagittal angulation of the drill guide–wand assembly will place the cursor in either disc space adjacent to that pedicle. Errors in axial angulation of the drill guide–wand assembly or selected entry point in the coronal plane will place the cursor outside the boundaries of the vertebral body or pedicle wall (Fig. 11-5).

CLINICAL APPLICATIONS

Image-guided spinal navigation was initially used for insertion of pedicle screws in the thoracic and lumbosacral spines of cadaver specimens. The accuracy of screw insertion using image-guided navigation was documented by plain film radiography and thin-section CT imaging of the instrumented levels. All inserted pedicle screws were satisfactorily placed.[18]

The application of image-guided spinal navigation to spinal surgery is directed by the complexity of the procedure and, specifically, by the need to visualize the unexposed component of a spinal segment. The spinal procedures that can be facilitated by image-guided navigation include most screw fixation procedures as well as selected spinal column neoplasms, fractures, and deformities. Image-guided navigation can be used with or without standard intraoperative imaging techniques (i.e., fluoroscopy). In either case, image-guided navigation improves the surgeon's orientation to the pertinent spinal anatomy, which subsequently facilitates the accuracy and effectiveness of the procedure.

Pedicle Fixation

In the past decade pedicle fixation of the spinal column has gained greater acceptance as improved instrumentation and clinical effectiveness have become apparent.[19] However, because of the complexity of the involved spinal anatomy as well as the need to individualize the instrumentation construct to each patient, pedicle screw fixation is associated with a significant learning curve. This results in varying incidences of neural injury and fixation failure secondary to suboptimal screw placement. These complications can be minimized if the surgeon is properly oriented to each pedicle to be instrumented prior to screw insertion.

The insertion of pedicle screws into the spinal column requires an understanding of the location and orientation of each pedicle to be instrumented. Generally the pedicle is not directly visualized by the surgeon prior to screw insertion. Instead, posterior bony landmarks (transverse process and facet joint) are used to estimate the approximate location of each pedicle. The diameter and axial angulation of each pedicle can be estimated from an analysis of radiographic studies and from a general understanding of the orientation of pedicles at each spinal level. Intraoperative imaging can then be used to help confirm screw positioning.

Two methods of intraoperative imaging are used to obtain anatomic orientation before pedicle screw placement. C-arm fluoroscopy provides real-time imaging of the appropriate spinal structures that the screws will traverse. However, the fluoroscopic views generated represent only two-dimensional images of a complex three-dimensional structure and can be easily misinterpreted. With manipulation of the fluoroscopic unit, the three dimensions can be visualized in a series of images, but these maneuvers can be cumbersome and time consuming. Other disadvantages include radiation exposure and the need to wear lead aprons during the procedure.

The second method of obtaining anatomic orientation in the spine is serial intraoperative radiography. Prior to screw insertion, metal pins are positioned in each pedicle and a lateral radiograph obtained to confirm the pins' relationship to the surrounding spinal column structures. If the position of the pins is not satisfactory, their trajectory is readjusted and a second radiograph obtained. Once the pins are satisfactorily positioned, they are removed, and the pedicle screws are inserted along the same trajectory. This technique can be time consuming and misleading in that only lateral radiographs are obtained. Oblique and anteroposterior views are difficult to acquire, and without these views, screws may be improperly positioned. Furthermore, the screw trajectory can change when the pins are removed and the screws inserted unless a cannulated screw system is used.

Although both of these intraoperative imaging techniques provide the surgeon with information regarding the parameters of pedicle screw insertion, neither technique demonstrates the relationship of a proposed screw trajectory to an axial image of the spine. It is this view that makes image-guided navigation superior to the two standard methods of intraoperative imaging.

A CT scan through the appropriate spinal segments is obtained preoperatively. The images consist of a three-dimensional volume data set of contiguous axial CT images. Scan parameters include a 2.0 mm slice thickness, a field of view of 25.6 cm, and a 512 × 512 pixel image matrix yielding an in-plane resolution of 0.5 mm. The images are pixel averaged in each plane and interpolated in the slice direction to yield a CT volume data set consisting of cubic 1.0 mm isotropic voxels. The image data are then transferred to the computer workstation via optical disc or a high-speed data link.

The patient is placed in the prone or kneeling position. A standard exposure of the spinal levels to be instrumented is performed. A lateral radiograph is obtained to confirm the appropriate level. The computer workstation and camera localizer are positioned following exposure of the appropriate spinal levels. The infrared camera detector is mounted near the foot of the table and aimed rostrally for thoracic and lumbosacral procedures. It is positioned at the head of the table and aimed caudally for cervical procedures.

Three to five reference points previously selected in the CT image set at a single spinal level are identified in the operative field and registered. The system will determine the millimetric error in registration that can be created by the surgeon's imprecise selection of registration points. If the computed error is significant (i.e., greater than 2.0 mm), the registration process is carefully repeated. Registration accuracy can also be assessed by placing the wand on several visualized anatomic landmarks (i.e., spinous process, transverse process, or facet joint) at the registered level. If the screen cursor localizes to the same points in the image data, the registration process is accurate. If the correlation is not precise, the registration process is repeated until accurate correlation is achieved.

Following registration, standard bony landmarks for pedicle localization are used to approximate the screw entry point (i.e., intersection of the midtransverse process line with the facet joint). A drill guide is placed on this entry point and the wand passed through the guide. The wand is activated, and the appropriate multiplanar CT images through the localized point are generated. The near-axial and near-sagittal views can be manipulated via a mouse or foot pedal control to show the "extension" of the wand through the selected entry point. This involves a lengthening of the trajectory line through each of the two views. The near-coronal view will adjust accordingly to show a cursor in the CT image set at the distal extent of the trajectory line.

The orientation of each pedicle to be instrumented can be assessed quickly and easily. Image manipulation occurs in near real time, with image updating eight times per second. The location of the trajectory line and screen cursor changes as the surgeon moves the wand through the surgical field. For each pedicle, an approximate screw entry point and trajectory are selected with the wand–drill guide assembly. Any errors in trajectory or entry point selection can be determined and corrected by minor adjustments of the wand–drill guide position.

After the wand–drill guide assembly is satisfactorily aligned with the optimal trajectory, the wand is removed and a drill (3.2 mm diameter) is positioned through the guide. The drill guide preserves the navigational information when the wand is removed. A pilot hole is drilled through the pedicle into the vertebral body. A pedicle sound instrument is placed in the hole to confirm satisfactory hole placement. The hole is tapped, and the appropriate length screw is inserted. The process is repeated for each pedicle to be instrumented. C-arm fluoroscopy or serial radiographs are not required.

When screws are placed at a second spinal level, a new set of registration points are selected at that level. This method, termed segmental registration, eliminates any discrepancy in anatomic orientation that may be related to a change in patient position between the preoperative CT scan and surgery. The spatial relationship of anatomic points at a single vertebral level is not affected by changes in body position.

Posterior C1-2 Transarticular Screw Fixation

The placement of screws across the C1-2 facet joints has gained acceptance as a reliable method of supplementing standard wire and bone graft fixation of the atlanto-axial complex. By providing rigid internal fixation, the transarticular screws reduce or eliminate the postoperative need for halo brace immobilization.

The procedure involves inserting a 3.5 or 4.0 mm diameter screw into the medial aspect of the C2 articular pillar and passing it in a rostral and ventral direction across the C1-2 facet joint and into the lateral mass of C1. The procedure is usually performed bilaterally and in conjunction with a C1-2 wire or cable and bone fixation.

The risks of inserting a screw into this region of the cervical spine include (1) injury to the vertebral artery if the screw trajectory is too lateral or ventral, (2) injury to the spinal cord if the screw trajectory is too medial, and (3) failure to engage the lateral mass of C1 if the screw trajectory is too ventral. The insertion of a screw on either side may be contraindicated if the transverse foramina of C2 is in an abnormally posterior and medial position (i.e., narrow pars interarticularis of C2).

The selection of the appropriate screw entry site and trajectory in both the sagittal and axial planes requires a thorough understanding of the atlanto-axial complex as well as a greater degree of precision than does pedicle screw insertion in the lumbosacral spine. Although fluoroscopic guidance can be helpful, it may not consistently offer the millimetric accuracy necessary for this technique.

The technique for applying image-guided navigation to posterior C1-2 screw fixation involves obtaining a preoperative CT scan extending from the lower occipital region to C3. The scans are obtained at 2.0 mm increments and can be combined with intravenous contrast media to better visualize the vertebral arteries. The image data are then transferred to the computer workstation.

A surgical planning software package can be used preoperatively to assess the safety of screw passage in relationship to the vertebral artery. A proposed entry point and target can be selected at the C2 and C1 levels, respectively. These two points are then connected by a trajectory line with a width proportional to a 4.0 mm diameter screw. The image data set can then be manipulated in multiple planes to demonstrate the position of a screw placed through the C2 pars interarticularis and its relationship to the corresponding transverse foramina. This information can be used preoperatively to determine the feasibility of safe screw placement. It allows the surgeon to plan for an alternative approach if the proposed screw trajectory intersects the path of the vertebral artery.

Positioning of the patient and exposure of the posterior C1-2 complex is performed using standard techniques. Three to five registration points are selected from the image data at the C2 levels. These points usually include the lateral margins of the C2-3 facet joints and the spinous process of C2. It is not necessary to register at the C1 level. Although the technique involves intersegmental screw passage, the primary difficulty of the procedure occurs at the C2 level. The proximity of the vertebral artery to a transarticular screw is greatest at the level of the narrow pars interarticularis of C2. The target (the lateral mass of C1) is relatively large and easily accessed provided the screw has been accurately passed through the C2 pars interarticularis. Consequently, the procedure is more of an intrasegmental technique with the precision of image-guided navigation directed at precise screw placement along the pertinent C2 anatomy. Although the relative positions of C1 and C2 in both the preoperative image set and in the surgical field are important, they are not critical enough to interfere with the process of image-guided navigation.

If there is a discrepancy in the position of C1 and C2, it is typically related to translation in the sagittal plane. This discrepancy will only affect the position of the screw tip in the lateral mass of C1. If there is an anterior translation of C1 intraoperatively (as compared with the preoperative images), the screw tip will be located more posteriorly in the lateral mass. If the translation of C1 is more posterior, the screw tip will have a more anterior location in the lateral mass. In either case the screw tip will reach the lateral mass of C1 provided accurate navigation through C2 has been achieved.

Following exposure of the posterior C1-2 complex, two separate stab incisions are made on either side of the midline at the C7-T1 level. A drill guide is placed through one of the stab incisions, passed through the paravertebral musculature, and brought out into the operative field. The registration points are selected, and the wand is passed through the drill guide so that its tip lies close to the proposed screw entry points. Intraoperative navigation and orientation of the C1-2 complex is performed and the precise screw entry point and trajectory confirmed (Fig. 11-6). The length of screws required will also be displayed by the system. The wand is then removed from the drill guide and a drill bit inserted. A hole is drilled along the selected trajectory, the hole tapped, and the appropriate length screw inserted. The procedure is repeated on the opposite side.

Cervical Lateral Mass Plate Fixation

Stabilization of the cervical spine using lateral mass plates involves the insertion of screws into the lateral articular pillar of the cervical spine. The screws are directed rostrally and laterally to avoid injuring the exiting nerve root and the vertebral artery. They measure approximately 12 to 16 mm in length.

Image-guided spinal navigation can be applied to this procedure to identify the optimal entry point and trajectory for each screw. Three to five registration

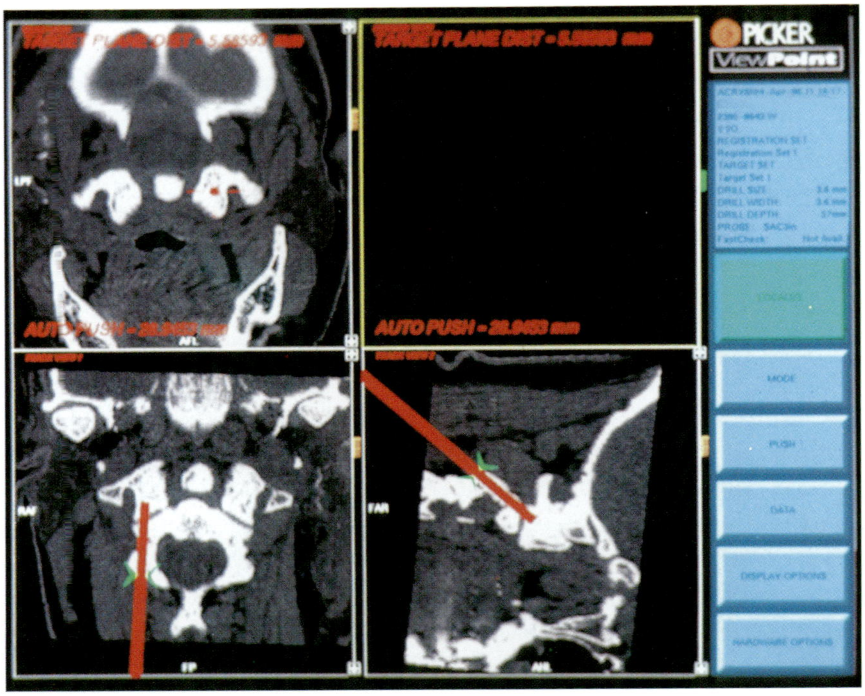

Figure 11-6. Workstation screen demonstrating a trajectory for insertion of a C1-2 transarticular screw. The image in the lower right screen quadrant shows the trajectory in the sagittal plane. The image in the lower left screen quadrant represents an orthogonal plane lying between the true axial and true coronal planes. It will demonstrate the medial-lateral direction of the selected trajectory. The upper left quadrant represents a plane that is perpendicular to the two other images. It demonstrates the location of a screw tip inserted along the selected trajectory at the indicated depth.

points are selected at each level to be instrumented. An approximate entry point over one lateral mass is selected. The entry point as well as the trajectory in the sagittal and axial planes can then be modified on the basis of the stereotactic images generated (Fig. 11-7).

When the C2 or C7 levels are included in the lateral mass plate construct, it may not be feasible to pass a screw into the lateral masses because of the obliquity or absence of a suitable lateral mass at these two levels. Under these circumstances, screws can be directly medially into the pars interarticularis of C2 or the pedicle of C7. Image-guided navigation can provide the surgeon with the appropriate medial and rostral trajectory for a C2 pars interarticularis screw and the medial and caudal trajectory for a C7 pedicle screw (Fig. 11-8).

Anterior Thoracic Screw Fixation

Anterior thoracic screw fixation involves the placement of fixation screws from one side of a vertebral body to the other. The screws pass under and nearly parallel to the floor of the spinal canal. Two screws generally are positioned into

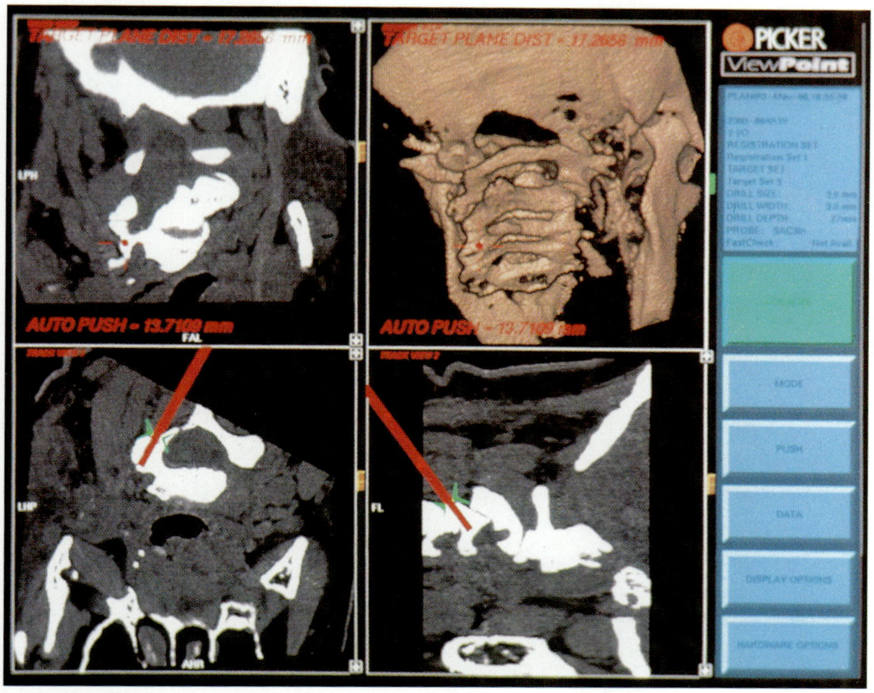

Figure 11-7. Workstation screen demonstrating the proposed trajectory of a lateral mass screw at the C3 level.

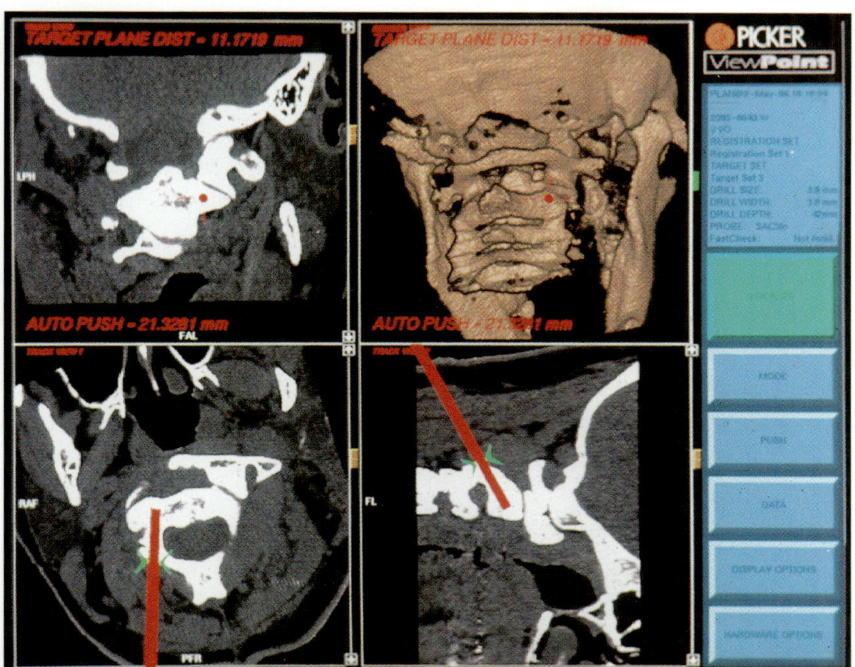

Figure 11-8. Workstation screen demonstrating the proposed trajectory of a screw to be placed through the C2 pars transarticularis.

each vertebra adjacent to a compromised segment of the spinal column. The screws are used to anchor a plate or rod system.

The parameters involved with screw insertion in the anterior thoracic spine involve the selection of the appropriate entry point, the trajectory in the axial and sagittal planes, and the depth of screw insertion. Each screw should ideally engage the distal vertebral cortex without injuring major vascular structures just beyond this cortex.

The selection of reference points for anterior spinal surgery is limited by the relative lack of prominent bony landmarks on the anterior aspect of the spinal column. However, reference points that can be used include the junction of the rib head with its adjoining disc space or pedicle, the disc space itself, or selected points on the vertebral body. Three to five registration points are used at each vertebral level. Following a thoracic corpectomy and reconstruction with a bone graft or prosthetic device, the reference points are registered and the appropriate screw entry points, trajectories, and lengths selected (Fig. 11-9).

Management of Spinal Neoplasms

A variety of neoplastic processes can involve the spinal column, producing varying degrees of spinal instability and/or neural compression. Tumors that extend out of the neural canal can dissect through the paravertebral soft tissues in a posterior, lateral, or anterior direction.

Neoplasms that lie adjacent to the spinal column and extend anteriorly are frequently approached from a posterior or posterolateral direction. This approach allows for a satisfactory decompression of the neural elements as well as posterior spinal stabilization at that level. However, the limitation of this approach is that the anterior and lateral extent of the paravertebral neoplasm may be difficult to assess because of the surrounding soft tissue structures. Image-guided spinal navigation can be used to identify these margins to optimize tumor removal.

The procedure is similar to other applications of image-guided spinal navigation. Standard bony landmarks on the posterior spinal column at the level of the neoplasm are selected and registered. As tumor removal proceeds, the wand can be placed within the cavity of the tumor or its exposed margin. The actual extent of tumor removal can be determined by noting the position of the wand tip on the images presented (Fig. 11-10). Although there is a potential for soft tissue shift during tumor removal, the relatively firm consistency of most paravertebral neoplasms minimizes this problem.

Localization of Fracture Fragments

Thoracolumbar fractures may involve retropulsion of fracture fragments into the anterior spinal canal. These fractures may be managed surgically through either an anterior or a posterior approach. If a posterior approach is used, precise localization of the retropulsed fracture fragment is necessary to prevent neural injury during decompression. Image-guided spinal navigation can be used to precisely localize these fragments prior to decompression (Fig. 11-11). It can be used to monitor the extent of fracture fragment removal. This is achieved by placing

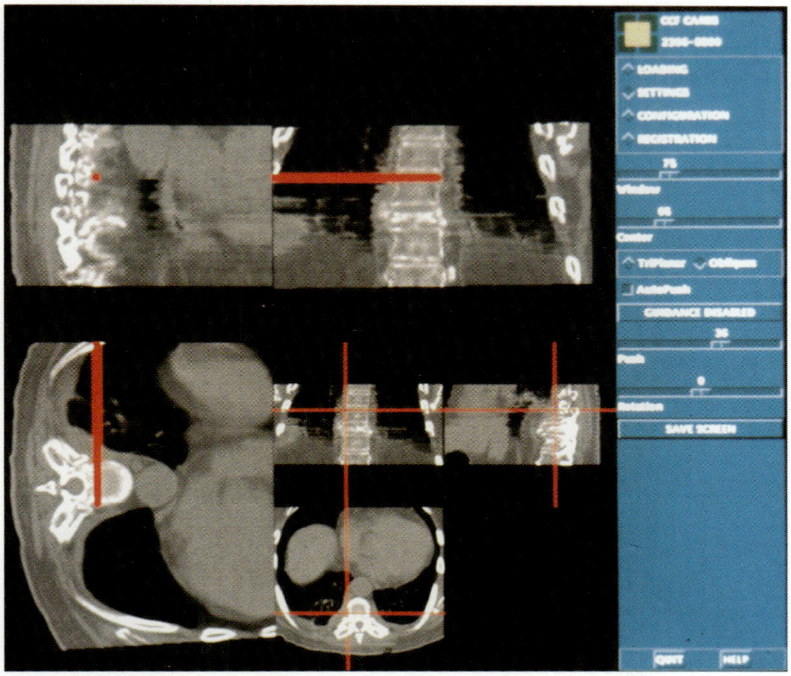

Figure 11-9. Workstation screen demonstrating the selected trajectory for insertion of an anterior thoracic screw. The images generated demonstrate the relationship of the proposed screw trajectory to the spinal canal, the adjacent disc spaces, and the distal vertebral cortex. The optimal screw length for bicortical screw fixation can also be determined.

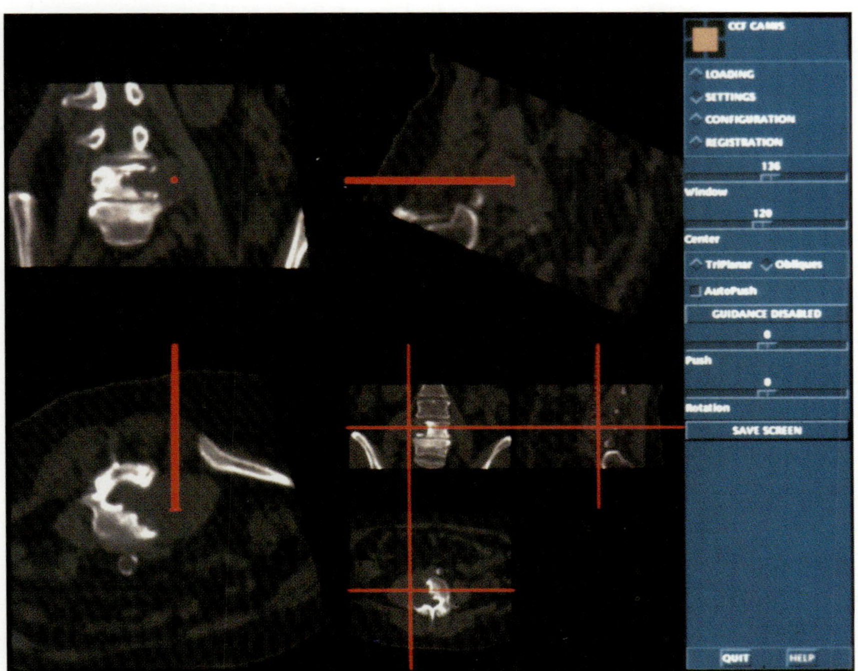

Figure 11-10. Workstation screen during removal of an L4 neurofibroma. Following partial removal of the neoplasm, the wand is placed into the tumor bed. The relative location of the tumor's anterior and lateral margins can be readily determined.

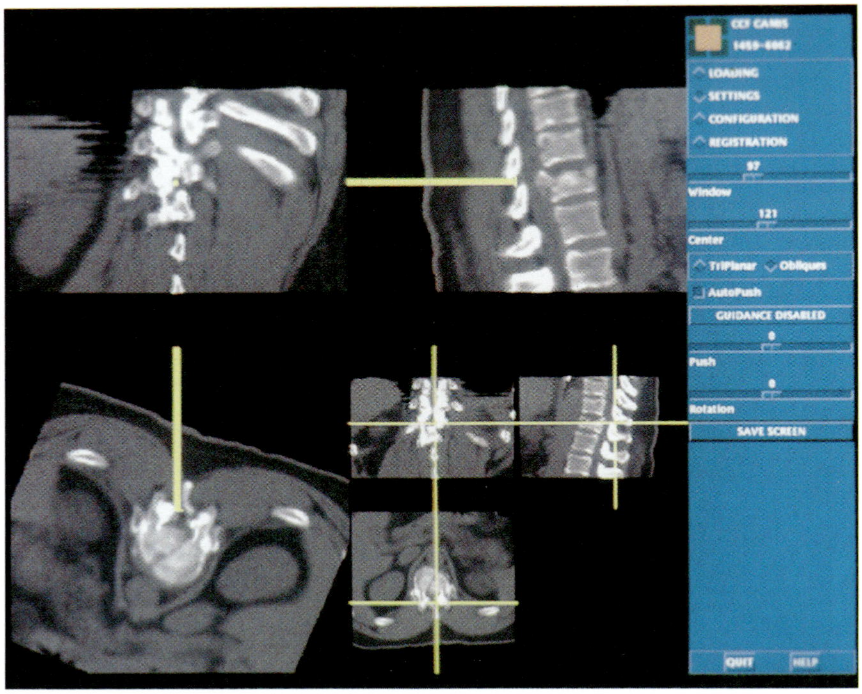

Figure 11-11. Workstation screen demonstrating a T12 burst fracture. The retropulsed fragment can be precisely localized prior to a decompression to minimize further neural injury.

the wand into the decompressed site and observing the relationship of the trajectory line to the fracture fragments in the preoperative image set. Following decompression, image guidance can be used for pedicle screw fixation of the injured spinal levels.

SUMMARY

Interactive surgical navigation technology has been successfully applied to spinal surgery. By linking digitized image data to spinal surface anatomy, it facilitates the surgeon's orientation to the unexposed spinal structures, thereby improving the precision and accuracy of the surgery. It is particularly effective for optimizing the placement of spinal fixation screws (Fig. 11-12) but can also be used to guide complex decompressive procedures. Ideally, the clinical application of this technology to spinal surgery should reduce operative time, morbidity, and costs as well as minimize or eliminate the need for standard intraoperative imaging (i.e., fluoroscopy).

However, image-guided spinal navigation is not a substitute for a thorough understanding of the pertinent spinal anatomy and the proper spinal stabilization techniques. Despite the presentation of optimal spinal imaging, the surgeon must still interpret the images and correlate them with his or her assessment of the exposed anatomy and the proposed surgical plan. The system functions primarily as

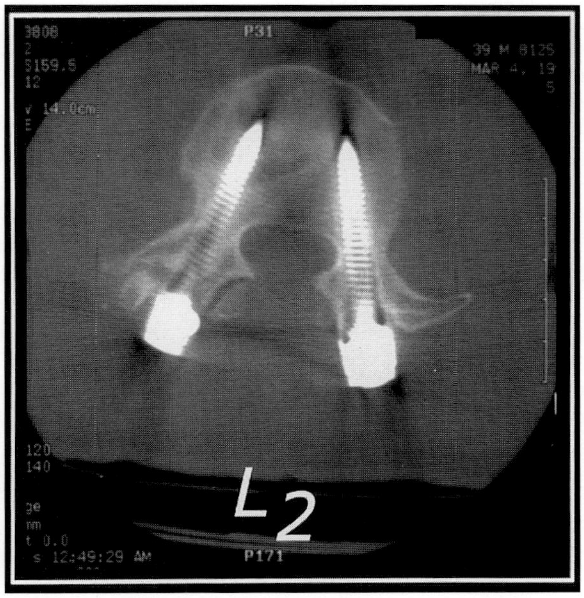

Figure 11-12. Postoperative CT scan showing satisfactory position of L2 pedicle screws.

a confirmatory tool, as does conventional intraoperative imaging, but with a greater degree of information provided to the surgeon.

The future of image-guided spinal navigation lies in the improvement of computer hardware systems, the development of more user-friendly and robust software, and the broadening of its clinical applications. However, the ultimate long-term success of this technology will depend on its expansion into other surgical disciplines to optimize its cost effectiveness.

References

1. Barnett GH, Kormos DW, Steiner CP, Weisenberger J. Use of a frameless, armless stereotactic wand for brain tumor localization with two-dimensional and three-dimensional neuroimaging. Neurosurgery 33: 674-678, 1993.
2. Barnett GH, Kormos DW, Steiner CP, Weisenberger J. Intraoperative localization using an armless, frameless stereotactic wand [Technical note]. J Neurosurg 78:510-514, 1993.
3. Bucholz RD, Heilbrun MP, McDurmont L. Use of an intraoperative optical digitizer in a system for free-hand stereotactic surgery. Presented at the Sixtieth Annual Meeting of the American Association of Neurological Surgeons. San Francisco, April 11-16, 1992.
4. Guthrie BL, Adler JR. Computer assisted pre-operative planning, interactive surgery and frameless stereotaxy. Clin Neurosurg 38:112-131, 1992.
5. Reinhardt HF, Horstmann GA, Gratzl O. Sonic stereometry in microsurgical procedures for deep-seated brain tumors and vascular malformations. Neurosurgery 32:51-57, 1993.
6. Roberts DW, Strohbehn JW, Hatch JF, Murray W, Kettenberger H. A frameless stereotaxic integration of computerized tomographic imaging and the operating microscope. J Neurosurg 65:545-549, 1986.
7. Tan KK, Grzeszczuk R, Levin DN, Pelizzari CA, Chen GT, Erickson RK, Johnson D, Dohrmann GJ. A frameless stereotactic approach to neurosurgical planning based on retrospective patient-image registration [Technical note]. J Neurosurg 79:296-303, 1993.
8. Watanabe E, Mayanagi Y, Kosugi Y, Manaka S, Takakura K. Open surgery assisted by the neuronavigator, a stereotactic articulated sensitive arm. Neurosurgery 28:792-800, 1991.

9. Zamorano L, Kadi AM, Dong A. Computer-assisted neurosurgery: Stimulation and automation. Stereotact Funct Neurosurg 59:115-122, 1992.
10. Dohrmann GJ, Rubin JM. Intraoperative ultrasonic imaging of the spinal cord: Syringomyelia, cysts, and tumors—A preliminary report. Surg Neurol 18:395-399, 1982.
11. George DC, Krag MH, Johnson CC, Van Hal ME, Haugh LD, Grobler LJ. Hole preparation technique for transpedicle screws: Effect on pull-out strength from human cadaveric vertebrae. Spine 16:181-184, 1991.
12. Gertzbein SD, Robbins SE. Accuracy of pedicle screw placement in vivo. Spine 15:11-14, 1990.
13. Weinstein JN, Spratt KF, Spengler D, Brick C, Reid S. Spinal pedicle fixation: Reliability and validity of roentgenogram-based assessment and surgical factors on successful screw placement. Spine 13:1012-1018, 1988.
14. Steinmann JC, Herkowitz HO, El-Kommos H, Wesolowski DP. Spinal pedicle fixation: Confirmation of an image-based technique for screw placement. Spine 18:1856-1861, 1993.
15. Brodwater BK, Roberts DW, Nakajima T, Friets EM, Strohbehn JW. Extracranial application of the frameless stereotactic operating microscope: Experience with lumbar spine. Neurosurgery 32:209-213, 1993.
16. Bryant JT, Reid JG, Smith BL, Stevenson JM. A method for determining vertebral body positions in the sagittal plane using skin markers. Spine 14:258-265, 1989.
17. Kalfas IH, Kormos DW, Murphy MA, McKenzie RL, Barnett GH, Bell GR, Steiner CP, Trimble MB, Weisenberger JP. Application of frameless stereotaxy to pedicle screw fixation of the spine. J Neurosurg 83:641-647, 1995.
18. Murphy MA, McKenzie RL, Kormos DW, Kalfas IH. Frameless stereotaxis for the insertion of lumbar pedicle screws. J Clin Neurosci 1:257-260, 1994.
19. Wiltse LL. History of pedicle screw fixation of the spine. Spine: State of Art Rev 6:1-10, 1992.

12

Epilepsy

David W. Roberts, M.D. • Terrance M. Darcey, Ph.D.

Surgical management of the patient with medically intractable epilepsy has increased greatly in the past decade. This has led to a growing number of medical centers with surgical epilepsy programs and number of patients being evaluated and treated. The impetus for these developments were the first and second international symposia held on the "Surgical Treatment of the Epilepsies" in 1986[1] and 1991,[2] respectively. Paralleling this phenomenon has been an extensive refinement of the diagnostic and therapeutic technologies that play prominent roles in the management of these patients. Image-guided surgical techniques are among the most important of these.

The goal of evaluation of the patient with intractable epilepsy is the identification and localization of the seizure focus; the complementary therapeutic intervention is the eradication of that same focus. These processes require accurate spatial localization during preoperative imaging and physiologic investigations as well as accurate co-registration of the preoperative database with the surgical field. It is an inherently stereotactic task.

This overview will look at the role of emerging interactive surgical navigation techniques for preoperative seizure evaluation, including intracranial electrode investigation, and then in surgical planning and surgical intervention.

PREOPERATIVE INVESTIGATION

Noninvasive Studies

The major advances in neuroradiology brought about by CT and MR imaging have had as great an impact on epilepsy management as on any other field of neurosurgery. With the advent of CT scanning, direct assessment of soft tissue volumes as well as potentially epileptogenic lesions became possible, and the improved soft tissue resolution of MRI has been even more revolutionary. Further, the imaging of physiologic substrates by PET, SPECT, and electromagnetic source imaging is currently providing new, nonstructural information. Finally, newly developed functional MRI allows us to visualize functionally significant cortical areas in direct relation to the anatomy.

The ability to co-register each of these modalities with the others underlies their value in trying to understand what is often a complex pathophysiology. This co-registration exploits the complementary strengths of each study, whether spatial fidelity or bony detail on CT, sulcal delineation on MRI, or relative regional blood flow on SPECT, by combining them into a single multimodal fused image set. To be optimally useful to the neurosurgeon, this data set must also be co-registered with the patient in the operating room. Neuroradiologists and neurosurgeons share common ground in establishing these spatial relationships since co-registration algorithms such as those designed by Pelizzari and Chen[3] for fitting CT and MR scans are also applicable to matching imaging studies and scalp contours intraoperatively.

Video-EEG recording of actual seizure events, a central component in the investigation of the seizure patient, yields an enormous amount of potentially valuable information for the central database as well. High-resolution digital EEG and/or magnetoencephalography may be considered an imaging modality, especially when co-registered and visualized along with anatomic and functional images, and display of their information to the investigator is an area of continued development. Techniques have evolved from schematic graphic presentations (e.g., BEAM) to spatially accurate representations and superimposed depictions of electrode or sensor locations and field maps of epileptiform spikes, seizures, and evoked potentials. With accurate electrode localization and anatomic detail, finite element modeling techniques may be applied to quantitatively estimate the sources of electrical activity in three dimensions.

Intracranial Studies

Depth Electrodes

In 1986 a survey of surgical epilepsy centers at the first Palm Desert Symposium showed that centers were fairly evenly divided between those inserting multi-contact depth electrodes by freehand techniques and those using stereotactic methodology.[1] Five years later a similar survey revealed that the great majority of centers used stereotactic techniques.[2] Driven by both the demand for the additional information that accurately placed depth electrodes can provide and by the facilitation of the stereotactic procedure by CT and MRI guidance, intracranial electrodes have enabled successful localization of more difficult seizure disorders and have a well-established role today.[4-10] In early analyses, Spencer[7] and Spencer et al.[10] demonstrated that a significant number of additional patients could be offered surgical treatment based on information made available only by such investigation, and conversely that many patients who otherwise would have been offered surgery could be spared what would ultimately be unsuccessful intervention. Although centers vary in their use of invasive recording, most use such recording techniques selectively today.

Depth electrode implantation by stereotactic technique offers the two advantages of increased accuracy in placement and increased safety. Direct visualization of the amygdala and hippocampus by MRI, coupled with an accuracy of several millimeters using frame-based stereotaxy, has enabled trajectories down the long axis of the temporal lobe that ensure implantation of critical mesial structures.

Preoperative planning at a graphics workstation allows renderings of proposed trajectories in triplanar display as well as in reformatted planes along the electrode course. In addition to the feasibility of achieving such trajectories, the methodology may be coupled with digital subtraction angiography or less invasive MR angiography to allow visualization of vascular structures to be avoided.[11-13]

Subdural Strip and Grid Electrodes

Since epilepsy is primarily a disease of the cerebral cortex in most patients, an additional method for evaluation when the results of the noninvasive workup are equivocal is subdural electrode recording.[5,8,9,14-24] Subdural strip electrodes consist of a linear array of stainless steel or platinum disclike recording contacts, commonly eight in number, evenly spaced a centimeter apart and embedded in a flexible Silastic strip. They are most commonly inserted through a burr hole and cruciate dural opening, with each entry accommodating placement of one or more electrodes. A tail containing the electrode leads is subcutaneously tunneled and brought out through a separate stab incision. Although commonly placed over the temporal and frontal convexity, they are often directed subtemporally, subfrontally, interhemispherically, and over the parietal and occipital lobes as well. Following placement, patients are monitored with continuous video-EEG recording in the epilepsy unit until a sufficient number of seizures have been recorded.

Studies of the EEG and clinical value of subdural and depth electrodes have variably concluded that depth electrodes are more accurate[8,19] and, alternatively, that depth and subdural electrodes can be of equal utility.[5,9,15-17] Subdural electrodes have the advantages of coverage of the cortical surface, easier placement operatively, and preservation of brain parenchyma integrity. On the negative side, they do not sample medial temporal structures as well as depth electrodes. The most critical factor in the reliability and usefulness of subdural strip electrodes is the accuracy of placement. The strategy employed by Awad et al.[25] is to insert strips beneath the temporal lobe and to the undersurface of the medial temporal lobe structures; if adjacent to these structures as intended, such electrodes will be sensitive to seizure activity arising mesially. In patients in whom invasive recording is desired to clarify the extent of the epileptogenic region associated with a subcortical structural lesion or to help determine which of multiple abnormalities may be responsible for a given seizure disorder, such electrodes may be directed over the pathologic area. With both medial temporal and subcortical lesions, accurate placement is essential, and while insertion is in general relatively easy, accurate placement cannot be taken for granted. Toward that end, interactive image-guided techniques may be useful.[26] Given the spatial limitations of intracranial recording contacts and the resultant insensitivity of contacts distant to seizure onset, there is a premium on accurate placement.

A stereotaxy frame is not generally used to guide the insertion of subdural electrodes, although it has on occasion been useful for assisting such electrode placement over lesions when it has already been placed on the patient for concurrent depth electrode placement. In such instances a frame's probe may serve simply as a pointer on the overlying scalp. Frameless stereotactic techniques, on the other hand, make such insertion guidance reasonable and accessible on a routine basis. At Dartmouth the SurgiScope stereotactic operating microscope system (Elekta AB, Stockholm, Sweden) has been used for this purpose in 25 procedures. With the patient awake but the head immobilized on a headrest and secured with tape, co-registration with preoperative MRI studies is accomplished using natural fiducials, including the tragus, lateral canthi, and nasion. The burr hole entry site and orientation points along the desired trajectory of each subdural strip electrode are then indicated by a laser light directed through the robotically driven operating microscope; the operating microscope itself is not optically used by the surgeon during the procedure. Although this has also been accomplished using the light-emitting diode (LED) hand-held probe that comes with the system, if the probe is moved until it matches the planned entry and trajectory reference points, the efficiency of noniterative, direct robotic guidance is particularly apparent in this multi-targeting procedure. In the manner described, preoperative electrode array plans have been executed with consistent placement of contacts over specific gyri, representing a clear improvement over our previous unguided technique. In all of our intracranial electrode placements the actual location of recording contacts is reconstructed from CT imaging following implantation, and thus interpretation of recorded data is not directly dependent on preoperative intentions.

Subdural grid electrodes are similar to strip electrodes but consist of a two-dimensional array of contacts (rows and columns) embedded in a Silastic or similar sheet. Although they are most commonly placed subdurally, they can be placed epidurally either routinely or in special instances of reoperation when subdural dissection may be difficult. They require a craniotomy for placement but sample a larger area than strip electrodes and can more accurately localize a seizure focus within that region. In addition, they provide the opportunity for more complete mapping of motor, language, and visual cortex through cortical stimulation techniques.[14,27,28]

Subdural grid electrodes, like subdural strip electrodes, are currently placed in most centers without stereotactic guidance. In most instances this approach may be fully adequate provided that very accurate placement is not required and that final electrode locations are determined by scanning after implantation. Ready access to frameless stereotactic guidance, however, has enabled its use in grid placement as well. Placement over possibly epileptogenic cortical or subcortical lesions such as tumors, cavernous angiomas, heterotopias, and schizencephalies has been unequivocally facilitated by image guidance in 13 of our patients. Placement of grids to facilitate functional mapping can also be accomplished in this manner.

In SurgiScope-assisted subdural grid placement, co-registration is performed following the administration of a general anesthetic and three-point pin fixation of the patient's head. The scalp flap and craniotomy are planned with the assistance of the SurgiScope's LED hand-held probe or with the microscope's directed laser light. Following elevation of the bone flap and opening of the dura, the robotic microscope is directed to show the surface locations of any pathologic areas identified on the images. Placement and orientation of the grid electrode may be accomplished in one of several ways. The most obvious and simplest manner of placement simply centers the grid over the already demonstrated area of suspected epileptogenicity. Alternatively, the grid's location may be planned preoperatively and the proposed location of at least two of the grid's contacts entered at a workstation prior to surgery. Intraoperatively, with the cortex exposed, the grid is moved over the surface of the brain until the identified contacts are aligned with the laser light or LED probe. Once positioned, the electrode leads from the grid are tunneled subcutaneously and brought out through separate incisions, as with strip electrodes. It has been possible to place such arrays within several millimeters of a preoperative plan, optimizing the ability to achieve successful recordings and to obtain desired functional mapping.

CT or MR images are obtained in all implanted patients prior to returning to the video-EEG monitoring unit following surgery. The documentation of exact electrode locations is critical, and prior to recent developments, assessment entailed conventional review of CT (for optimal electrode visualization) or MR (for optimal neuroanatomic detail) images. Automated electrode recognition algorithms and co-registration techniques to enable interactive display of CT-derived electrode locations on a prior high-resolution MR scan (Darcey TM, Battiston J, Roberts DW, Williamson PD, unpublished data) have facilitated and improved this process and are now part of standard protocol at our institution.

THERAPEUTIC PROCEDURES

Lesionectomy

Although interactive surgical navigation systems have been used most often for the resection of tumors, their adaptation to epilepsy surgery has been equally useful and similar in practice (Figs. 12-1 and 12-2). Surgical treatment of seizure disorders associated with structural lesions has been highly successful in producing seizure-free outcomes. In the combined series survey generated from the Second Palm Desert International Conference on the Surgical Treatment of Epilepsies, lesionectomy achieved a seizure-free result in 66.6% of 293 cases, with improvement noted in an additional 21.5%.[29] These are comparable to seizure-outcome results achieved with temporal lobe resections and considerably better than can be expected with nonlesional extratemporal resections.

In the intractable epilepsy population the most common structural pathologies have been developmental abnormalities (most commonly neuronal migration disorders), tumors (notably ganglioglioma, astrocytoma, dysembryoplastic neuroepithelial tumor, and oligodendroglioma), vascular malformations (cavernous hemangiomas and arteriovenous malformations), and posttraumatic gliotic scars. The tremendous advances that have taken place in neuroimaging over the past decade, particularly MRI, have led to a much higher recognition of such pathologies in the seizure patient population.

Although the relationship between these structural abnormalities and the actual seizure disorder remains incompletely understood, this relationship has significant implications for surgical intervention. In a retrospective analysis of 47 patients who underwent surgery for epilepsy associated with structural lesions, Awad et al.[25] explored this question. Seventeen of eighteen patients who had complete lesion resection independent of the extent of seizure focus excision became seizure free; five of six patients who had complete focus resection but in-

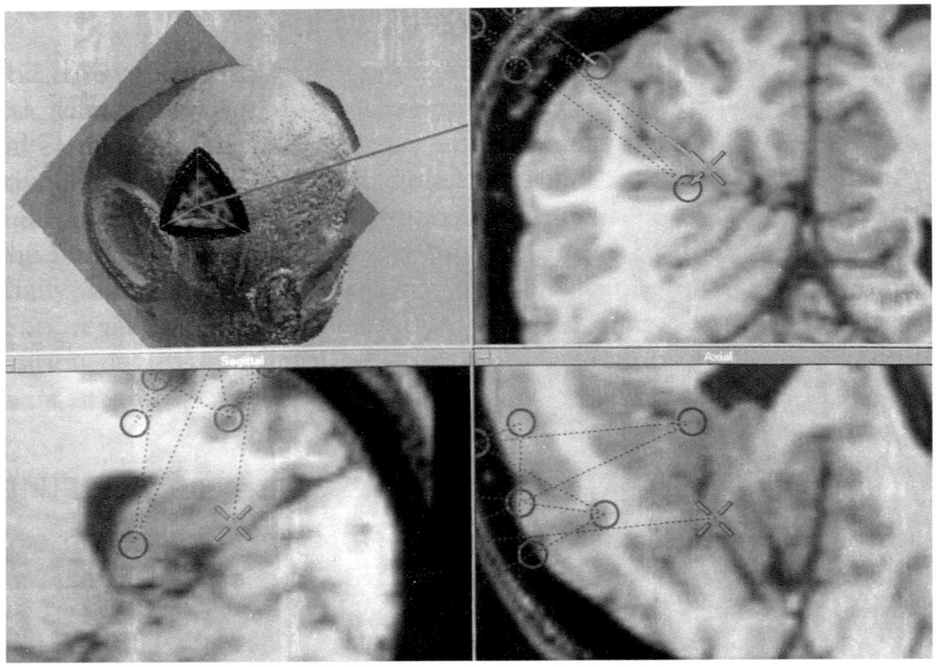

Figure 12-1. The position of the operating microscope's focal point (represented by a large X) relative to the preoperative MRI scan can be followed in this dissection down a large schizencephalic cleft. The triplanar display in this figure shows traditional coronal, axial, and sagittal planes. (From Roberts DW, Darcey TM. The evaluation and image-guided surgical treatment of the patient with a medically intractable seizure disorder. Neurosurg Clin N Am 7:215-227, 1996.)

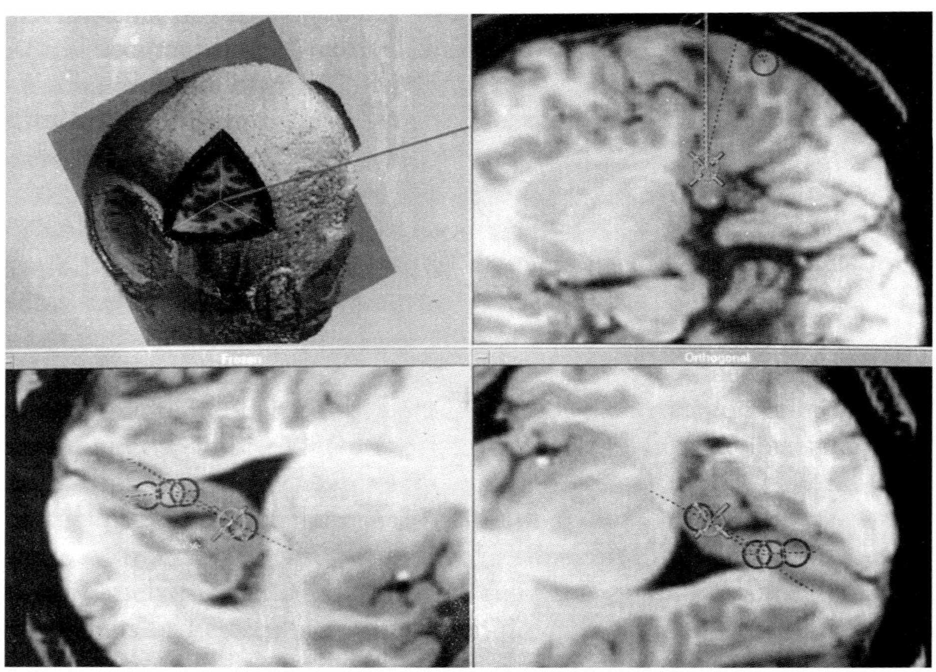

Figure 12-2. The microscope's focal point (represented by a large X within a circle) has now been directed to a portion of the deep heterotopia (same patient as in Fig. 12-1). In this instance the surgeon has selected a display showing a plane corresponding to the focal plane of the microscope (bottom right) and a plane perpendicular to the focal plane (top right). (From Roberts DW, Darcey TM. The evaluation and image-guided surgical treatment of the patient with a medically intractable seizure disorder. Neurosurg Clin N Am 7:215-227, 1996.)

complete lesion resection had a similar outcome. In only 12 of 23 patients with incomplete resection of both the lesion and the focus was seizure control achieved. Statistical analysis of the series showed the importance of completeness of lesion resection, but the study was not prospective.[25] Piepgras et al.[30] reported a series of 102 patients with arteriovenous malformations who had had at least one preoperative seizure and found 83% seizure free at long-term follow-up. Montes et al.[31] recently reported 16 of 18 children with lesional epilepsy free of seizure following lesionectomy alone.

Limitations to a structural approach alone have been suggested by other studies. Cascino et al.[32] reported their findings in a series of 23 patients with intractable partial epilepsy and foreign tissue lesions treated by stereotactic lesionectomy, finding 74% of patients had a ≥90% reduction, but only 56% had a class I outcome. A nonrandomized comparative study from the same center looking at anterior temporal lobectomy vs. stereotactic lesionectomy for medically intractable lesional epilepsy showed less morbidity with the latter but considerably poorer success in achieving a seizure-free outcome (50% vs. 90%).[33] In a recent retrospective review, Jooma et al.[34] reported 3 of 16 (18.8%) patients seizure free following lesionectomy alone compared with 13 of 14 (92.8%) patients seizure free with EEG definition of the seizure focus and wider resection.

These clinical studies do not definitively resolve the question of the optimal extent of resection or the means of achieving that resection, but collectively they do illustrate the complexity of epileptogenicity as it relates to multiple factors, including the anatomic lobe involved, the duration of seizures, and the number of preoperative seizures.[25,30,32,35,36]

One may conclude that there remains an important role for the multidisciplinary epilepsy team in the evaluation and management of these patients and that significantly better surgical outcomes may be achieved when intervention planning considers a broader database than imaging alone. The ability to seamlessly integrate multiple three-dimensional information data sets, including structural imaging, functional imaging, and electrophysiologic data, is becoming a necessity for surgical epilepsy centers and will soon be a standard feature of intraoperative surgical navigation systems.

Anterior Temporal Lobectomy

Navigational guidance may be useful at several points during anterior temporal lobe resection. In determination of the lines of cortical resection near the beginning of the procedure and in orientation during removal of medial structures, correlation of the surgical field with imaging studies can improve the accuracy of the resection as well as shorten operative time. Established practice commonly dictates resecting 4.5 cm back from the temporal pole, along the middle temporal gyrus, on the language-dominant side, and approximately 1 cm farther back on the nondominant side. Language function on the dominant side more anterior than 4.5 cm in some individuals has been demonstrated by Ojemann et al.,[37] who have consequently cautioned against the use of such arbitrary guidelines in favor of individualized functional mapping. Regardless of whether functional mapping is employed, however, the surgical team typically orients itself to the operative field following dural opening by measuring distances to the temporal pole and middle fossa floor. Given the curvature of both the temporal lobe and of the irregular middle fossa, these measurements can be imprecise and not necessarily concordant with the actual volumetric anatomy of the brain. In this determination intraoperative guidance systems have enhanced surgical precision[11,12,26] by allowing convenient preoperative measurement of the imaged temporal lobe and identification of the proposed line of resection for subsequent display during surgery.

When language or sensorimotor mapping has been performed preoperatively, guidance systems can easily incorporate that information at the time of surgical planning and do not require that the electrodes be left in place. Even if the electrode grid has been previously removed or demonstrated to have shifted during reexposure, the localized information from functional mapping is unaffected, provided that scans after implantation with electrodes in place are used to plan and execute the surgery. In those instances in which the grid has remained in place (a useful navigational guide in conventional epilepsy surgery), the transfer of that grid's localizing information to the underlying cortex becomes transparent and automatic with the capability of memorizing and returning to selected locations in the surgical field.

Removal of medial structures follows the above-described anterolateral resection step in the majority of temporal lobe resections for nonlesional epilepsy. The approach to the anterior portion of the temporal horn may be straightforward for those with experience, but directional assistance to that structure may be appreciated by both younger and older surgeons. Whether a hand-held probe or microscope focal point is used as a guide, the temporal horn is visualized much as any other structure or lesion (Fig. 12-3). Once the ventricular system has been entered and the hippocampus exposed, a guidance system may continue to be useful. In our experience this has been in demonstrating the superior extent of desired amygdala resection, where natural reference guidelines are less available, and in assuring resection of the desired length of hippocampus. The latter can always be directly measured intraoperatively, but with a guidance method already functioning in the previous stages of the operation, its continued application at this point adds no additional time or effort.

Selective Medial Temporal Resection

With recognition of the primary importance of medial temporal structures in the great majority of patients with complex partial epilepsies and with increasing confidence in the ability to localize seizure disorders to those structures in selected patients, there has been increasing interest in the procedure of selective amygdalo-hippocampectomy. The original description of the procedure by Weiser and Yasargil[38] entailed exposure of that anatomy through the anterior sylvian fissure. A number of centers have followed the lead of a more selective resection in certain patients but have accomplished this through minimization of the anterolateral neocortical resection; a posterior line of resection 3.5 cm from the temporal pole, for example, provides sufficient access to the hippocampus. Alternatively, selective resection of medial temporal structures can be accomplished

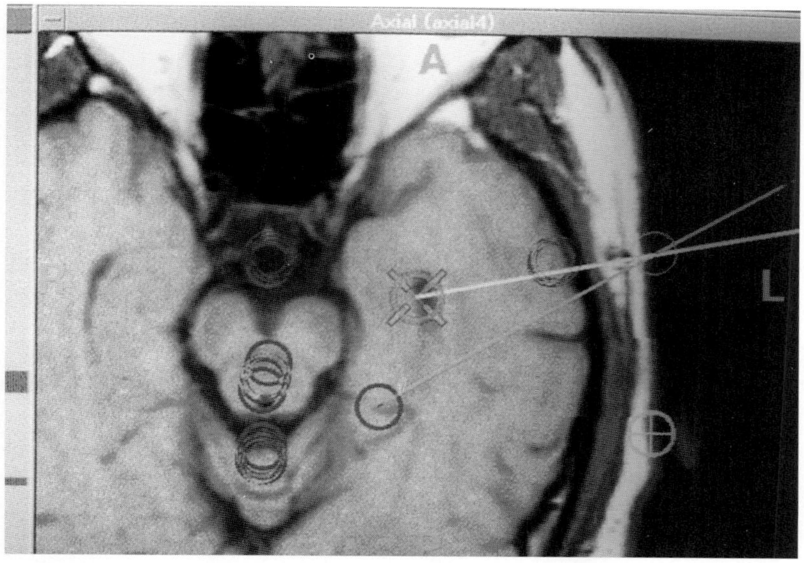

Figure 12-3. This display for a left anterior temporal resection demonstrates the position of the microscope's focal point (the lighter X in a circle) on the anterior hippocampus as well as the optical axis (the lighter oblique line). The microscope can be robotically driven to such a predetermined point and trajectory.

through a lateral corticotomy without the need for neocortical resection. Interactive surgical navigation techniques can be of considerable assistance in this last procedure.

Selective amygdalo-hippocampectomy through a lateral corticotomy is performed at our institution in the following manner. The anesthetized patient is placed on the operating room table in the supine position with the head secured in three-point fixation and turned approximately 30 degrees to the contralateral side. The microscope's laser pointer is then directed along the preoperatively planned trajectory, which lies approximately 15 mm anterior to the pinna and is directed at the hippocampus approximately 10 mm posterior to its anteriormost extent. The middle temporal gyrus is exposed through a 4 cm linear incision that begins just above the level of the zygoma and a free-bone flap measuring approximately 2.5 cm in greatest diameter. The draped microscope is now brought into the field, and following the laser guide, a 2 cm cortical incision can be made in either the middle temporal gyrus or immediately inferior sulcus. The dissection is carried directly down to the temporal horn, following either the laser guide or the progress of the microscope's focal point as depicted on the adjacent monitor. A user-selected panel of images, including triplanar and three-dimensional rendered formats, is displayed on this monitor, and reference to a high-magnification coronal image is sometimes especially helpful.

After the temporal horn is entered, self-retracting narrow brain ribbons are placed, and with the microscope in a spherical mode (rotating around the microscope's maintained focal point on the hippocampus), the exposure of the medial structures is examined. A subpial dissection is begun just lateral to the anterior hippocampus and carried down to the pia of the parahippocampal gyrus, although

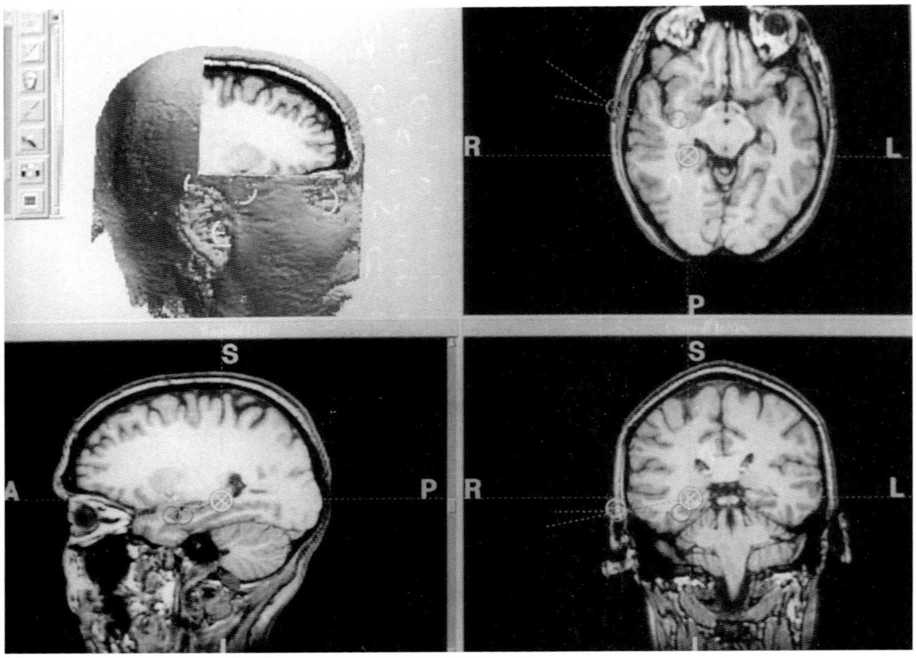

Figure 12-4. During preoperative planning for a selective right amygdalo-hippocampectomy a landmark point on the posterior hippocampus (depicted by a light-colored X within a circle) has been selected on this triplanar display. A target point on the anterior hippocampus (depicted as a darker circle) as well as trajectories (shown as oblique dotted lines) to both of these points have also been chosen.

alternatively the dissection may be performed down the lateral occipitotemporal (fusiform) gyrus if desired. The dissection is now carried anteriorly and medially around the hippocampus to the region of the uncus, and the amygdala is then dissected. As previously described, guidance along the superior plane of the amygdala resection is available if needed.

Directing attention posteriorly, the subpial dissection parallel to the hippocampus is carried back the length of the planned hippocampal resection (Fig. 12-4) by measurement as well as by stereotactic guidance provided by both laser light and monitor. In those instances in which previous evaluation has included depth electrode recording along the length of the hippocampus, the extent of hippocampal resection to ensure removal of epileptogenic tissue as well as the relationship between previous electrode contact positions and the exposed surgical field are clear to the surgeon during the procedure. The hippocampus is now transected, and opening of the exposed choroidal fissure begins posteriorly. The vascular pedicles to the hippocampus and parahippocampal gyrus are sequentially identified, coagulated, and divided. Anteriorly the dissection is carried across the uncinate fasciculus and the fibers of the anterior commissure, arriving at the previously dissected region of the amygdala. The hippocampus and adjacent parahippocampal tissue are delivered en bloc. Closure and postoperative management follow standard practice.

Neocortical Resection

Among the most challenging of intractable seizure disorders are those involving nonlesional, extratemporal cortex. Such resections generally follow careful demarcation of the epileptogenic zone by a subdural grid and strip electrode recording and frequently incorporate functional mapping and/or evoked potential information as well. The distribution of these seizure foci and their subsequent resection are individualized to the patient to an even greater degree than in mesial temporal lobe epilepsy. Based on primarily ictal video-EEG findings and motor and language mapping information, a preoperative resection plan is developed jointly with the multidisciplinary surgical epilepsy team to achieve the goal of maximally resecting the responsible seizure focus while preserving critical cortex.

The actual cortical resection is usually performed at the time of grid electrode removal. The grid itself may serve as a valuable, although sometimes inconvenient, guide during resection of underlying cortex, but with the availability of image guidance, the limits of the cortical resection can be visualized directly on the cortical surface. The cortical resections in which such guidance has been most helpful have been those in which the cortical surface is not widely exposed as it would be on the convexity. In particular, resections of the supplementary motor area and of the subfrontal regions have been facilitated to the greatest degree. The corticectomy itself is carried out in standard fashion once the lines of cortical resection in the surgical field have been determined.

Corpus Callosum Section

The reported clinical experience with navigational assistance during commissurotomy remains anecdotal but positive.[39-42] Inadvertently incomplete or (in the instance of partial callosal section) insufficient division of the commissure was not uncommon in the early experience with corpus callosotomy for the treatment of intractable generalized seizure disorders without an identifiable, resectable seizure focus. As more recent analyses have shown a correlation between length of callosal section and seizure outcome, the surgeon's ability to precisely execute a given length of callosal section has become more important.[41] Methodologies to address this have evolved that use radiographic or stereotactic feedback regarding the length of section,[41,43,44] but obtaining an intraoperative film or employing a stereotaxy frame may encumber an otherwise straightforward procedure. Currently emerging frameless stereotactic systems, on the other hand, provide this feedback easily. As dissection along the corpus callosum proceeds, the ability to monitor the extent of section either by graphics on an adjacent screen or superposed through the optics of the operating microscope can be a useful adjunct.

Reoperation

There is increasing evidence that reoperation can be worthwhile in many patients who respond suboptimally to initial epilepsy surgery.[21,45,46] Reevaluation and consideration of further surgery in selected individuals are highly appropriate. In this regard, perhaps no surgery for epilepsy is better assisted by navigational assistance than reoperation. All of the potential advantages that interactive image guidance can bring to first-time surgery apply at reoperation, but in the setting of postsurgical resection cavities, scarring, and adhesions that can obscure normal anatomic landmarks, such assistance can prove invaluable. In addition to the now obvious aid in orientation and location that can assist the surgeon intraoperatively, there is the additional advantage that information from previous evaluations can be integrated into the current workup.

If intracranial electrode recording and/or functional mapping has been performed previously, that information can be incorporated with the most recent recordings or imaging. Although some plasticity and reorganization of functional cortex are possible, it is entirely reasonable in most instances not to repeat mapping of speech and motor cortex. Unlike the initial surgery in which an orienting grid electrode may still be present at the time of cortical resection and provide an alternative to navigational assistance, reoperation may be greatly aided by the display of that previous grid on a recent co-registered study. Attention to any invalidating degree of subsequent shift of remaining brain tissue is in this instance clearly appropriate.

FUTURE DEVELOPMENTS

Few areas of neurosurgery are as complicated physiologically as that for epilepsy, and the role of image guidance in seizure surgery will only increase. Ever more sophisticated, complementary localizing techniques permit surgical intervention in a larger number of patients with improved outcome prospects, but they require computerized databases and co-registered surgery. It is likely that future surgical intervention will benefit from a number of new developments, including accurate noninvasive source localization based on realistic head models derived from individual scan data. Stereotactic correlation will benefit from increasingly transparent and accurate noncontact co-registration methodologies, and modeling, prediction, and tracking of brain deformations and shifts during surgery will help maintain the validity of that registration. High-end visualization, including real-time electrophysiology (e.g., electrocorticography) and timely analysis in the operating room, will be commonplace. Multimodal heads-up displays will inform the operating surgeon, whose tools will include, among other advances, refined endoscopic techniques, robotically driven instruments at both the macro and micro level, and various ablative devices such as focused radiation and other high-energy sources. Computer-assisted navigational surgery already has found a welcome place in the treatment of medically intractable epilepsy, and in the future it will be essential.

References

1. Engel J Jr, ed. Surgical Treatment of the Epilepsies. New York: Raven Press, 1987.
2. Engel J Jr, ed. Surgical Treatment of the Epilepsies. New York: Raven Press, 1993.
3. Pelizzari CA, Chen GTY. Registration of multiple diagnostic imaging scans using surface fitting. In Proceedings of the Ninth International Conference on the Use of Computers in Radiation Therapy. Amsterdam: Elsevier Science, 1987.

4. McCarthy G, Spencer DD, Riker RJ. The stereotaxic placement of depth electrodes in epilepsy. In Lüders H, ed. Epilepsy Surgery. New York: Raven Press, 1991, pp 385-393.
5. Smith JR, Flanigin HF, King DW, et al. Analysis of a four-year experience with depth electrodes and a two-year experience with subdural electrodes in the evaluation of ablative seizure surgery candidates. Appl Neurophysiol 50:380-385, 1987.
6. So NK. Depth electrode studies in mesial temporal epilepsy. In Lüders H, ed. Epilepsy Surgery. New York: Raven Press, 1991, pp 371-384.
7. Spencer SS. Depth electroencephalography in selection of refractory epilepsy for surgery. Ann Neurol 9:207-214, 1981.
8. Spencer SS. Depth versus subdural electrode studies for unlocalized epilepsy. J Epilepsy 2:123-127, 1989.
9. Spencer SS, Spencer DD, Williamson PD, et al. Combined depth and subdural electrode investigation in uncontrolled epilepsy. Neurology 40:74-79, 1990.
10. Spencer SS, Spencer DD, Williamson PD, et al. The localizing value of depth electroencephalography in 32 patients with refractory epilepsy. Ann Neurol 12:248-253, 1982.
11. Olivier A, Germano IM, Cukiert A, et al. Frameless stereotaxy for surgery of the epilepsies—Preliminary experience [Technical note]. J Neurosurg 81:629-633, 1994.
12. Olivier A, Lacertee D, Cukiert A, et al. Frameless stereotactic craniotomies in the surgical treatment of epilepsy: Preliminary experience in 70 patients. Presented at the Sixty-second Annual Meeting of the American Association of Neurological Surgeons, San Diego, 1994, p 352.
13. Watson V, Xei J, Wilson C, et al. MR stereotactic procedure planning with vascular and cortical guidance: Comparison and correlation of MRA, 3-D MRI, digital subtraction angiography (DSA), and intracerebral electrodes. Presented at the Sixty-second Annual Meeting of the American Association of Neurological Surgeons, San Diego, 1994.
14. Arroyo S, Lesser RP, Awad IA, et al. Subdural and epidural grids and strips. In Engel J Jr, ed. Surgical Treatment of the Epilepsies. New York: Raven Press, 1993, pp 377-386.
15. Blom S, Flink R, Hetta J, et al. Interictal and ictal activity recorded with subdural electrodes during preoperative evaluation for surgical treatment of epilepsy. J Epilepsy 2:9-20, 1989.
16. Devinsky O, Sato S, Kufta CV, et al. Electroencephalographic studies of simple partial seizures with subdural electrode recordings. Neurology 39:527-533, 1989.
17. Lüders H, Han JF, Lesser RP, et al. Basal temporal subdural electrodes in the evaluation of patients with intractable epilepsy. Epilepsia 30:131-142, 1989.
18. Rosenbaum TJ, Laxer KD, Vessely M, et al. Subdural electrodes for seizure focus determination. Neurosurgery 19:73-81, 1986.
19. van Veelen CWM, Debets RMChr, van Huffelen AC, et al. Combined use of subdural and intracerebral electrodes in preoperative evaluation of epilepsy. Neurosurgery 26:93-101, 1990.
20. Wyler AR. Subdural strip electrodes in surgery of epilepsy. In Lüders H, ed. Epilepsy Surgery. New York: Raven Press, 1991, pp 395-398.
21. Wyler AR, Hermann B, Richey ET. Results of reoperation for failed epilepsy surgery. J Neurosurg 71:815-819, 1989.
22. Wyler AR, Ojemann GA, Lettich E, et al. Subdural strip electrodes for localizing epileptogenic foci. J Neurosurg 60:1195-1200, 1984.
23. Wyler AR, Walker G, Somes G. The morbidity of long-term seizure monitoring using subdural strip electrodes. J Neurosurg 74:734-737, 1991.
24. Wyler AR, Wilkus RJ, Blume WT. Strip electrodes. In Engel J Jr, ed. Surgical Treatment of the Epilepsies. New York: Raven Press, 1993, pp 387-397.
25. Awad IA, Rosenfeld J, Ahl J, et al. Intractable epilepsy and structural lesions of the brain: Mapping, resection strategies, and seizure outcome. Epilepsia 32:179-186, 1991.
26. DeSalles AAF, Hoebel B, Bhenke E, et al. Frameless stereotaxy validation in general neurosurgery. Presented at the Sixty-second Annual Meeting of the American Association of Neurological Surgeons, San Diego, 1994.
27. Lesser RP, Gordon B, Fisher R, et al. Subdural grid electrodes in surgery of epilepsy. In Lüders H, ed. Epilepsy Surgery. New York: Raven Press, 1991, pp 399-408.
28. Uematsu S, Lesser RP, Gordon B, et al. Total resection of perioccipital epileptogenic area with preservation of visual function: The advantage of preoperative subdural grid mapping. Presented at the Sixty-second Annual Meeting of the American Association of Neurological Surgeons, San Diego, 1994.
29. Engel J Jr, Van Ness PC, Rasmussen TB, et al. Outcome with respect to epileptic seizures. In Engel J Jr, ed. Surgical Treatment of the Epilepsies. New York: Raven Press, 1993, pp 609-621.

30. Piepgras DG, Sundt TM Jr, Ragoowansi AT, et al. Seizure outcome in patients with surgically treated cerebral arteriovenous malformations. J Neurosurg 78:5-11, 1993.
31. Montes JL, Rosenblatt B, Farmer J-P, et al. Lesionectomy of MRI-detected lesions in children with epilepsy. Pediatr Neurosurg 22:167-173, 1995.
32. Cascino GD, Kelly PJ, Sharbrough FW, et al. Long-term follow-up of stereotactic lesionectomy in partial epilepsy: Predictive factors and electroencephalographic results. Epilepsia 33:639-644, 1992.
33. Moore JL, Cascino GD, Trenerry MR. A comparative study of lesion resection with corticectomy with stereotactic lesionectomy in patients with temporal lobe lesional epilepsy. Epilepsia 33(Suppl 3):96, 1992.
34. Jooma R, Yeh H-S, Privitera MD, et al. Lesionectomy versus electrophysiologically guided resection for temporal lobe tumors manifesting with complex partial seizures. J Neurosurg 83:231-236, 1995.
35. Cohen DS, Zubay BA, Goodman RR. Seizure outcome after lesionectomy for cavernous malformations. J Neurosurg 83:237-242, 1995.
36. Yeh H-S, Tew JM, Gartner M. Seizure control after surgery on cerebral arteriovenous malformations. J Neurosurg 78:12-18, 1993.
37. Ojemann GA, Sutherling WW, Lesser RP, et al. Cortical stimulation. In Engel J Jr, ed. Surgical Treatment of the Epilepsies. New York: Raven Press, 1993, pp 399-414.
38. Weiser HG, Yasargil MG. Selective amygdalohippocampectomy as surgical treatment of mediobasal limbic epilepsy. Surg Neurol 17:445-457, 1984.
39. Bucholz RD, Baumann CK. The use of image-guided frameless stereotaxy during epilepsy surgery. Presented at the Sixty-second Annual Meeting of the American Association of Neurological Surgeons, San Diego, 1994.
40. Bucholz RD, Smith KR. A comparison of sonic digitizers versus light emitting diode-based localization. In Maciunas R, ed. Interactive Image-Guided Neurosurgery. Park Ridge, Ill.: American Association of Neurological Surgeons, 1993, pp 179-200.
41. Roberts DW, Reeves AG, Nordgren RE. The role of posterior callosotomy in patients with suboptimal response to anterior callosotomy. In Reeves AG, Roberts DW, eds. Epilepsy and the Corpus Callosum. New York: Plenum Press, 1995, pp 183-190.
42. Roberts DW, Rayport M, Maxwell RE, et al. Corpus callosotomy. In Engel J Jr, ed. Surgical Treatment of the Epilepsies. New York: Raven Press, 1993, pp 519-526.
43. Awad IA, Wyllie E, Lüders H, et al. Intraoperative determination of the extent of corpus callosotomy for epilepsy: Two simple techniques. Neurosurgery 25:102-106, 1990.
44. Roberts DW, Strohbehn JW, Hatch JF, et al. A frameless stereotaxic integration of computerized tomographic imaging and the operating microscope. J Neurosurg 65:545-549, 1986.
45. Awad IA, Nayel MH, Lüders H. Second operation after failure of previous resection for epilepsy. Neurosurgery 28:510-518, 1991.
46. Polkey CE, Awad IA, Tanaka T, et al. The place of reoperation. In Engel J Jr, ed. Surgical Treatment of the Epilepsies. New York: Raven Press, 1993, pp 663-667.

13

Hydrocephalus

Mark G. Luciano, M.D., Ph.D. • R.L. Patrick Rhoten, M.D. • Gene H. Barnett, M.D.

Although neuroendoscopic procedures have been performed since the early 1900s, the last decade has witnessed increased interest in the use of the endoscope in neurosurgery.[1-4] This popularity stems from the growing demand for less invasive surgical techniques as well as the advances in endoscopic technology. Fiber optics, for example, have allowed visualization through smaller diameter scopes and also some flexibility in the instruments. Because of its many applications in the treatment of hydrocephalus, such as in shunt placement, catheter retrieval, third ventriculostomy, and fenestrations, endoscopy has become an essential tool in the treatment of more complex problems encountered in patients with hydrocephalus and has renewed interest in older treatments such as third ventriculostomy and choroid plexus coagulation.[3,5-14] In addition, the endoscope is finding broader application in surgery of the spine and cisterns and for management of cysts, abscesses, hemorrhages, and tumors.[2,15-20]

The use and indications for neuroendoscopy are undoubtedly expanding; however, the surgeon's experience and the present technology pose limitations that must be considered. Problems of visibility, tissue manipulation, coagulation, orientation, and navigation remain to be addressed.

Although standard visually guided neuroendoscopy is often adequate for catheter placement and for most third ventriculostomies, orientation and navigation become more problematic when orienting landmarks are not present, when targets are small, or when fluids are not clear. In the case of hydrocephalus the ventricles are often easily accessible with a single pass, and once the surgeon is oriented, targeting is immediate based on ventricular anatomy such as the choroid plexus and foramen of Monroe. However, in loculated hydrocephalus, for example, targeting and orientation in multiple cysts may be difficult because of the absence of normal landmarks. From the inside many cysts look alike, and the optimal site of fenestration to avoid structures on the other side or to align the scope for subsequent fenestrations is not possible based on the endoscopic view alone.

A portion of this work was presented at the Annual Meeting of the Joint Section of Pediatric Neurosurgeons, St. Louis, December, 1994.

Potential Indications for Neuroendoscopy

- Hydrocephalus
  - Optimal catheter placement
  - Foreign body retrieval
  - Third ventriculostomy
  - Membrane fenestration
    - Arachnoid cyst
    - Multicompartmental hydrocephalus
    - Septum pellucidum
  - Ablation of choroid plexus
- Cyst aspiration
  - Abscess
  - Tumor
  - Hematoma
- Tumor biopsy or resection
- Microvascular decompression, trigeminal neuralgia
- Craniosynostosis release
- Endoscopic-assisted microsurgery
- Spinal surgery
  - Sympathectomy
  - Discectomy
  - Syringomyelia drainage

As with stereotactic procedures, accurate endoscope trajectories are required to safely reach critical areas and small targets. Even "flexible" fiber-optic endoscopes act as essentially rigid systems that require a specific planned trajectory for minimal tissue injury and proper visualization of the target. Unlike stereotactic surgery, in which lateral probe movement is rarely considered after insertion into the brain, such a "rowing" movement is often performed with the endoscope when visual feedback is available. Obviously, since structures lateral to the scope are unseen, excessive or blind movement is dangerous.

Visual guidance alone is not adequate in opaque fluids such as hematomas and abscesses. In these cases endoscopic visualization may be used as an adjunct to stereotactic drainage and becomes more useful as the drainage is near completion and an open cavity created.[15,16] Finally, ventricular or periventricular lesions may be better visualized by contrast-enhanced imaging than by the endoscope alone. In these cases the use of endoscopy is limited and additional guidance is needed.

SOLUTIONS TO ENDOSCOPIC GUIDANCE

Clearly, better navigation would improve the efficacy and safety of neuroendoscopy. An ideal guidance system would provide real-time visualization of the endoscope's movement through accurately depicted brain structures. MRI would provide the best anatomic resolution, and "open" MRI systems may allow such imaging during procedures. With the advancements in "open" MRI technology, including improvement in working space, acquisition time, and image resolution, and with the development of MRI-compatible endoscopes and instruments, this method may eventually prove to offer optimal endoscopic navigation.

Ultrasound may also be useful in neuroendoscopic guidance. This existing technology is relatively inexpensive and has the advantage of true real-time imaging. In addition, color Doppler imaging may have the ability to identify major blood vessels so they can be avoided, and the flow of cerebrospinal fluid may be visualized after fenestrations. One major disadvantage is the inability to image through bone. Ultrasound imaging may be performed noninvasively in infants through an open fontanel. However, a separate or extended craniotomy is needed in adults. Another disadvantage is the low resolution of ultrasound in comparison to MRI or even CT imaging.

STEREOTACTIC GUIDANCE

Although real-time imaging is ideal, the widespread use and documented efficacy of stereotactic procedures demonstrate the utility of preoperative images for guidance. Stereotactic guidance is readily available, familiar, relatively inexpensive, and accurate; however, errors can be introduced with intraprocedural tissue shifts. Such shifts can be expected with any mass removal and with ventricular drainage in hydrocephalus. Although techniques to minimize the effect of intraoperative shifts are helpful,[21,22] this limitation remains an important factor.

Stereotaxy frames have been adapted for endoscopic guidance.[23] They are especially helpful in trajectory planning and targeting and holding the endoscope in a fixed position. However, when multiple targets are needed or when movement of the scope under visual guidance is also desired, these systems become quite cumbersome. Thus the system is useful for the initial approach but not for intraoperative use.

As described in other chapters, frameless stereotactic systems have the advantage of being much less cumbersome and more flexible while retaining adequate accuracy. Although several systems have been devised for localization in space using mechanical arms and light and sound emitters, we employed the Picker sonic system developed at The Cleveland Clinic and already in use for tumor localization. This system was mechanically linked to a rigid endoscope, which was already used routinely. We call this the computer-assisted neuroendoscopy, or CANE, system.[24]

INSTRUMENTATION

A detailed description of the principles and characteristics of the image-guided stereotactic Viewpoint wand and the techniques of reference fiducial placement have been previously published and discussed in more detail in other chapters of this book.[25-27] Briefly, the operative hardware consists of a rigid wand with two ultrasonic sound emitters, a panel fixed to the operative table with an array of four microphones, and a computer station (computer type) with a video screen.

The accuracy of frameless stereotactic systems is subject to several variables, including the nature of the three-dimensional digitizer, the use of scalp- or cranium-fixed fiducials, and the registration scheme. The overall accuracy of frameless stereotactic systems is generally comparable to that achieved with conventional frames. When the wand tip is in the optimal position, the reproducibility of this particular system is ± 0.6 mm (standard deviation) and demonstrates a broad range of orientations that maintain error at ±1.0 mm. The mean linear error when measuring distances within a 1000 cm^3 volume is 1.1 ± 1.1 mm (1.01 ± 0.7%).[25-28]

Endoscope Coupling

Because the stereotactic guidance system depends on line-of-sight between the emitter and sensor, calculation of the endoscope tip depends on a fixed and rigid system. For this reason, a rigid Gaab endoscope is coupled to the stereotactic wand via the working port of the endoscope. This scope has a 4.5 mm diameter access channel with a glass rod lens for excellent image quality and working ports for irrigation and instrumentation.

The physical linkage between the endoscope and the Viewpoint wand system was created in two ways to allow its use in both planning and performing the target approach with the obturator and subsequent relocalization during the endoscopic procedure itself. First, the standard Gaab obturator was fitted at the distal end with a screw thread, which can be attached to the standard Viewpoint probe (Fig. 13-1). The calculations for endoscope tip location were programmed to allow

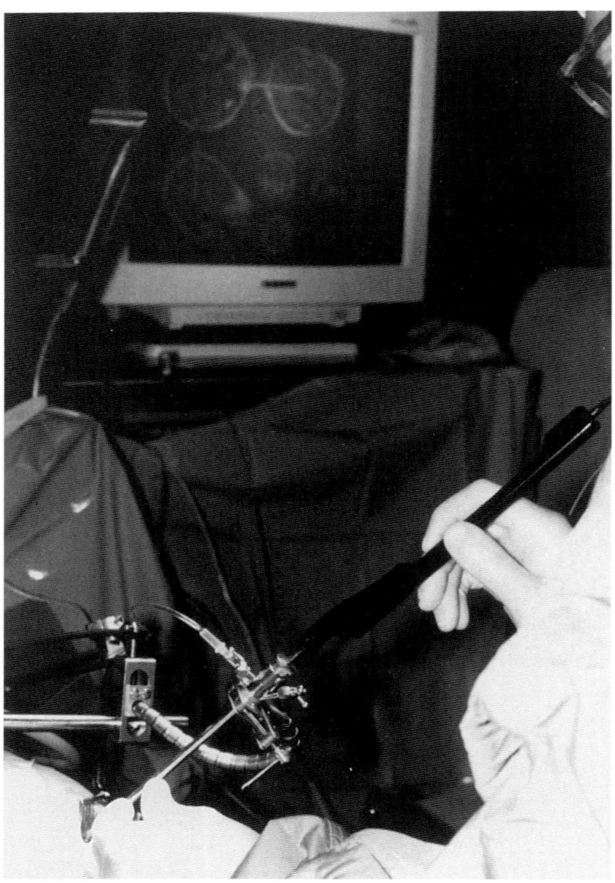

Figure 13-1. The CANE system. The sonic wand (in black) is attached to the obturator of the endoscope sheath.

for this longer configuration. This link allowed the use of the Viewpoint navigator in trajectory planning to ventricles or other targets.

The localizing wand is also coupled to the endoscope itself; when the obturator is removed and the endoscope placed into the rigid working channel, image guidance can proceed during the procedure. This link used a custom-manufactured 2-inch adapter that screws into the end of the wand system (as did the obturator) and has a cylindric proximal end designed to fit the distal working port channel and to lock in that position (Fig. 13-2).

PREOPERATIVE PREPARATION

Use of the CANE system was considered for any patient in whom the Gaab rigid endoscope would ordinarily be indicated. The guidance system is used when additional orientation and navigation are desirable.

Imaging

Before imaging, six to eight fiducials were glued to the scalp in standardized positions with underlying scalp tattoos. Fiducials consisted of staples or plastic spheres for CT or MRI, respectively. Images were performed 1 to 3 days before the operation and data from volumetric CT or MRI were collected and loaded into a portable computer workstation by a magnetic tape network such as Ethernet. The imaging studies were performed with the patient in the same position selected for surgery in an attempt to reduce the effective range shift error.

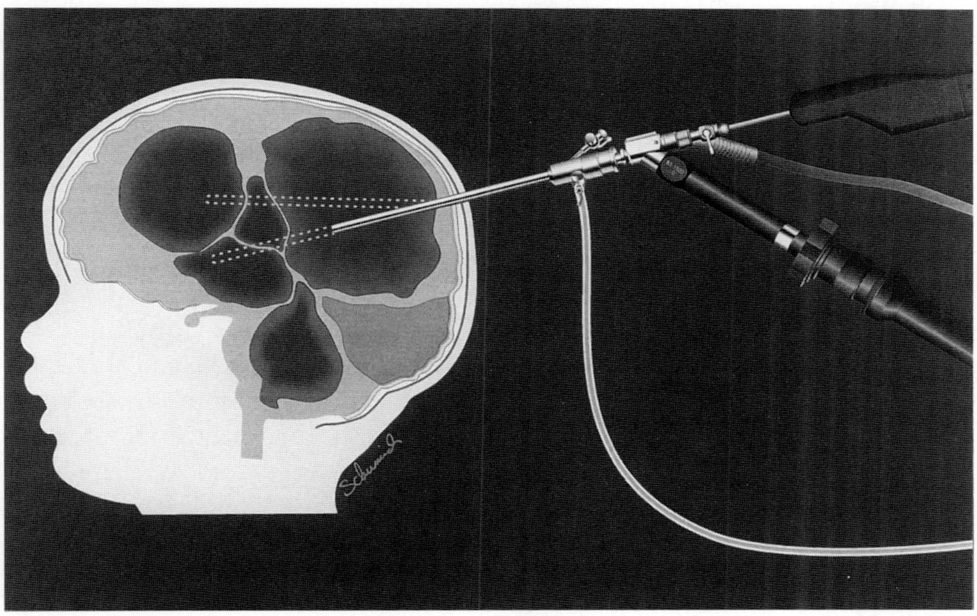

Figure 13-2. Use of the CANE system in a patient with multiloculated hydrocephalus.

Setup

This system involves a localized wand of known geometric proportions that emits ultrasonic pulses that are then detected by a detector array of microphones fixed to the operating room table near the surgical field (Fig. 13-3). The patient's head is in pin fixation. In the operating room the equipment is set up with the endoscopic and image-guidance video screen adjacent to each other, a comfortable viewing position for the endoscopic neurosurgeon. After head fixation the stereotactic fiducials are registered with a three-dimensional sonic digitizer adapted for operating room use.

TRAJECTORY PLANNING AND INTRAOPERATIVE GUIDANCE

The unmodified Viewpoint localizer wand is used to register patient data and to plan the optimal location of the burr hole site. Surgical preparation and draping are performed in a routine fashion for a burr hole in the chosen location. A sterile wand is connected to the Gaab neuroendoscope sheath and obturator, which is in turn placed into the Gaab working sheath and locked into place. This whole system is stabilized with a Greenberg retractor system (see Fig. 13-1).

For precise trajectory planning, the three-dimensional image data obtained may be presented in conventional orthogonal planes or oblique planes referenced to the axis of the endoscope. These oblique views are particularly useful when coupled to target and trajectory guidance software, allowing the endoscope to be directed along preplanned trajectories or to preselected targets. In addition, the oblique views graphically demonstrate the anatomic structures that will be traversed by the scope and are along the 0% optical axis of the endoscope (Fig. 13-4). A foot pedal control is used to track the trajectory and progress of the tip of the obturator before and during insertion to the target point. After the insertion is complete, the obturator is removed, and in the case of ventricular access, egress of cerebrospinal fluid is often observed. The system is fixed in position with both the Greenberg clamps and by hand.

The working Gaab endoscope is then placed into the channel and secured. The localized wand fitted with the endoscope coupler is, in turn, secured to the distal end. At this point the view from the endoscope and the endoscope tip position can be simultaneously viewed on the adjacent video screens. Continuous irrigation with warmed lactated Ringer's solution is used to maintain a clear visual field and to prevent collapse of the operative fluid space. Use of the wand localizer does not interfere with endoscopic visualization during the procedure, and the system may be activated with a foot switch to initiate localization at any time during the procedure. However, at the present time the wand localizer uses the distal working port of the endoscope and therefore must be removed when other instruments such as the biopsy forceps or coagulation devices are being used. After the endoscopic procedure is completed, the endoscope and sheath are removed and the burr hole closed in a routine fashion.

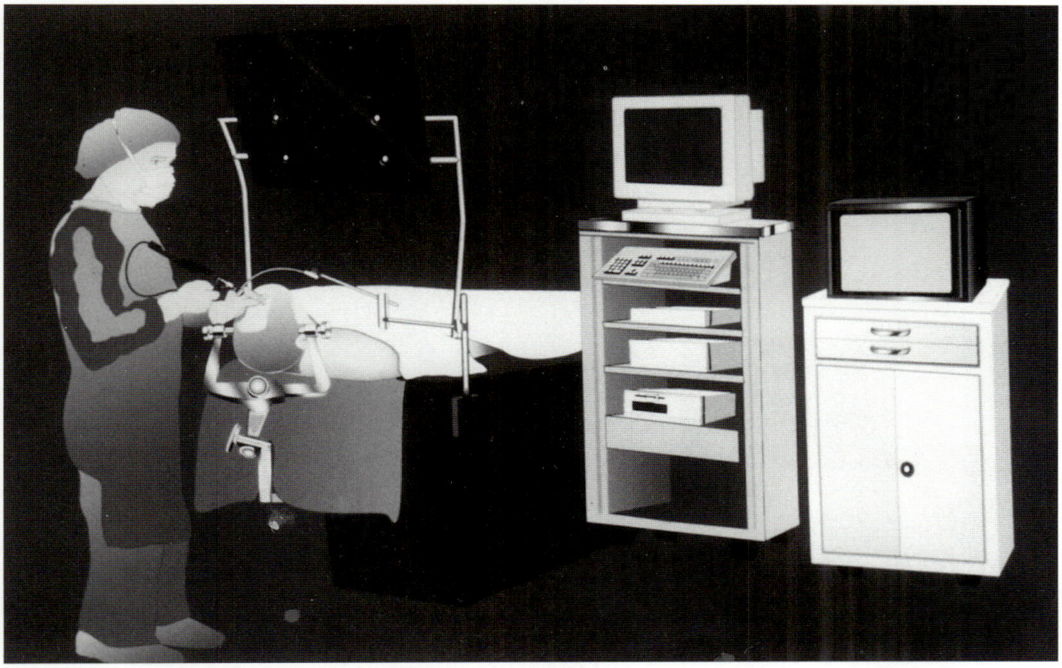

Figure 13-3. Intraoperative setup of the CANE system.

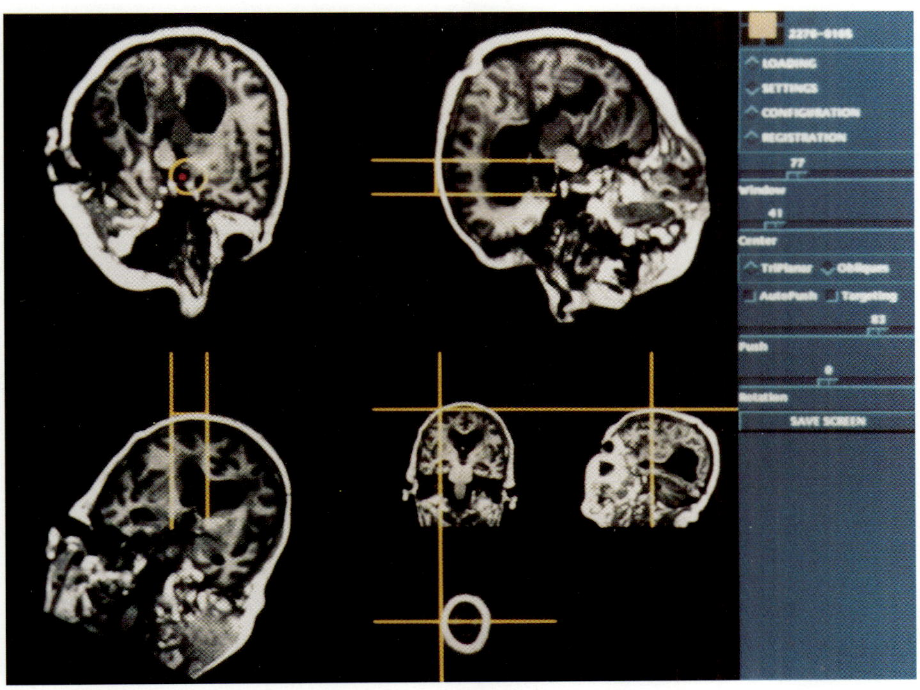

Figure 13-4. Transverse, sagittal, and coronal planes with two-dimensional and three-dimensional representations along the CANE trajectory during third ventriculostomy.

Table 13-1. Patient Population

Sex/Age (yr)	Diagnosis	Procedure
F/5	Multicompartmental hydrocephalus	Ventricular fenestration with shunting
F/1.5	Multicompartmental hydrocephalus	Ventricular fenestration with shunting
M/1.2	Multicompartmental hydrocephalus	Ventricular fenestration with shunting
M/21	Germinoma lining ventricular system	Endoscopic biopsy
M/7	Pineal region teratoma	Third ventriculostomy
F/13	Tectal mass	Third ventriculostomy
F/38	Pineocytoma	Third ventriculostomy
M/25	Aqueductal stenosis	Third ventriculostomy/shunting
F/70	Aqueductal stenosis	Third ventriculostomy
F/45	Aqueductal stenosis	Third ventriculostomy
M/18	Aqueductal stenosis	Third ventriculostomy
M/21	Aqueductal stenosis	Shunting

SURGICAL TECHNIQUE AND CLINICAL EXPERIENCE

Use of the CANE system is illustrated in 12 cases: three patients with multiloculated hydrocephalus, eight patients with obstructive hydrocephalus, and one patient with hydrocephalus and a periventricular lesion (Table 13-1). All patients showed clinical improvement following surgery with the exception of a single patient who later required shunting after failure of a third ventriculostomy. No deaths and no morbidity were related to surgery.

Multicompartmental Hydrocephalus

In patients with multicompartmental hydrocephalus and a history of meningitis and intraventricular hemorrhage, clinical and radiographic findings were consistent with multiloculated progressive hydrocephalus.[29-32] Standard treatments for this condition include placement of multiple catheters that increase the morbidity and failure rate, blind multihole catheter placement in an attempt to drain several cysts with a single trajectory, or open craniotomy and loculation fenestration. Converting a multicystic ventricle into a unilocular cavity is usually beneficial in these patients since it greatly simplifies the drainage system.[33-35] Although this has been performed as an open procedure with success, the endoscope permits a less invasive operation.[13,32] Nonetheless, multicompartmental hydrocephalus can be one of the most challenging endoscopic procedures with the potential for disorientation, hemorrhage, missed cysts, and reclosure of fenestrations. The added guidance afforded by the CANE system should provide better orientation, avoid missed cysts, decrease dangerous endoscope movement, and facilitate the production of larger optimally placed fenestrations.

After a single burr hole is placed, the endoscope is passed into the superficial cyst and progressively inserted into each septum. The CANE system is used to plan the optimal trajectory, identify each cyst and septum, and help determine the optimal area of fenestration before performing the septostomy as well as trajectory and burr hole planning (see Fig. 13-2). If possible, trajectories are planned so that the endoscope will enter all of the compartments in a single pass with the least lateral movement. Fenestrations are made with a combination of unipolar coagulation and sharp and blunt dissection. A 1 to 2 cm diameter is preferred. Vascular and neuronal structures are identified with a combination of visual and image data.

Endoscopic inspection of the cysts as well as postoperative imaging are used to confirm the communication between the cavities after fenestration. Bilateral or other multiple trajectories are sometimes required for communication of all cavities. All fenestrations to date have required only simplified drainage systems, although a greater number of patient follow-up visits are necessary to determine the persistence of these fenestrations.

Obstructive Hydrocephalus

Percutaneous and endoscopic third ventriculostomies have been well described.[19,30,36-45] Currently this is the most common application of the neuroendoscope, but complication rates and long-term efficacy have not been documented. Initially patients with aqueductal stenosis or obstruction were the primary candidates for this procedure, but the success rate in other forms of hydrocephalus such as in patients with myelomeningocele are also being investigated. Ventricles must be large enough to accommodate the endoscope. Many groups, including our own, have performed the procedure successfully in patients with either small or slit ventricles after acute preoperative expansion. Although visual guidance is often adequate to perform the third ventriculostomy safely, in cases of abnormal anatomy such as occurs in patients with myelomeningocele who have an abnormal third ventricle floor and large mass intermedin, additional guidance is helpful. Even in patients with large ventricles the system can ensure a straight trajectory from the burr hole, through the foramen of Monroe, and to the appropriate site on the floor. It can also help avoid an unseen basilar artery or its branches on the other side.

Patients selected for treatment with the CANE system fulfilled standard criteria for third ventriculostomy candidates.[41,46,47] Preoperative planning permitted ideal trajectories that allowed a direct unobstructed entrance through the foramen of Monroe into the third ventricle (see Fig. 13-4). As has been previously described, an area anterior to the mammillary bodies and just caudal to the infundibular recess is selected for fenestration when this area is appropriately thinned.[41-43,46,48] By making the floor of the ventricle the target point and the foramen of Monroe the "entry site," we could compute the ideal entry location on the skull via computer extrapolation. After insertion under obturator wand guidance, the endoscope is introduced and localization confirmed visually and by computer image before fenestration. An opening is made bluntly with a closed forceps and widened with a Fogarty balloon catheter.

Since in most of these cases the anatomic landmarks of the floor of the third ventricle were clear, this final check is primarily used to test the accuracy of the guidance system in this region after ventricular entry and partial drainage. At least under these conditions tissue shift with respect to the floor of the third ventricle after ventricular access does not disrupt the system's accuracy.

Success was measured by clinical improvement and cine-MRI cerebrospinal

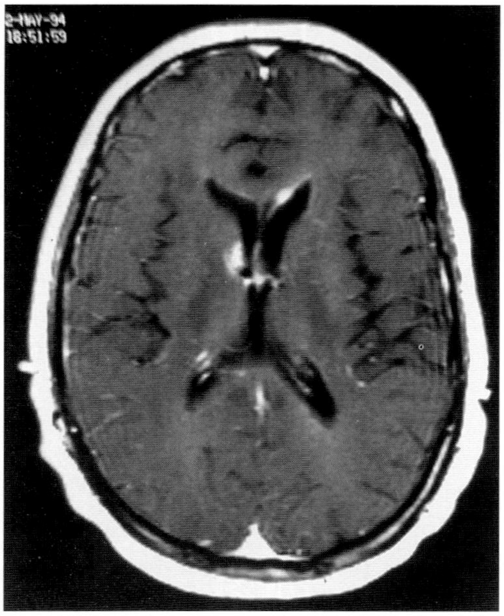

Figure 13-5. MR image of a patient with periventricular lesions.

fluid flow studies. Our overall success rate with third ventriculostomies has been 70%; the success rate with the endoscope improved to 86%. However, this rate difference reflects surgical experience, patient selection, and other instrumentation, not necessarily the use of the CANE system alone.

Tumor Biopsy

Often ventricular and periventricular masses can be biopsied using visual guidance alone to direct the endoscope. Endoscopic techniques for tumor biopsy or resection have been well described.[20,47,49-53] For example, in a patient who underwent a CANE-assisted tumor biopsy, conventional stereotactic techniques were not believed to be a viable alternative because of the size of the tumor nodules and their periventricular location (Fig. 13-5). This patient had negative cerebrospinal fluid cytologic findings and underwent a biopsy of the tumor nodule at the level of the right foramen of Monroe. The CANE system was useful in locating a subependymal nodule that was not readily apparent with the endoscope. The final pathologic report revealed a germinoma, and the patient underwent radiation therapy. Thus, in this case involving a small subependymal tumor, the CANE system was beneficial in guiding us to the tumor and allowing for a successful biopsy despite a normal overlying ependymal lining.

DISCUSSION

Neurosurgeons have long recognized the potential applicability of endoscopy.[2,54-56] However, lack of instrumentation and significantly high morbidity and mortality rates limited its clinical usefulness. The incidence of morbidity and mortality associated with neuroendoscopic procedures is now relatively small compared with the early 1900s.* With the technologic advances in optics, microsurgical instrumentation, and endoscopes and the heightened public interest in minimally invasive surgery because of reduced morbidity and hospital stay, neuroendoscopy has become increasingly more common.[47,58,60-63] Neuroendoscopy is undoubtedly a useful tool, but visualization alone can have its limitations.[34,47,64] Therefore we combined the technologies of computer-assisted, image-guided neurosurgery with minimally invasive neuroendoscopy to enhance the safety and accuracy of ventriculoscopy.

The efficacy of standard stereotactic guidance in the planning, localization, and resection of brain tumors has been well reported.[21,22,65-67] Frame stereotaxy combined with endoscopy has recently been performed to permit image-guided localization.[51,53,58,64,68] Many surgeons find frame stereotaxy to be logistically cumbersome and nonintuitive, and when the time required for frame application and imaging studies are considered, it can actually lengthen the overall procedure.[25-28] Frameless stereotactic techniques have become increasingly more common and are now being used for numerous neurosurgical procedures.[25-28,69-73] We have previously described our early experience with the CANE system and find it a useful adjunct in more complex cases.

The CANE system, as described here, is a readily available and useful system to improve the safety and efficacy of neuroendoscopy through stereotactic navigation. We found the system to be useful in all patients for preoperative planning of burr hole placement and localizing the ideal trajectory. Planning the ideal trajectory and continuous computer updates of the endoscope or obturator tip position allow us to change their position before actually penetrating structures and prevent unnecessary movement in the penetrated white matter and cortex, which should enhance safety.[58] Other solutions such as intraoperative ultrasound or MRI will also need to be explored further.

There are limitations that must be considered. Currently we are restricted to rigid endoscopes. For the tip to be accurately localized, rigid hardware is needed to calculate the relationship between the emitters and the tip of the endoscope. Although rigid head fixation is not usually a problem, difficulty could arise when performing CANE procedures on infants less than 1 year of age. The youngest patient we have operated on was 14 months, and we found that with adequate protection, rigid fixation of the head is safe in this age group. Another limitation that exists is that the wand coupling device uses the working endoscope port in the present system, so that the wand has to be removed for placement of instruments into this port. We are currently working on incorporating the emitters on the endoscope to solve this problem. Furthermore, as with any image-guided system, brain shifts are a possibility. Kelly[21] and Kelly et al.[22] have addressed issues that may minimize these distortions, including thin image slices and the smallest bony opening feasible. Finally, the wand/endoscope combination is somewhat lengthy and cumbersome. We are currently working on streamlining the system.

---

*See references 1, 38, 39, 44, 46, 54, 57-59.

SUMMARY

Ventriculoscopy in the face of abnormal anatomy can be difficult even with direct visualization. Although the CANE system may not always be necessary, correlation of the endoscope tip location with an intraoperative MR image should enhance the safety and efficacy of neuroendoscopy.

References

1. Cohen AR. The history of neuroendoscopy. In Manwaring KH, Crone KR, eds. Neuroendoscopy. New York: Mary Ann Liebert, 1992, pp 3-8.
2. Geiger M, Cohen AR. The history of neuroendoscopy. In Cohen AR, Haines SJ, eds. Minimally Invasive Techniques in Neurosurgery. Concepts in Neurosurgery, vol 7. Philadelphia: Williams & Wilkins, 1995, pp 1-5.
3. Fukushima T, Ishijima B, Hirakawa K, Nakamura N, Sano K. Ventriculofiberscope: A new technique for endoscopic diagnosis and operation [Technical note]. J Neurosurg 38:251-256, 1973.
4. Vries JK. Endoscopy as an adjunct to shunting for hydrocephalus. Surg Neurol 13:69-72, 1980.
5. Milhorat TH. Failure of choroid plexectomy as treatment for hydrocephalus. Surg Gynecol Obstet 139: 505-508, 1974.
6. Milhorat TH, Hammock MK, Chien T, Davis DA. Normal rate of cerebrospinal fluid formation five years after bilateral choroid plexectomy. Case report. J Neurosurg 44:735-739, 1976.
7. Oka K, Ohshiro S, Go Y, Kin Y, Tomonaga M, Mannoji H, Daikuzono N. New surgical therapy for hydrocephalus—Percutaneous flexible endoneurosurgical choroid plexus coagulation. In Matsumoto S, Tamaki N, eds. Hydrocephalus—Pathogenesis and Treatment. Tokyo: Springer-Verlag, 1991, pp 692-698.
8. Kleinhaus S, Germann R, Sheran M, Shapiro K, Boley SJ. A role for endoscopy in the placement of ventriculoperitoneal shunts. Surg Neurol 18:179-180, 1982.
9. Bucholz RD, Pittman T. Endoscopic coagulation of the choroid plexus using the Nd:YAG laser: Initial experience and proposal for management. Neurosurgery 28:421-426, 1991.
10. Griffith HB. Endoscopic choroid plexus coagulation and cerebrospinal fluid perfusion in the treatment of infantile hydrocephalus. In Manwaring KH, Crone KR, eds. Neuroendoscopy. New York: Mary Ann Liebert, 1992, pp 91-96.
11. Griffith HB, Jamjoom AB. The treatment of childhood hydrocephalus by choroid plexus coagulation and artificial cerebrospinal fluid perfusion. Br J Neurosurg 4:95-100, 1990.
12. Pittman T, Bucholz RD. Endoscopic choroid plexectomy. In Manwaring KH, Crone KR, eds. Neuroendoscopy. New York: Mary Ann Liebert, 1992, pp 97-102.
13. Powers SK. Fenestration of intraventricular cysts using a flexible, steerable endoscope. Acta Neurochir Suppl 54:42-46, 1992.
14. Scarff JE. The treatment of nonobstructive (communicating) hydrocephalus by endoscopic cauterization of the choroid plexuses. J Neurosurg 33:1-18, 1970.
15. Hellwig D, Bauer BL, Dauch WA. Stereotactic endoscopic treatment of brain abscesses. In Cohen AR, Haines SJ, eds. Minimally Invasive Techniques in Neurosurgery. Concepts in Neurosurgery, vol 7. Philadelphia: Williams & Wilkins, 1995, pp 66-72.
16. Auer LM. Endoscopic evacuation of intracerebral hemorrhage. High-tech surgical treatment—A new approach to the problem? Acta Neurochir 74:124-128, 1985.
17. Huewel N, Perneczky A, Urban V, Fries G. Neuroendoscopic technique for the operative treatment of septated syringomyelia. Acta Neurochir Suppl 54:59-62, 1992.
18. Kao MC. Video endoscopic sympathectomy using a fiberoptic CO_2 laser to treat palmar hyperhidrosis. Neurosurgery 30:131-135, 1992.
19. Manwaring KH. Endoscopic ventricular fenestration. In Manwaring KH, Crone KR, eds. Neuroendoscopy. New York: Mary Ann Liebert, 1992, pp 79-90.
20. Otsuki T, Jokura H, Yoshimoto T. Stereotactic guiding tube for open-system endoscopy: A new approach for the stereotactic endoscopic resection of intra-axial brain tumors. Neurosurgery 27:326-330, 1990.
21. Kelly PJ. Volumetric stereotactic surgical resection of intra-axial brain mass lesions. Mayo Clin Proc 63: 1186-1198, 1988.
22. Kelly PJ, Kall BA, Goerss SJ. Results of computed tomography-based computer-assisted stereotactic resection of metastatic intracranial tumors. Neurosurgery 22:7-17, 1988.
23. Zamorano L, Chavantes C, Jiang Z, Kadi AM. Stereotactic neuroendoscopy. In Cohen AR, Haines SJ, eds. Minimally Invasive Techniques in Neurosurgery. Concepts in Neurosurgery, vol 7. Philadelphia: Williams & Wilkins, 1995, pp 49-65.

24. Rhoten RL, Luciano MG, Barnett GH. Computer-assisted endoscopy for neurosurgical procedures [Technical note]. Neurosurgery 40:632-638, 1997.
25. Barnett GH, Kormos DW, Steiner CP. Frameless stereotaxy using a sonic digitizing wand: Development and adaptation to the Picker ViStar Medical Imaging System. In Maciunas RJ, ed. Interactive Image-Guided Neurosurgery. Park Ridge, Ill.: American Association of Neurological Surgeons, 1993, pp 113-119.
26. Barnett GH, Kormos DW, Steiner CP, Weisenberger J. Intraoperative localization using an armless, frameless stereotactic wand [Technical note]. J Neurosurg 78:510-514, 1993.
27. Barnett GH, Kormos DW, Steiner CP, Weisenberger J. Use of a frameless, armless stereotactic wand for brain tumor localization with two-dimensional and three-dimensional neuroimaging. Neurosurgery 33: 674-678, 1993.
28. Barnett GH, Steiner CP. Image-guided neurosurgery using sonic digitizers. In Gildenberg PL, Tasker RR, eds. Textbook of Stereotactic and Functional Neurosurgery. New York: McGraw-Hill, 1995.
29. Albanese V, Tomasello F, Sampaolo S. Multiloculated hydrocephalus in infants. Neurosurgery 8:641-646, 1981.
30. Albanese V, Tomasello F, Sampaolo S, Picozzi P. Neuroradiological findings in multiloculated hydrocephalus. Acta Neurochir 60:297-311, 1982.
31. Schultz P, Leeds NE. Intraventricular septations complicating neonatal meningitis. J Neurosurg 38:620-626, 1973.
32. Lewis A, Crone K. Endoscopic management of loculated hydrocephalus. In Cohen AR, Haines SJ, eds. Minimally Invasive Techniques in Neurosurgery. Concepts in Neurosurgery, vol 7. Philadelphia: Williams & Wilkins, 1995, pp 25-32.
33. Heilman CB, Cohen AR. Endoscopic ventricular fenestration using a "saline torch." J Neurosurg 74: 224-229, 1991.
34. Manwaring KH. Endoscope-guided placement of the ventriculoperitoneal shunt. In Manwaring KH, Crone KR, eds. Neuroendoscopy. New York: Mary Ann Liebert, 1992, pp 29-40.
35. Rhoton AL Jr, Gomez MR. Conversion of multilocular hydrocephalus to unilocular. Case report. J Neurosurg 36:348-350, 1972.
36. Cohen AR, Shucart WA. Ventriculoscopic management of colloid cysts of the third ventricle. In Manwaring KH, Crone KR, eds. Neuroendoscopy. New York: Mary Ann Liebert, 1992, pp 109-117.
37. Dalrymple SJ, Kelly PJ. Computer-assisted stereotactic third ventriculostomy in the management of noncommunicating hydrocephalus. Stereotact Funct Neurosurg 59:105-110, 1992.
38. Drake JM. Ventriculostomy for treatment of hydrocephalus. Neurosurg Clin N Am 4:657-666, 1993.
39. Jones RF, Teo C, Stening WA, Kwok BCT. Neuroendoscopic third ventriculostomy. In Manwaring KH, Crone KR, eds. Neuroendoscopy. New York: Mary Ann Liebert, 1992, pp 63-78.
40. Jones RF, Stening WA, Kwok BC, Sands TM. Third ventriculostomy for shunt infections in children. Neurosurgery 32:855-859, 1993.
41. Kelly PJ. Stereotactic third ventriculostomy in patients with nontumoral adolescent/adult onset aqueductal stenosis and symptomatic hydrocephalus. J Neurosurg 75:865-873, 1991.
42. Kelly PJ, Goerss S, Kall BA, Kispert DB. Computed tomography-based stereotactic third ventriculostomy [Technical note]. Neurosurgery 18:791-794, 1986.
43. Sainte-Rose C. Third ventriculostomy. In Manwaring KH, Crone KR, eds. Neuroendoscopy. New York: Mary Ann Liebert, 1992, pp 47-62.
44. Vries JK. An endoscopic technique for third ventriculostomy. Surg Neurol 9:165-168, 1978.
45. Jack CR Jr, Kelly PJ. Stereotactic third ventriculostomy: Assessment of patency with MR imaging. AJNR 10:515-522, 1989.
46. Jones RF, Stening WA, Brydon M. Endoscopic third ventriculostomy. Neurosurgery 26:86-91, 1990.
47. Walker ML, MacDonald J, Wright LC. The history of ventriculoscopy: Where do we go from here? Pediatr Neurosurg 18:218-223, 1992.
48. Cohen AR. Endoscopic laser third ventriculostomy. N Engl J Med 328:552, 1993.
49. Cohen AR. Ventriculoscopic surgery. Clin Neurosurg 41:546-562, 1994.
50. Fukushima T. Endoscopic biopsy of intraventricular tumors with the use of a ventriculofiberscope. Neurosurgery 2:110-113, 1978.
51. Hor F, Desgeorges M, Rosseau GL. Tumour resection by stereotactic laser endoscopy. Acta Neurochir Suppl 54:77-82, 1992.
52. Powell MP, Torrens MJ, Thomson JL, Horgan JG. Isodense colloid cysts of the third ventricle: A diagnostic and therapeutic problem resolved by ventriculoscopy. Neurosurgery 13:234-237, 1983.
53. Zamorano L, Chavantes C, Dujovny M, Malik G, Ausman J. Stereotactic endoscopic interventions in cystic and intraventricular brain lesions. Acta Neurochir Suppl 54:47-52, 1992.
54. Dandy WE. An operative procedure for hydrocephalus. Bull Johns Hopkins Hosp 33:189-190, 1922.

55. Mixter WJ. Ventriculoscopy and puncture of the floor of the third ventricle. Preliminary report of a case. Boston Med Surg J 188:277-278, 1923.
56. Putnam TJ. Treatment of hydrocephalus by endoscopic coagulation of the choroid plexus: Description of a new instrument and preliminary report of results. N Engl J Med 210:1373-1376, 1934.
57. Auer LM, Holzer P, Ascher PW, Heppner F. Endoscopic neurosurgery. Acta Neurochir 90:1-14, 1988.
58. Caemaert J, Abdullah J. Diagnostic and therapeutic stereotactic cerebral endoscopy. Acta Neurochir 124:11-13, 1993.
59. Pamir MN, Ozer AF, Siva A, Ozek MM, Kansu T. "Upside down" reversal of vision after third ventriculostomy. J Neuroophthalmol 10:271-272, 1990.
60. Hellwig D, Bauer BL. Minimally invasive neurosurgery by means of ultrathin endoscopes. Acta Neurochir Suppl 54:63-68, 1992.
61. Karakhan VB. Endofiberscopic intracranial stereotopography and endofiberscopic neurosurgery. Acta Neurochir Suppl 54:11-25, 1992.
62. Walker ML, Petronio J, Carey C. Ventriculoscopy. In Cheek W, American Society of Pediatric Neurosurgeons, Section of Pediatric Neurosurgery of the AANS, eds. Pediatric Neurosurgery: Surgery of the Developing Nervous System. Philadelphia: WB Saunders, 1994, pp 572-581.
63. Yamakawa K, Kondo T, Yoshioka M, Takakura K. Application of superfine fiberscope for endovasculoscopy, ventriculoscopy, and myeloscopy. Acta Neurochir Suppl 54:47-52, 1992.
64. Hellwig D, Bauer BL. Endoscopic procedures in stereotactic neurosurgery. Acta Neurochir Suppl 52:30-32, 1991.
65. Hassenbusch SJ, Anderson JS, Pillay PK. Brain tumor resection aided with markers placed using stereotaxis guided by magnetic resonance imaging and computed tomography. Neurosurgery 28:801-805, 1991.
66. Kelly PJ, Kall BA, Goerss S, Earnest F IV. Computer-assisted stereotaxic laser resection of intra-axial brain neoplasms. J Neurosurg 64:427-439, 1986.
67. Moore MR, Black PM, Ellenbogen R, Gall CM, Eldredge E. Stereotactic craniotomy: Methods and results using the Brown-Roberts-Wells stereotactic frame. Neurosurgery 25:572-577, 1989.
68. Goodman RR. Magnetic resonance imaging–directed stereotactic endoscopic third ventriculostomy. Neurosurgery 32:1043-1047, 1993.
69. Friets EM, Strohbehn JW, Hatch JF, Roberts DW. A frameless stereotaxic operating microscope for neurosurgery. IEEE Trans Biomed Eng 36:608-617, 1989.
70. Guthrie BL, Adler JR. Frameless stereotaxy: Computer interactive neurosurgery. Perspect Neurol Surg 2(1):1-19, 1991.
71. Roberts DW, Strohbehn JW, Friets EM, Kettenberger J, Hartov A. The stereotactic operating microscope: Accuracy refinement and clinical experience. Acta Neurochir Suppl 46:112-114, 1989.
72. Roberts DW, Strohbehn JW, Hatch JF, Murray W, Kettenberger H. A frameless stereotaxic integration of computerized tomographic imaging and the operating microscope. J Neurosurg 65:545-549, 1986.
73. Watanabe E, Watanabe T, Manaka S, Mayanagi Y, Takakura K. Three-dimensional digitizer (neuronavigator): New equipment for computed tomography-guided stereotaxic surgery. Surg Neurol 27:543-547, 1987.

14

Skull Base Neurosurgery

Troy D. Payner, M.D.

Although skull base approaches to intracranial lesions were developed before frameless stereotactic technology became available, these operations now serve as one of the most useful applications of this technology. Skull base procedures typically require deep exposures that result in limited peripheral visibility within and around the targeted lesion. An analogy can be drawn by comparing skull base surgery to reading a road map through a dime-sized hole. You may know which road you are on but are uncertain about which direction leads to your destination. Frameless surgical navigation provides a broad view of the map in the form of a CT or MRI slice with a marker that says, "You are here." Experienced skull base surgeons developed their skills without the benefit of this technology. Today the learning curve for residents and other neurosurgeons to successfully operate in the skull base region can be significantly shortened by its use. Surgical navigation can reduce the incidence of complications, increase the extent of resections, and shorten the duration of procedures.

The greatest value and versatility of surgical navigation in skull base surgery is that it provides guidance in planning the incision, determining the size of the craniotomy flap, and assessing the extent of bone resection at the skull base. Additionally, surgical navigation orients the surgeon intraoperatively by assessing the extent of the target lesion. Various pathologic targets, including bone lesions, tumors, and vascular anomalies, can be localized. Lesions within and attached to the bone of the skull base are ideal for surgical navigation because the bone remains fixed in relation to the fiducial landmarks used to calibrate the equipment. This relative fixation maintains the accuracy of surgical navigation systems (SNSs) throughout the operation and reduces the error related to brain shift from retraction, hyperventilation, cerebrospinal fluid drainage, or mannitol administration.

This chapter reviews the indications for and limitations of surgical navigation in skull base surgery. Its use for identifying landmarks, guiding approaches, localizing specific lesions, and estimating the extent of resection are reviewed for several types of skull base approaches. Case illustrations are presented from an analysis of our first 50 cases using this technology.

INDICATIONS FOR SURGICAL NAVIGATION

Placement of the Incision and Craniotomy

One of the fundamental functions of surgical navigation, not unique to skull base surgery, is the identification of underlying surface structures. The skin incision must be placed to allow access to the essential surface area of the skull for each approach. Surgical navigation eliminates insufficient exposure of the skull because of anatomic variations among patients. This same advantage applies to planning the craniotomy, thus avoiding injury to vital underlying structures while drilling. For example, the bone overlying the transverse sinus is intentionally traversed when performing combined middle and posterior fossa craniotomies. The bone covering the sigmoid sinus is then removed as part of the transpetrosal exposure. Advanced knowledge of the precise location of the sinuses can reduce the potential complications associated with their inadvertent injury or sacrifice. Burr holes can be placed to straddle the transverse sinus, enabling unroofing with a punch rather than a drill or separation of the sinus dura from the bone prior to drilling across it.[1] The surgeon can adequately expose both the middle and posterior fossa as necessary for each case and improve the safety of this exposure.

Approaches to the anterior skull base may require a bifrontal craniotomy with or without opening the frontal sinus. Since there are no reliable surface landmarks to identify the frontal sinus, surgical navigation provides the necessary intraoperative guidance to avoid unintentional opening of the frontal sinus, thus avoiding the potential for cerebrospinal fluid leak and infection. Additional operative time, which would have been necessary to reconstruct or cranialize the sinus had it been opened, is eliminated.

These two examples of the utility of surgical navigation in identifying superficial structures support its benefit in preventing potential complications and reducing the operative time. The availability of immediate localization of a surface landmark by radiographic images in three planes is an added assurance for experienced neurosurgeons. This same benefit is amplified for residents and less experienced neurosurgeons.

Identification of Skull Base Landmarks

A thorough knowledge of the bony anatomy of the skull is prerequisite, especially for approaches involving the petrous bone and for those to the cavernous sinus, clivus, and anterior foramen magnum. Skull base surgeons who are very knowledgeable about this anatomy, however, at times will experience uncertainty. For transpetrosal approaches, an SNS produces reliable images to localize the mastoid air cells, antrum, semicircular canals, petrous carotid artery, internal auditory canal, and petrous apex. It shortens the time needed to obtain adequate exposure by avoiding drill injury of vital bony landmarks and by reducing the amount of drilling necessary once the desired trajectory to the target lesion is provided by the SNS. Improved outcome should result, especially hearing preservation because the vital structures for hearing can be anticipated and visualized before actual exposure. Studies are under way to evaluate the effect of surgical navigation on hearing preservation.

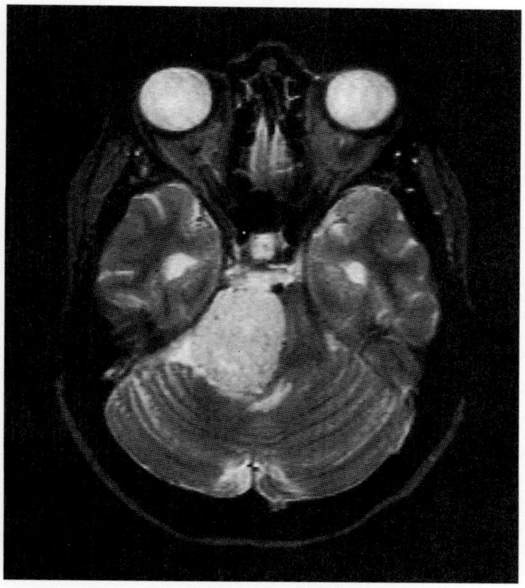

Figure 14-1. An axial MR image after contrast shows the close relationship of the basilar artery to the medial side of the tumor. Surgical navigation enables the surgeon to anticipate when this artery is near before it can be directly visualized.

For anterior approaches in a normal skull, structures easily identified by the SNS include the sphenoid and ethmoid sinuses, superior orbital fissure, optic foramen, anterior clinoid, foramen ovale, foramen spinosum, and foramen rotundum. However, aggressive meningiomas and malignant tumors involving the skull base often erode, invade, or distort the normal bony anatomy. In these cases even the most experienced surgeons will value surgical navigation for localizing vital structures such as the optic nerve and carotid artery.

Other useful bony landmarks include the transverse foramen at C1 and the occipital condyle for far lateral approaches to the anterior foramen magnum region. An SNS can also identify the midline, which is an essential orientation in transfacial approaches to the clivus and upper cervical spine. Cadaver studies show that surgical navigation can detail specific landmarks that can be localized in various skull base approaches.[2,3]

Localization of the Boundaries of the Lesion

Circumferential visualization of skull base tumors is usually difficult; therefore internal debulking of larger tumors is usually necessary. However, there is always uncertainty as to how much of the tumor remains and when the other side of the tumor is near. Surgical navigation makes this information immediately available, thus preventing injury to vital structures (e.g., brainstem) that result from debulking beyond the limits of the tumor. For example, when coagulating across the dural attachment of a clival meningioma, it is useful to know when the other side is near, especially if the basilar artery borders the medial side of the tumor (Fig. 14-1).

Because circumferential visualization of skull base tumors is usually difficult, surgical navigation can confirm the location of a certain border. For example, during resection of a large tumor at the petrous apex, it may appear that the most inferior limit of the tumor has been reached. However, surgical navigation may show that another lobule of tumor remains and that further dissection is necessary. Likewise, if the inferior extent of the tumor is reached but is not recognized, additional dissection may risk unnecessary neurologic injury. SNS guidance could prevent excessive retraction and exposure beyond the limits of the tumor.

Estimation of the Extent of Resection

Most skull base tumors are removed in sections; one portion may be debulked and then its capsule dissected from surrounding structures. Surgical navigation allows identification of these poles of the tumor so that the extent of resection can be assessed. Usually an inferior or superior pole of the tumor is resected and some normal anatomic structures identified. By informing the surgeon how large that pole of the tumor is, surgical navigation provides an estimate of the remaining lesion. Frequently a resected pole of a large skull base tumor is far smaller than anticipated. Some tumors such as epidermoids can have projections into crevices that may go unrecognized. Although surgical navigation can only demonstrate the preoperative status of the tumor, this usually is sufficient to identify projections that may not be recognized intraoperatively.

SNSs are especially valuable when subtotal resection is planned, for example, brainstem decompression in an elderly patient or hearing preservation in a patient with neurofibromatosis type 2. In these cases it is often difficult to estimate how much tumor has been removed. However, an SNS pinpoints the location within the tumor and allows an accurate assessment of the remaining lesion. This accuracy improves the likelihood of sufficient decompression of the tumor and preservation of vital surrounding structures while the tumor capsule may be intentionally left unresected.

TYPES OF LESIONS TARGETED

Surgical navigation has a variety of indications in neurosurgery, with most reported cases involving applications for tumors.[4-7] A review of our first 50 consecutive cases shows a variety of pathologies: 36 cases involved tumors, six were for shunt procedures, three were for vascular malformations or aneurysms, two were for odontoid resections in rheumatoid patients, and two were for decompression of the optic nerve after a traumatic skull fracture. One patient underwent biopsy of a small skull lesion that proved nondiagnostic (Table 14-1). Meningiomas were by far the most common lesion for which surgical navigation was used; however, other surgeons have used surgical navigation more commonly for the treatment of gliomas.[5]

This technology is useful for a variety of lesions, especially those at the skull base, because they are intimately associated with bony structures that remain in a fixed position. Most of these tumors are meningiomas; chordomas, acoustic and trigeminal neuromas, esthesioneuroblastomas, squamous cell carcinomas, and adenocystic carcinomas are also included. The strongest advantage in these lesions as opposed to tumors with a glial origin is their attachment to the skull base.

Table 14-1. Types of Lesions Among 50 Consecutive Cases Using Surgical Navigation

Lesion	Cases*
Meningioma	16
Astrocytoma	7
Shunt	6
Miscellaneous	5
Chordoma	4
Metastasis	3
Trigeminal neuroma	2
Acoustic neuroma	1
Aneurysm	1
Arteriovenous malformation	1
Cavernous malformation	1
Colloid cyst	1
Epidermoid	1

*One patient with a small skull lesion had a biopsy that was nondiagnostic.

There should be less error associated with the use of surgical navigation for lesions secured to bone than those within the brain substance that can "move" during resection as well as with the use of hyperventilation, diuretics, and cerebrospinal fluid drainage. The accuracy is reliant on preoperative calibration using fiducial markers. The spatial orientation of these markers is expected to reflect the position of targets fixed to bone better than brain. New techniques are being developed to recalibrate intraoperatively using ultrasound guidance or even CT or MRI. To my knowledge this has not been applied to skull base surgery.

TECHNICAL CONSIDERATIONS

Preoperative Selection of an Imaging Modality

Details of the procedure necessary for fiducial placement and preoperative imaging as well as image transfer to the computer are discussed elsewhere in this book. However, in skull base surgery, choosing the appropriate imaging modality (i.e., CT or MRI) is essential to obtain maximal benefit from the technology. During the initial phase of the operation in which the skull base is exposed, bony anatomy is most critical, and CT provides the most detailed images. However, when tumor resection is performed, MRI is generally more useful. Careful review of the preoperative CT and MR images is necessary to determine which will be most useful intraoperatively. If the surgeon is confident in performing the exposure without optimal bony detail provided by SNSs, then MR images can be used to guide the resection of the tumor. If the tumor can be adequately seen on CT images, then this modality can be sufficient for exposure and resection. The newer frameless systems allow changes in the windowing of the images during the operation without recalibration. This allows use of a bone window to guide the exposure and a soft tissue window to guide tumor resection. There is now technology available offering image fusion of CT and MR images, which can then be seen superimposed on each other, perhaps providing the ultimate detail for both exposure and resection of skull base lesions.

Positioning the Equipment

The use of SNSs in skull base surgery is certainly an asset; however, this cannot be at the expense of sterile technique and an unobstructed operative field. Two basic SNSs available today include a mechanical arm system and a light-emitting diode/camera system (as described in other chapters). In skull base surgery there are unique considerations for positioning the equipment in relation to the patient and to the other operating room equipment. A mechanical arm has the advantages of being used in the operative field without concern for obstructing the line-of-sight of other equipment and personnel in the room and without the need for a reference frame. Once the mechanical arm is positioned and calibrated at the start of the procedure, its base cannot be moved in relation to the head without recalibration. Therefore it is important that the arm with the probe attached can be brought into the field and moved in any direction necessary within the anticipated operative exposure. The arm must also be manipulated so that the probe reaches all of the fiducials used for calibration. Additionally, the arm must be flexible enough to be removed from the field, thus allowing unobstructed access to the operative field by the surgeon, assistant, and scrub personnel. The arm must not interfere with retraction devices (e.g., Budde halo) or with other equipment (e.g., operating microscope).

In my experience a mechanical arm is best mounted to the left of the patient's head except when a right-sided posterior fossa lesion is approached in the park bench position. The base of the arm should be as low as possible to allow the probe tip at the end of the arm access to the entire field (Fig. 14-2). This requirement usually results in the base of the arm being level to the midposition of the head. It is essential that the arm be tested to reach all desired trajectories before

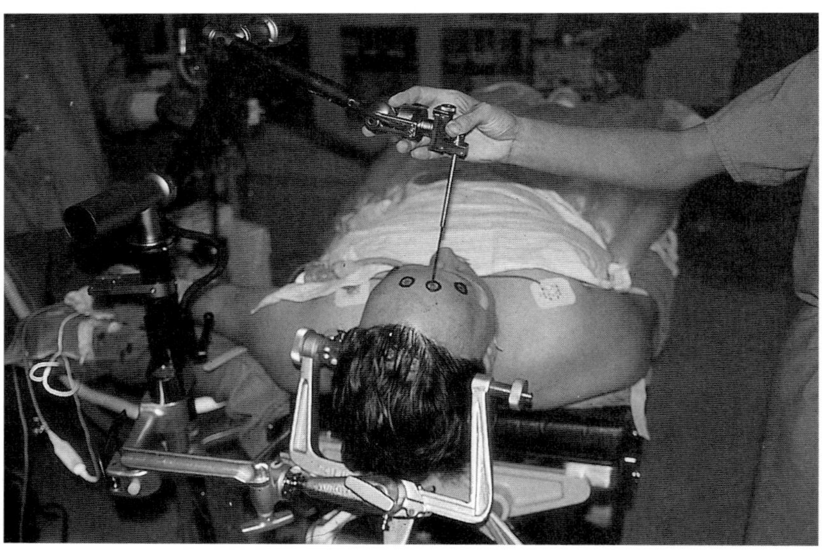

Figure 14-2. Positioning of the arm-based frameless stereotactic system in relation to the patient's head prior to calibration. Note the probe can be directed into the field when needed but can be completely removed when not in use so as to avoid interfering with access to the operative field by the surgeon, surgical assistant, scrub personnel, and other equipment.

committing to the final arm position and proceeding with the calibration. Because the operating microscope is usually brought in from the left, the computer monitor for viewing the SNS images is positioned to the right and slightly behind the surgeon. This configuration of the equipment neither obstructs the view nor interferes with the preservation of or access to the surgical field by the surgeon, scrub personnel, and surgical assistant.

Camera-based systems have several advantages over the mechanical arm. The probe can be completely removed from the operative field when not in use, eliminating interference with the surgeon or equipment. Unlike a mechanical arm, the probe is more freely manipulated within the field because it is not attached to a series of joints. These advantages of a camera-based system are offset by several limitations. All camera systems require an unobstructed line-of-sight to the probe and to a reference frame that must be mounted next to or around the patient's head. This limitation requires that operating personnel be positioned out of this line. The probe must be held in such a way that exposure of the diodes to the cameras is maintained. The retraction systems, microscope, sterile drapes, and surgeon cannot interfere with the reference frame, which must always remain in complete view of the cameras.

In my experience, similar to a mechanical arm, the reference frame for a camera system is best mounted to the left of the patient's head except for a right-sided posterior fossa lesion that is approached in the park bench position. During calibration, fiducial markers on the back of the head must allow simultaneous visualization of the probe and the reference frame. Thus the cameras are best positioned at the foot of the patient. As with an arm-based system, the computer monitor showing the radiographic images is positioned to the right and slightly behind the surgeon.

SKULL BASE APPROACHES

SNS guidance has been most useful for four basic skull base approaches. These include transpetrosal approaches to lesions of the middle fossa, posterior fossa, or both; transfacial approaches to lesions in the anterior midline involving the sella, clivus, and upper cervical spine; extradural resection of the anterior clinoid process for lesions along the proximal internal carotid artery, medial sphenoid wing, and cavernous sinus; and far lateral approaches to lesions of the anterior foramen magnum and lower clivus. Among the first 50 cases in our series, 22 were skull base lesions, 22 were nonskull base lesions, and six were for shunt procedures. The most common skull base approach using SNS guidance was transpetrosal. Case examples are provided for each of these approaches.

Transpetrosal approaches

Transpetrosal approaches accounted for 9 of the 22 skull base lesions in this series. Surgical navigation was useful for positioning the patient, planning the incision, placing burr holes for the craniotomy, providing landmarks for the otologist during petrosectomy, and localizing landmarks within and around the lesions during neurosurgical resection.

Case Illustration. A 47-year-old woman presented with facial numbness and balance difficulties. MR images showed a large enhancing mass in the region of Meckel's cave that extended to both the middle and posterior fossa; the brainstem was distorted and compressed (Fig. 14-3, *A* and *B*). A transpetrosal approach was selected and the SNS provided localization of the surface landmarks and bony anatomy necessary to obtain adequate exposure. Because of the large size of this tumor, it was removed in small pieces. Surgical navigation was used to estimate the extent of the resection and guide the direction of the tumor removal. Vital structures such as the brainstem were anticipated and visualized before they were encountered. The limits of the inferior pole of the tumor were assessed to ensure preservation of both the seventh and eighth cranial nerve complex at the internal auditory canal as well as the ninth through eleventh cranial nerve complex exiting the jugular foramen. The final portion of the tumor was within the posterior cavernous sinus and surgical navigation helped to ensure preservation of the carotid artery. This tumor proved to be a trigeminal neuroma. A postoperative MR image shows the extent of the tumor resection, and a CT scan shows the removal of bone achieved for this exposure while preserving the patient's hearing postoperatively (Fig. 14-3, *C* and *D*). Although our series is too small to obtain statistically significant data, surgical navigation likely improved the safety and speed of this transpetrosal approach during the exposure and resection of the tumor.

Transfacial Approaches

Anterior or transfacial approaches have been significantly improved by the use of surgical navigation. Historically, these approaches required intraoperative fluoroscopy, usually oriented in a lateral position. Identification of the midline is essential during the exposure but can be misleading if the usual landmarks (e.g., nasal septum or vomer) are eccentrically positioned. Although an anteroposterior radiographic view can be obtained to identify the midline, it may obstruct the working area, particularly if a microscope is used. Anteroposterior fluoroscopy may also increase the risk of contamination. Surgical navigation can eliminate the use of fluoroscopy completely by identifying the midline during the exposure and guiding the extent of resection in the axial, coronal, and sagittal planes. Transfacial approaches account for 5 of the 22 skull base cases in this series.

Case Illustration. A 49-year-old man presented with diplopia and underwent a transsphenoidal partial resection of a clival chordoma at another institution. Resection was followed by external beam radiation. Recurring diplopia was caused by a sixth nerve palsy. MR images showed a large clival mass (Fig. 14-4, *A* and *B*). Resection of this mass required a Le Fort I osteotomy using an exposure from the floor of the sella down to the foramen magnum. In this case surgical navigation was vital because of the distorted anatomy from the previous surgery, particularly the deviated septum and scarring. The safest way to perform this resection is to accurately identify the midline and monitor the depth and the extent (i.e., superior, inferior, and lateral) of the tumor. It is essential to avoid injury

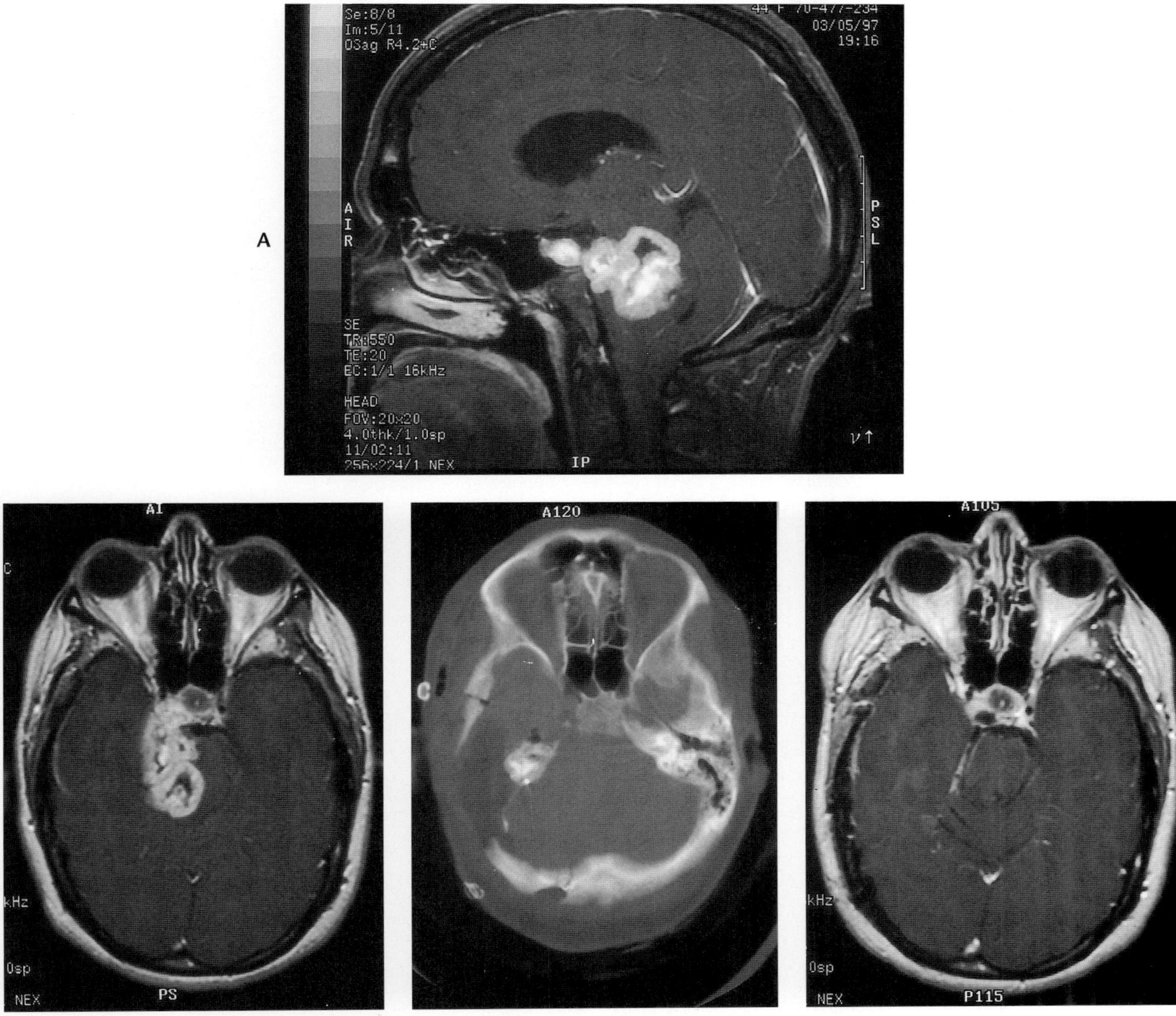

A

B C D

Figure 14-3. A 47-year-old woman presented with facial numbness and balance difficulties. **A,** A preoperative sagittal MRI scan shows a large enhancing mass extending from the posterior fossa to the middle fossa. **B,** An axial view shows severe distortion of the brainstem and anterior displacement of the right internal carotid artery. **C,** A postoperative CT shows how surgical navigation helped guide maximal bone resection with preservation of the semicircular canals and other structures necessary to preserve hearing. **D,** A postoperative MR image shows reexpansion of the brainstem after removal of the tumor, although a small portion of tumor may remain in the cavernous sinus abutting the carotid artery.

A

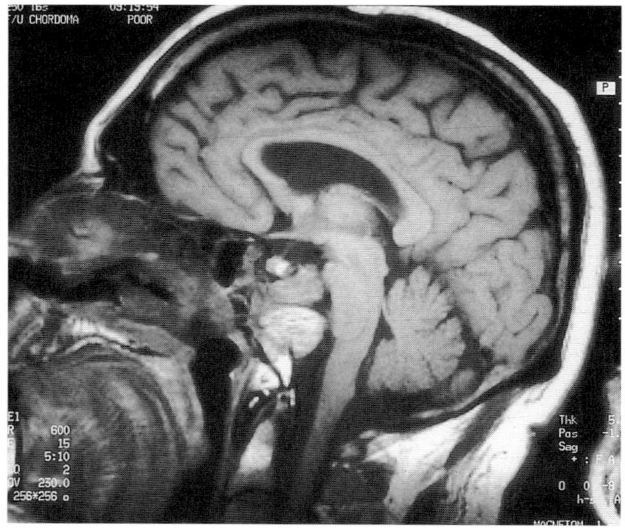

B

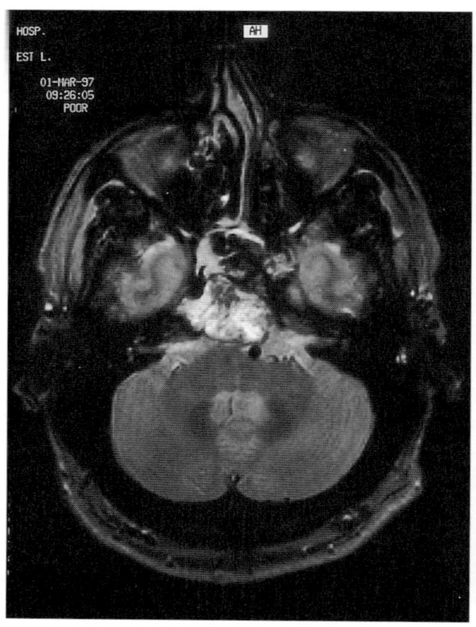

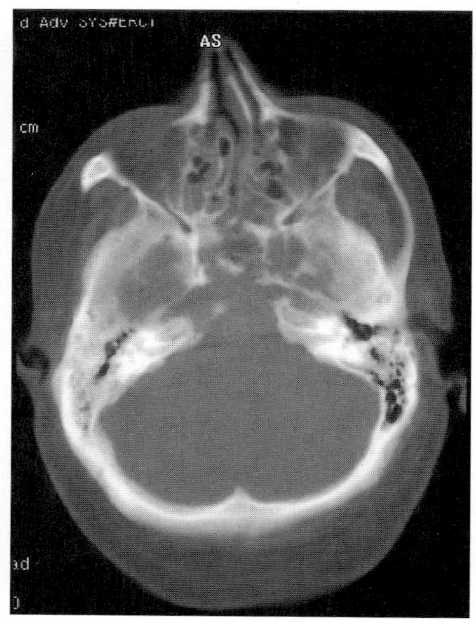

C

Figure 14-4. A 49-year-old man presented with recurrent diplopia 6 years after partial resection and radiation of a clival chordoma. **A,** A sagittal MR image shows a large clival mass extending from just below the sella to near the tip of the clivus. Some brainstem distortion is present. **B,** An axial MR image shows the relation of the tumor to both internal carotid arteries and the basilar artery. Deviation of the nasal septum and scarring from previous surgery are also evident. **C,** A postoperative CT image shows the bony margins of the tumor bed after resection.

to the petrous segment of the internal carotid arteries that border the tumor on both sides. Surgical navigation can provide this information quickly and accurately with minimal operative field interference. A postoperative CT shows the bony detail of the tumor bed after resection of the tumor (Fig. 14-4, C).

Extradural Resection of the Anterior Clinoid Process

Cavernous sinus and medial sphenoid wing approaches have been enhanced by the extradural bony resection of the anterior clinoid process as described by Dolenc.[8] This approach aids exposure of tumors, vascular anomalies, and bony lesions in this region and accounts for 4 of the 22 skull base cases in this series. Surgical navigation is especially useful when the normal anatomy is distorted.

Case Illustration. A 32-year-old man suffered a fracture of the orbital roof with bony compromise of the optic foramen in a motor vehicle accident. This injury was confirmed by a CT scan that showed the site of the fracture (Fig. 14-5). He had partial visual loss that further deteriorated despite high-dose steroid treatment. Frontotemporal craniotomy with extradural resection of the orbital roof was performed, the optic foramen was opened, and the anterior clinoid process was removed. Since the location of the fracture was identified by surgical navigation, the risk of further injury to the optic nerve was reduced. A more precise assessment of the extent of decompression could be performed intraoperatively by placing the probe circumferentially around the exposed nerve sheath to ensure that there was no additional compromise of the foramen. In addition, surgical navigation helped ensure that the ethmoid sinuses were not entered unintentionally and expose the patient to the risk of cerebrospinal fluid leak. An objective improvement in the patient's vision was noted on follow-up.

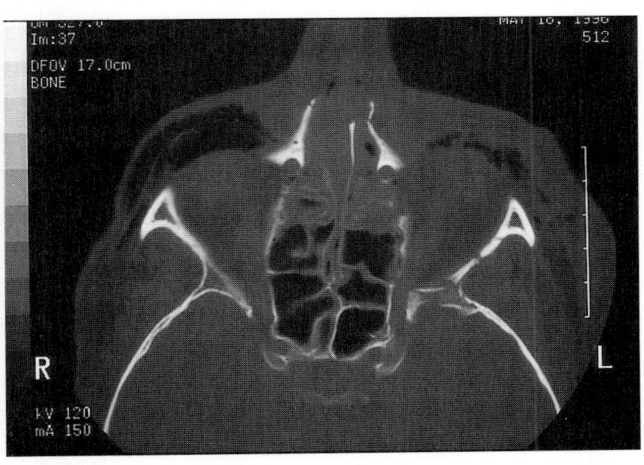

Figure 14-5. An axial CT image shows a fracture along the lateral optic canal that distorted the optic nerve and caused visual deterioration in a 32-year-old man involved in a motor vehicle accident. Surgical navigation was used to localize the fracture, identify the optic foramen extradermally, and prevent inadvertent entry into the ethmoid sinuses.

Far Lateral Approaches

In this series the far lateral skull base approach accounted for only 4 of the first 22 skull base cases. Perhaps the limited number of cases makes the use of surgical navigation even more valuable. Far lateral approaches are used for vascular lesions or tumors near the anterior foramen magnum up to the internal auditory canal. In each case the exposure was modified to meet the specific trajectory necessary to reach the target lesion.

Case Illustration. A 53-year-old man presented with headaches and ataxia that became progressively worse over a 3-month period. A cerebral aneurysm at the pontomedullary junction anteriorly was suspected based on an MR image and was confirmed by angiography (Fig. 14-6, *A*). A far lateral approach was taken from the left side. Surgical navigation was useful in identifying the vertebral artery, particularly at the transverse foramen of the atlas. However, the most useful advantage of this technology is during the drilling of the lateral mass of the atlas and the occipital condyle. Anatomic landmarks in the occipital condyle are lacking to determine the limit of resection until the hypoglossal canal is encountered; however, this may risk injury of the nerve. Surgical navigation can provide an immediate assessment of the trajectory toward the target lesion as the condyle is drilled. Once the desired trajectory is reached, additional drilling becomes unnecessary and the risk of complications is reduced. In this case surgical navigation was valuable during the approach but was not necessary during dissection and clipping of the aneurysm. Postoperative CT scans show the extent of the bone resection that enabled safe clipping of this aneurysm (Fig. 14-6, *B* and *C*).

COMPLICATIONS AND LIMITATIONS

In the 50 cases of this series there were no complications related to the use of surgical navigation. In two patients scheduled for skull base applications, the CT data could not be transferred to the computer and the use of surgical navigation was aborted; these two cases are excluded from the data. In all cases the maximal accepted error was less than 5 mm but was determined to be less than 3 mm in most. The accuracy of some of the SNSs are reported elsewhere in this book. However, in our series in no case did the degree of error result in injury to a patient. It is imperative for neurosurgeons to have a thorough knowledge of the anatomy encountered during skull base approaches and not to rely on surgical navigation as a substitute.

Although surgical navigation has been a tremendous asset to skull base surgeons, there are definite limitations. In skull base approaches there are frequently deep exposures that become quite small at their depth, much like a cone. Arm-based systems have a probe that must be directed into this exposure. However, the surgeon must be able to precisely visualize where the tip of the probe is to make use of the SNS computer image that pinpoints an anatomic landmark. Even at their tips, these probes may be several millimeters in diameter, reducing their precision. Because of this, the probe may identify the general vicinity but not an exact anatomic marker. In most of the camera systems the selection of a probe can be almost any instrument the surgeon desires. Instruments such as a dissector or bipolar forceps can be calibrated after attachment of the diodes to the instrument for the cameras to identify. These instruments may serve as a more accurate probe by defining a smaller target. However, in both the arm-based and camera systems the surgeon looks first at the operative field where the probe is touching an anatomic landmark and then looks to see that landmark displayed in three planes of view on the computer monitor. To do this, the surgeon must

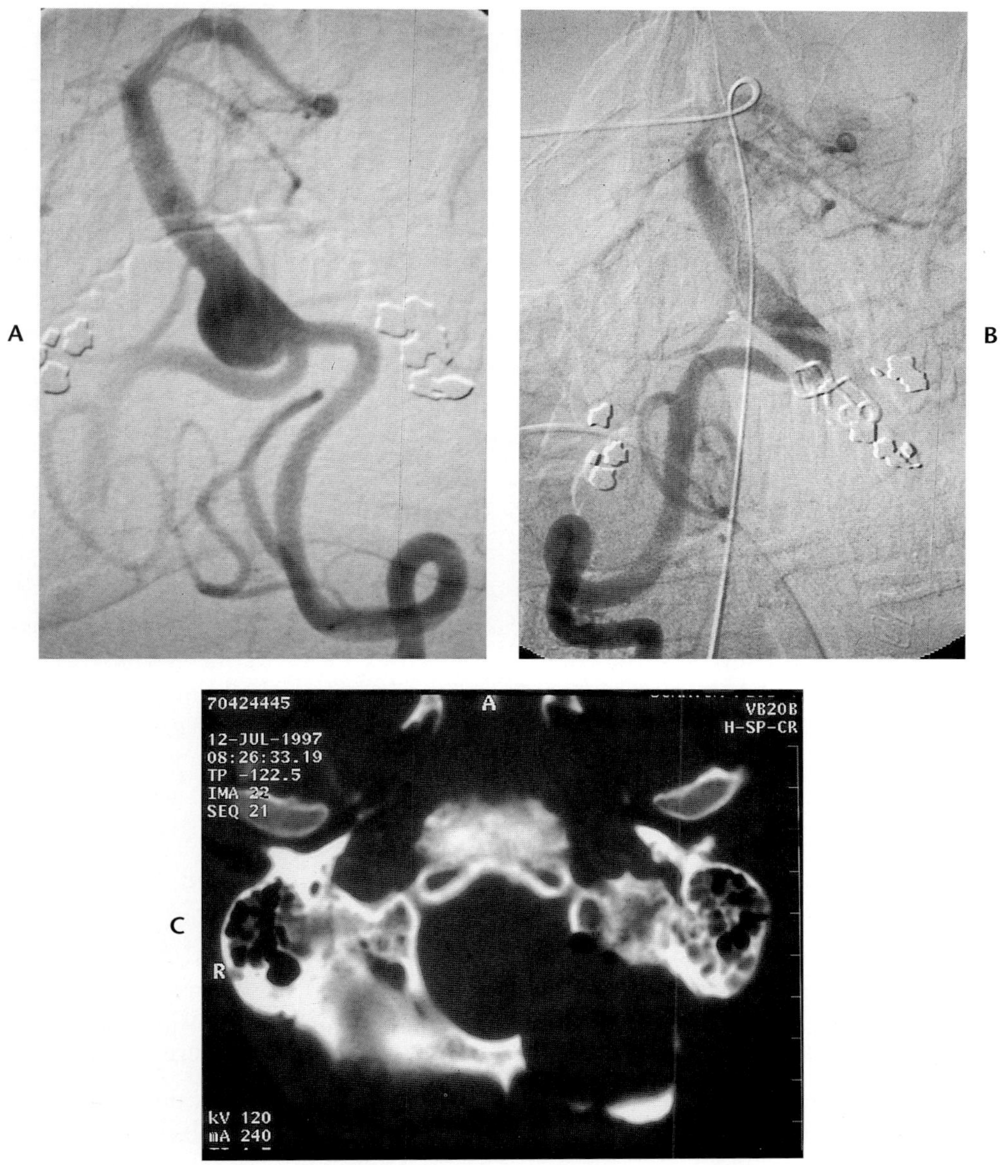

Figure 14-6. A 53-year-old man presented with headaches and ataxia. **A,** A preoperative left vertebral artery angiogram shows a large broad-necked aneurysm arising just beyond the vertebrobasilar junction. **B,** An intraoperative right vertebral artery angiogram confirms the patency of this artery through the fenestration of two clips and obliteration of the aneurysm. **C,** A postoperative CT scan shows the extent of the bone resection after a far lateral exposure using surgical navigation guidance.

stop operating to check his or her position on the SNS. Some systems have a heads-up display in the microscope field of view that shows the preselected outline of the target and the relation of the probe tip to that target. The microscope display does not show the three planes of view with the probe's selected landmark. Therefore it remains necessary for the surgeon to look away from the field to identify these landmarks. In my opinion this lessens the advantage of calibrating other instruments to use as probes because the surgeon cannot continue to operate while looking away from the field regardless of which instrument he chooses as a probe.

LEARNING CURVE

As with most new instrumentation, there is a learning curve associated with the use of surgical navigation in general and for skull base approaches in particular. This learning curve involves the proper placement of the fiducials to cover a sufficient area around the head while maintaining easy access to these fiducials during the calibration process. As discussed earlier in this chapter, experience also improves the surgeon's ability to position the equipment to avoid interference during the operation. Perhaps the greatest learning curve relates to knowing when the SNS is useful and when it is superfluous. Early in my experience I frequently used the probe to confirm exposed anatomy that I already recognized. The more familiar I have become with skull base approaches, the fewer interruptions have been needed during the operation to confirm the exposed anatomy. Surgical navigation is now most useful for invasive tumors and redo operations in which the anatomy may be distorted or when scarring obscures the normal structural landmarks. It is also more useful for large skull base tumors, particularly at the petrous apex and clivus with brainstem compression in which simultaneous circumferential exposure is limited. In these cases more frequent SNS localizations allow safer and faster resection of these tumors by preventing resection beyond the limits of the tumor into vital brain structures.

SUMMARY

Surgical navigation serves many purposes in neurosurgery and will become an essential component of modern practices. It has a special niche in skull base surgery. Although most of the skull base techniques were developed prior to the advent of this technology, parallel advances in both areas have enabled their integration. Future advancements will increase the accuracy and the resolution of SNSs, perhaps enabling individual cranial nerves and small arteries to be localized around tumors to further ensure their preservation. Accuracy may be enhanced by intraoperative imaging, which can provide updated data to reflect partial resection of tumors and account for brain shift related to hyperventilation, mannitol administration, and cerebrospinal fluid drainage. Advancements in computer technology may enable computer-assisted exposure and resection of tumors to supplement the localization features that already exist.

References

1. Tew JM, van Loveren HR. Atlas of Operative Microneurosurgery. Philadelphia: WB Saunders, 1994, pp 44-53.
2. Bumpous JM, Curtin HD, Prokopakis EP, Janecka IP. Applications of image-guided navigation in the middle cranial fossa: An anatomic study. Skull Base Surg 6:187-190, 1996.
3. Fernandez PM, Zamorano L, Nolte L, Jiang Z, Kadi AM, Diaz F. Interactive image guidance in skull base surgery using an opto-electronic device. Skull Base Surg 7:15-21, 1997.
4. Carrau RL, Curtin HD, Snyderman CH, Bumpous J, Stechison M. Practical applications of image-guided anterior craniofacial resection. Skull Base Surg 5:51-55, 1995.
5. Golfinos JG, Fitzpatrick BC, Smith LR, Spetzler RF. Clinical use of a frameless stereotactic arm: Results of 325 cases. J Neurosurg 83:197-205, 1995.
6. McDermott MW, Gutin PH. Image-guided surgery for skull base neoplasms using the ISG viewing wand: Anatomic and technical considerations. Neurosurg Clin N Am 7:285-295, 1995.
7. Robinson JR, Golfinos JG, Spetzler RF. Skull base tumors: A critical appraisal and clinical series employing image guidance. Neurosurg Clin N Am 7:297-311, 1996.
8. Dolenc VV. Anatomy and Surgery of the Cavernous Sinus. Vienna: Springer-Verlag, 1989, pp 233-256.

PART

III

Technologic Applications

15

Brain Biopsy and Related Procedures

Gene H. Barnett, M.D. • David W. Miller, M.D.

Brain biopsy was among the first clinical applications of image-guided frame stereotaxy[1-5] and remains the most common procedure performed with frame technology today. This relationship is ideal since biopsy requires targeting and guidance to a point in space, at times along a defined trajectory, and image-guided frame stereotaxy performs these functions using common imaging modalities with reasonable accuracy. Although readily applied to related procedures such as cyst or clot aspiration,[6-10] brachytherapy,[11,12] depth electrodes,[13,14] and functional procedures,[15-18] adaptation to craniotomy required elaborate computer systems or tedious procedures to achieve more than point stereotaxy guidance.[19-26]

The development of surgical navigation systems (SNSs) has been a major advancement in many areas because of its more intuitive nature, simplified logistics, and interactivity.[27-35] Although SNSs are well suited to providing localization and orientation information, only recently have robust means of target and trajectory guidance suitable for brain biopsy been devised (see Chapter 3). Our initial experience with SNS-guided brain biopsy is presented.

We reviewed all cases of brain biopsies and similar procedures performed from June 1994 through September 1997 at The Cleveland Clinic Foundation in which a frameless SNS alone was used to provide blind guidance. Procedures in which similar guidance was used for the purpose of biopsy through an open craniotomy were excluded. Data were recorded prospectively in a database and supplemented with retrospective material as required.

HARDWARE

We set out to devise a method of brain biopsy that would be potentially adaptable to most common SNSs, uses readily available components, allows for a wide variety of biopsy instruments without the need for modification of each device, and provides a rigid platform to support the probe throughout the procedure. Instrument support was provided by an extra-large Greenberg instrument holder system to which a stereotactic guide block capable of holding a wide variety of stereotactic instruments is attached (Fig. 15-1). This multiarticulated arm allows for facile orientation of the localizing wand, yet when tightened, provides

A

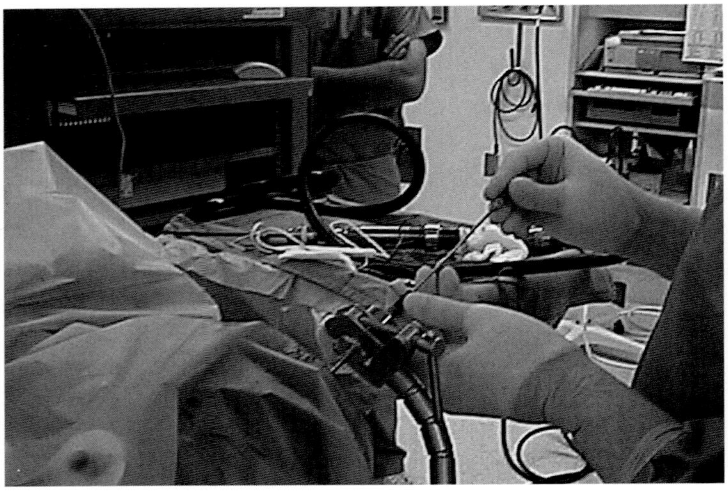

B

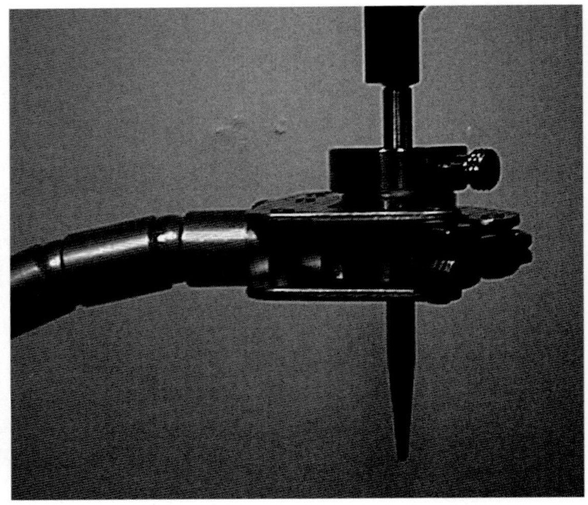

Figure 15-1. A, Extra-large Greenberg instrument holder provides support and maintains alignment throughout biopsy process. **B,** Stereotactic guide block capable of holding drills and reducing tube is held in jaws of Greenberg device.

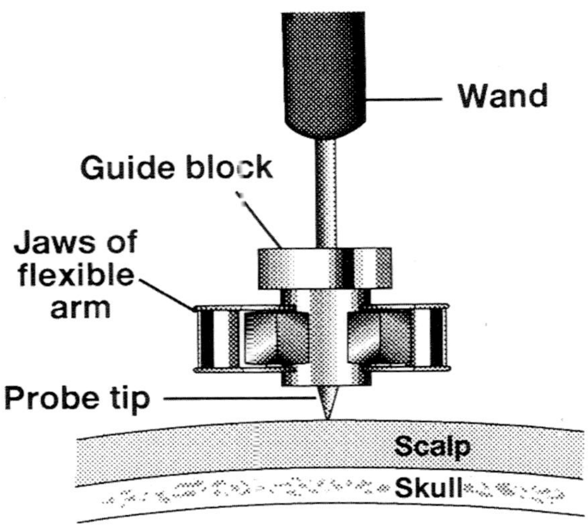

Figure 15-2. Tip of SNS localizing wand is designed so that it fits snugly in guide block and has a tapered tip that can engage in the twist drill hole.

rigid fixation that withstands even the stresses applied during drilling through the skull.

The localizing tip of a standard SNS wand was replaced with one specially designed for biopsy (Fig. 15-2). Its diameter allows a snug fit within the guide block, and its tapered, blunt tip allows it to be safely engaged into twist drill or burr holes. Although the computer could be given the actual length of this tip when computing target depth information, we have found that using a virtual probe length of zero or 100 mm is more convenient for calculation purposes.

The SNS used in this series of patients initially had a sonic digitizer[28,29]; this has subsequently been replaced with a light-emitting diode (LED) system tracked by dual charge-coupled device two-dimensional cameras. The system was capable of target and trajectory guidance as presented in Chapter 3.

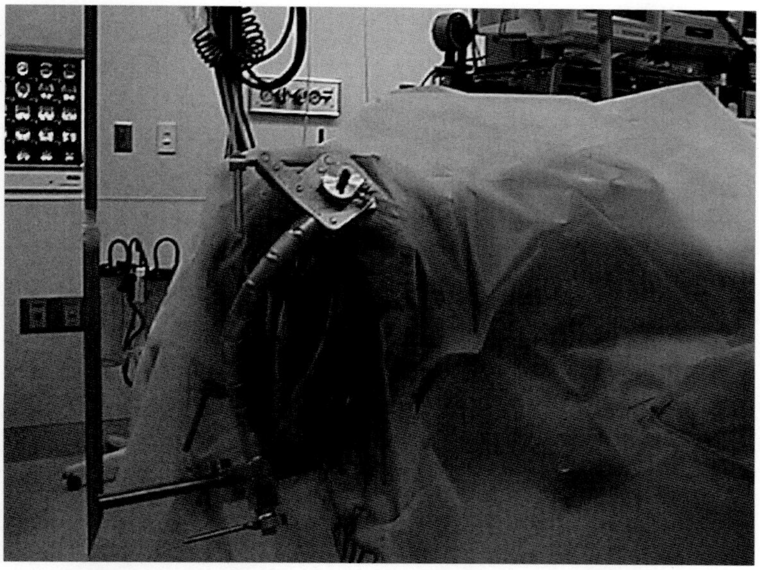

Figure 15-3. A sterile eye drape covers the operative field. The sterile Greenberg apparatus is then clamped over the drape to the underlying Mayfield three-point device.

PREOPERATIVE PREPARATION

Imaging, Registration, and Patient Setup

Multiple scalp fiducials are placed to allow flexibility of head positioning and use of best-fit algorithms that may increase accuracy over simple three-point transformations. Volumetric CT or MRI data sets are acquired resulting in 1.25 × 1.25 × 3 mm and 1.25 × 1.25 × 2 mm voxel sizes, respectively, that are interpolated to 1.25 mm cubes. Target and, optionally, entry points are identified on triplanar (coronal, sagittal, and transverse) images and stored.

At surgery the patient's head is immobilized, typically using a three-point fixation device. A tracking body secured to the fixation device detects head movement when using the LED digitizer. The fiducial sites are then touched with a wand and the necessary fitting and transformations performed transparently by the SNS. When a satisfactory registration has been obtained, the wand is manually rotated and translated so that the bore of the guide block becomes colinear with the target and, if selected, the entry point. The scalp is then marked, and the patient's head shaved and prepared with antiseptic solutions. A semitransparent eye drape is placed and the sterile Greenberg mounting hardware attached to the fixation device, leaving a completely sterile field (Fig. 15-3).

SURGICAL TECHNIQUE

The Greenberg arm is positioned over the previously marked entry point and the wand biopsy tip inserted into the bore of the guide block. This assembly is maneuvered as previously described until the bore of the guide block is colinear with the target and entry point. The arm is then tightened and the wand trajectory again confirmed and corrected if necessary (Fig. 15-4).

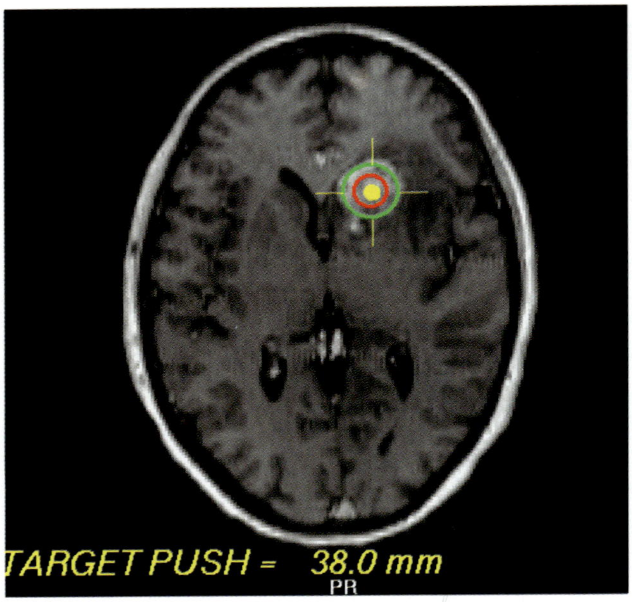

Figure 15-4. Concentric circles of target guidance system denote that surgical trajectory is "on target" and depth is presented by which position of biopsy instruments may be calculated.

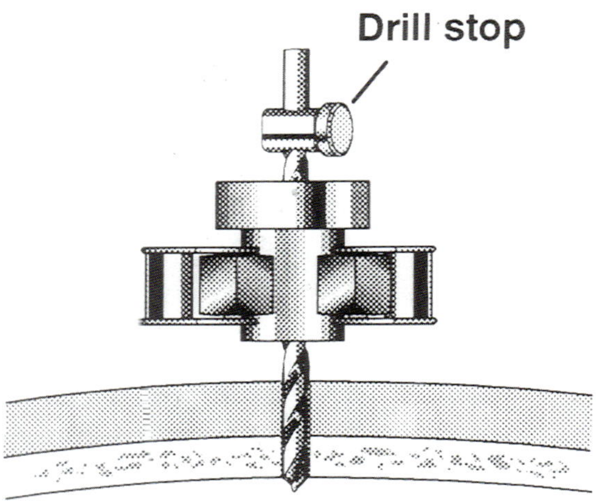

Figure 15-5. Twist drill hole (4.5 mm) is fashioned along surgical trajectory.

Typically, a twist drill hole is fashioned using the appropriate hardware secured in the guide block (Fig. 15-5). Care should be taken not to apply rotational or horizontal forces to the drill that could move the guide block off trajectory. The wand is replaced in the guide block and its tip engaged in the bony opening. Proper orientation is confirmed, or if reorientation is required, the engaged tip ensures that the probe will pass through the hole (Fig. 15-6) en route to the target (the trajectory may need to be compromised, however). The distance between the guide block and the shank of the wand (wand offset) is measured.

The depth presented by the SNS (SNS depth) is that from the target to the shank of the probe less the virtual probe length (VPL). The wand is removed, the

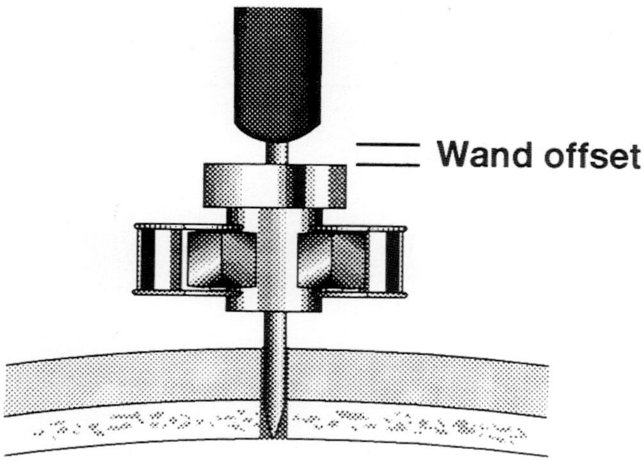

Figure 15-6. Tip of wand is engaged in twist drill hole, and any realignment with the target is performed as necessary. This step ensures the instrument will pass freely through the hole.

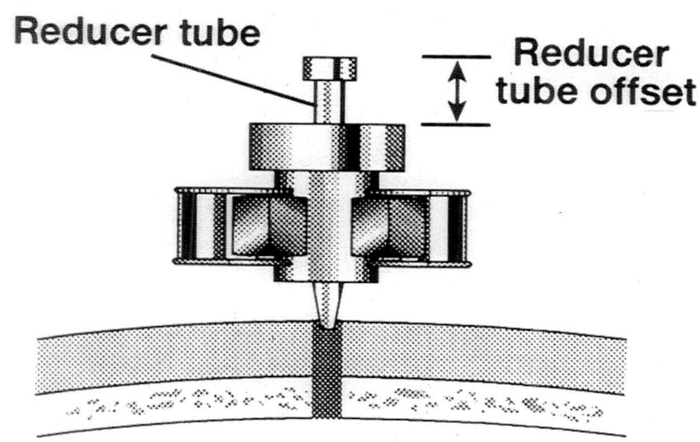

Figure 15-7. The required depth for the instrument to reach the target is the SNS depth + RT offset − wand offset.

dura perforated, and the appropriate reducing tube for the biopsy instrument (or catheter, etc.) placed in the guide block. The offset depth of the end of the reducing tube (RT offset) to the guide block is measured. The final depth to which the probe should be set (Fig. 15-7) is then determined by the formula:

$$\text{Final depth} = \text{SNS depth} + \text{VPL} + \text{RT offset} - \text{Wand offset}$$

When VPL = 0,

$$\text{Final depth} = \text{SNS depth} + \text{RT offset} - \text{Wand offset}$$

Ventricular catheters, brachytherapy catheters, depth recording electrodes, endoscopes,[36] and similar devices are also placed in this manner.

RESULTS

A total of 200 patients underwent 220 biopsies or related procedures in 207 surgical sessions using this SNS (Table 15-1). The most common procedure was brain biopsy (172 cases) followed by cyst aspiration with or without placement of an Ommaya reservoir (21 cases). The average age of patients was 55 years (range 1 to 90 years, median 58 years). The procedures were performed by seven sur-

Table 15-1. Percutaneous Procedures Performed Using the SNS

Procedure	Alone	Combined	Total
Third ventriculostomy	1	1	2
Abscess drainage	2		2
Biopsy	156	16	172
Brachytherapy	3	7	10
Cingulotomy	4		4
Cyst aspiration	2	4	6
Endoscopy	2	1	3
Depth electrode placement	2		2
Ommaya reservoir	15		15
Thrombolysis	4		4
	191	29	220

Table 15-2. Number of Cases Per Surgeon

Surgeon	Cases
A	125
B	4
C	4
D	3
E	1
F	19
G	51
	207

geons (Table 15-2) with individual contributions ranging from 1 to 125 operations.

Lesion locations are listed in Table 15-3. Most procedures involved the frontal or parietal lobes, and procedures were divided more or less equally between both sides. Guidance imaging consisted of CT in 101 cases with MRI in the remainder. Lesion dimensions were available in 153 cases. Maximum lesion diameter averaged 41.1 mm (median 39.7 mm, range 5.4 to 76.4 mm), whereas minimum lesion diameter averaged 28.6 mm (median 26.9 mm, range 5.4 to 63.8 mm). Measurements of depth from the scalp to the target were available in 30 cases and averaged 35.6 mm (median 33 mm, range 21 to 77 mm).

All but three biopsies (98%) were diagnostic (gliosis, astrocytosis, and lymphoma vs. vasculitis). Diagnoses are listed in Table 15-4. There were two (1.2%) infectious complications (abscess and meningitis) and two (1.2%) symptomatic hemorrhages in the biopsy series, resulting in sustained deficits in two patients. Both infections occurred before the described draping scheme was devised. In three cases catheter placements required revision when the catheter failed to puncture the target's wall in two cases and was placed beyond the cyst lumen in another case due to technical error. A subdural hematoma requiring craniotomy occurred after cingulotomy in one patient as a result of a thermal injury to a cortical artery. The patient made a full recovery, and the pain caused by cancer resolved. There were no surgically related deaths.

Table 15-3. Lesion or Target Locations

Location	Left	Midline	Right	Total
Basal ganglia	1		1	2
Brainstem		2		2
Cavum vergae		1		1
Cerebellopontine angle			1	1
Cerebellum	3	1	1	5
Cingulum	4		6	10
Corpus callosum		2		2
Falx		1		1
Frontal	37		48	85
Frontoparietal	2		3	5
Frontotemporal	1		1	2
Lateral ventricle	1			1
Midbrain	1			1
Occipital	5		7	12
Parasagittal	1		3	4
Paraventricular			1	1
Parietal	17		10	27
Parietal occipital			5	5
Septum pellucididum		1		1
Sphenoid wing	1		1	2
Suprasellar		4		4
Temporal	7		8	15
Temporal occipital	1			1
Temporal parietal	6		2	8
Thalamus	9		4	13
Third ventricle		2		2
	97	14	102	213

Table 15-4. Diagnoses Obtained by Biopsy in 172 Cases

Abscess	3
Amyloid	1
Anaplastic astrocytoma	22
Anaplastic oligodendroglioma	5
Astrocytosis	1
Blood clot	1
Brainstem glioma	1
Craniopharyngioma	1
Demyelination	7
Ependymoma	1
Glioblastoma	48
Gliosis	1
Infarct	4
Juvenile pilocytic astrocytoma	2
Low-grade astrocytoma	18
Low-grade oligodendroglioma	6
Lymphoma	11
Lymphoma vs. vasculitis	1
Malignant astrocytoma	1
Meningioma	8
Metastasis	18
Mixed glioma	3
Progressive multifocal leukodystrophy	1
Radiation necrosis	2
Schwannoma	1
Vasculitis	4
	172

DISCUSSION

The initial clinical applications of SNSs focused on their ability to provide near instantaneous localization and orientation information. Only with maturation of the technology did guidance to targets along predefined trajectories become possible. Such guidance has allowed facile, accurate use of SNS alone for blind guidance to intracranial targets.

The design philosophy of this technique of biopsy was to develop an approach that was portable to most SNSs with sufficient accuracy, flexibility, and target and trajectory guidance. Although the SNS provides guidance for these procedures, the Greenberg instrument holder provides stabilization and rigidly maintains the surgical trajectory. It is critical to use only the extra-large Greenberg because smaller versions of the instrument holder are not sufficiently unyielding. An important feature of the wand tip is that it will engage in the twist drill hole, allowing redirection should there be any skipping of the bit during drilling.

Of course, more complicated means of performing biopsy could be devised, such as placing emitters on the Greenberg arm, on the guide block, or on a microdrive or mating them to the instrument directly. Such an approach would allow the biopsy trajectory to be tracked in real time without the need for placing, removing, and replacing the wand in the guide block. We have developed two related instruments to streamline the biopsy process. The first is a guide block equipped with LEDs that allow direct tracking of the trajectory of the instruments it holds as well as provide a real-time reference of the distance from its top to the target plane (Fig. 15-8). Universal adapters allow real-time tracking of the biopsy instrument as it is passed to the target (Fig. 15-9). A combination of these devices will yield maximum guidance information throughout the biopsy procedure.

Regardless of the biopsy methodology, an interesting aspect of this project has been that scalp fiducials provide adequate accuracy for biopsy of targets a centimeter or more in minimum diameter despite their mobility. Careful attention to fiducial location and placement of skull fixation pins is required, however, to maintain freedom from error. Scalp fiducial placement for posterior fossa cases, however is more problematic because the overlying skin is more mobile than the scalp above the nuchal line. The number of posterior fossa biopsies or procedures in this series is small and likely reflects this situation. Skull-implantable fiducials are likely to improve the use of SNSs in the posterior fossa since they provide overall system accuracy that rivals or exceeds that attained by image-guided frame stereotaxy[37,38] and will be required for some functional procedures such as pallidotomy, thalamotomy, and deep brain stimulation.

The morbidity in this series of patients was actually lower than that in a previously reported frame stereotaxy series at this institution.[3] Two factors likely explain this difference. First, SNSs allow for visualization of the biopsy trajectory on three-dimensional data sets and in relationship to cortical and vascular anatomy. The frame systems used in our previous series either provided no trajectory information or did so only on a slice-by-slice basis. A second factor is probably related to the fact that the learning curve for performing stereotactic brain biopsy and related procedures is similar whether using a frame or not. Even though the surgeons in this report had an extensive background in frame stereotaxy, nearly two dozen procedures were performed employing both SNS and conventional stereo-

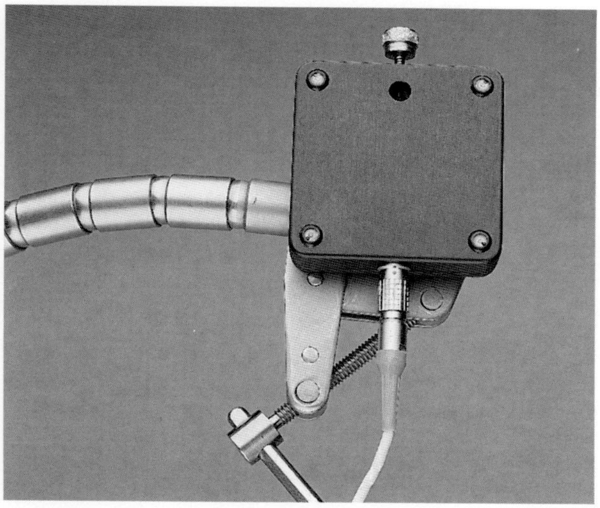

Figure 15-8. Guide block equipped with LEDs allows tracking of instrument trajectory throughout procedure.

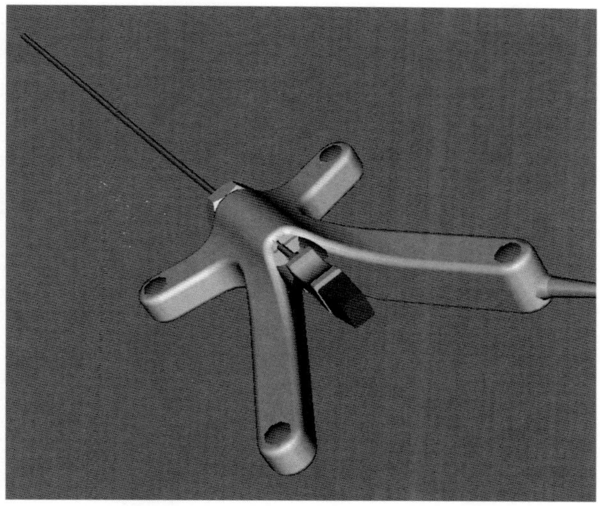

Figure 15-9. Universal adapter allows visualization of instrument trajectory and location as it is advanced to the target site.

taxy systems prior to embarking on using the SNS alone as reported in this series. It is suggested that surgeons new to SNS-assisted biopsy use a similar approach.

It is important that surgeons not experienced in frame stereotaxy brain biopsy learn the general principles of target and trajectory selection.[39] In general we prefer to target the center of enhancing lesions or the center of the lesion if it enhances only at the periphery or not at all. As such, the surgeon does not aim for the edge of ring-enhancing lesions; rather, after impaling the lesion at its core, the biopsy instrument is advanced or withdrawn by 5 or 10 mm intervals until frozen section reveals a diagnostic specimen. The principal consideration when selecting a trajectory is avoidance of vascular structures. Other important factors include (1) avoiding eloquent brain, (2) optimizing diagnostic yield, (3) avoiding crossing multiple pial and/or ependymal planes, and (4) minimizing the intracranial course.

SUMMARY

With adequate attention to detail, SNSs can provide simple, accurate guidance for image-guided brain biopsy and similar procedures without the need for stereotaxy frames. Surgeons with limited experience with frame stereotaxy biopsy should master the basic principles of brain biopsy when applying SNSs to these procedures.

References

1. Apuzzo MLJ, Chandrasoma PT, Cohen D, et al. Computed imaging stereotaxy: Experience and perspective related to 500 procedures applied to brain masses. Neurosurgery 20:930-937, 1987.
2. Chandrasoma PT, Smith MM, Apuzzo MLJ. Stereotactic biopsy in the diagnosis of brain masses: Comparison of results of biopsy and resected surgical specimen. Neurosurgery 24:160-165, 1989.
3. Gomez H, Barnett GH, Estes ML, et al. Stereotactic and computer-assisted neurosurgery at the Cleveland Clinic: Review of 501 consecutive cases. Cleve Clin J Med 60:339-410, 1993.
4. Lunsford LD, Martinez AJ. Stereotactic exploration of the brain in the era of computed tomography. Surg Neurol 22:222-230, 1984.
5. Mundinger F, Ostertag CB, Birg W, et al. Stereotactic treatment of brain lesions: Biopsy, interstitial radiotherapy (iridium-192 and iodine-125) and drainage procedures. Appl Neurophysiol 43:198-204, 1980.
6. Backlund EO, Von Holst H. Controlled subtotal evacuation of intracerebral hematomas by stereotactic technique. Surg Neurol 9:99-101, 1978.
7. Bosch DA, Rahn D, Backlund EO. Treatment of colloid cysts of the third ventricle by stereotactic aspiration. Surg Neurol 9:15-18, 1978.
8. Dyste GN, Hitchon PW, Menezes AW, et al. Stereotaxic surgery in the treatment of multiple brain abscesses. J Neurosurg 69:15-18, 1978.
9. Matsumoto K, Hondo H. CT-guided stereotactic evaluation of hypertensive intracerebral hematomas. J Neurosurg 61:440-448, 1984.
10. Rogers LR, Barnett GH. Percutaneous aspiration of brain tumor cysts via the Ommaya reservoir system. Neurology 41:279-282, 1991.
11. Bernstein M, Gutin PH. Interstitial irradiation of brain tumors: A review. Neurosurgery 9:741-750, 1981.
12. Gutin PH, Phillips PL, Wara WM, et al. Brachytherapy of recurrent malignant brain tumors with removable high-activity iodine-125 sources. J Neurosurg 60:61-68, 1984.
13. Lunsford LD, Latchaw RE, Vries JK. Stereotactic implantation of deep brain electrodes using computed tomography. Neurosurgery 13:280-286, 1983.
14. Pillay PK, Barnett GH, Awad IA. MRI-guided placement of depth electrodes in temporal lobe epilepsy: A comparison of CRW and BRW arc systems. Br J Neurosurg 6:47-53, 1992.
15. Gildenberg PL. Functional neurosurgery. In Schmidek HH, Sweet WH, eds. Operative Neurosurgery, vol 2. New York: Grune & Stratton, 1982, pp 993-1043.
16. Hassenbusch SJ, Pillay PK, Barnett GH. Radiofrequency cingulotomy for intractable cancer pain using stereotaxis guided by magnetic resonance imaging. Neurosurgery 27:220-223, 1990.
17. Kelly PJ, Ahlskog JE, Goerss SJ, et al. Computer-assisted stereotactic ventralis lateralis thalamotomy with microelectrode recording control in patients with Parkinson's disease. Mayo Clin Proc 62:655-664, 1987.
18. Rosenfeld JV, Barnett GH, Palmer J. CT stereotactic thalamotomy using the Brown-Roberts-Wells system for non-Parkinsonian movement disorders [Technical note]. Stereotact Funct Neurosurg 56:184-192, 1991.
19. Barnett GH, Ramos L, McKenzie RL. Non-volumetric stereotaxy-assisted craniotomy. Results in 50 cases. Stereotact Funct Neurosurg 61:80-95, 1993.
20. Hariz MI, Fodstad H. Stereotactic localization of small subcortical brain tumors for open surgery. Surg Neurol 28:345-350, 1987.
21. Hassenbusch SJ, Anderson JS, Pillay PK. Brain tumor resection aided with markers placed using stereotaxis guided by magnetic resonance imaging and computed tomography. Neurosurgery 28:801-806, 1991.
22. Kelly PJ. Volumetric stereotactic surgical resection of intra-axial brain mass lesions. Mayo Clin Proc 63:1186-1198, 1988.
23. Kelly PJ. Stereotactic resection: General principles. In Tumor Stereotaxis. Philadelphia: WB Saunders, 1991, pp 268-295.
24. Kelly PJ. Computer-assisted stereotaxis: New approaches for the management of intracranial intra-axial tumors. Neurology 36:535-541, 1986.

25. Kelly PJ, Kall BA, Goerss SJ. Computer-interactive stereotactic resection of deep-seated and centrally located intraaxial brain lesions. Confin Neurol 50:107-114, 1987.
26. Moore MR, Black PM, Ellenbogen R, et al. Stereotactic craniotomy: Methods and results using the Brown-Roberts-Wells stereotactic frame. Neurosurgery 25:572-577, 1989.
27. Barnett GH, Kormos DW, Steiner CP, et al. Frameless stereotaxy using a sonic digitizing wand: Development and adaptation to the Picker ViStar Medical Imaging System. In Maciunas RJ, ed. Interactive Image-Guided Neurosurgery. Park Ridge, Ill.: American Association of Neurological Surgeons, 1993, pp 113-119.
28. Barnett GH, Kormos DW, Steiner CP, et al. Intraoperative localization using an armless, frameless stereotactic wand. J Neurosurg 78:510-514, 1993.
29. Barnett GH, Kormos DW, Steiner CP, et al. Use of a frameless, armless stereotactic wand for brain tumor localization with 2-D and 3-D neuroimaging. Neurosurgery 33:674-678, 1993.
30. Friets EM, Strohbehn JW, Hatch JF, et al. A frameless stereotaxic operating microscope for neurosurgery. IEEE Trans Biomed Eng 36:608-617, 1989.
31. Guthrie BL, Adler JR. Frameless stereotaxy: Computer interactive neurosurgery. Perspect Neurol Surg 2(1):1-19, 1991.
32. Maciunas RJ, Galloway RL Jr, Fitzpatrick JM, et al. A universal system for interactive image-directed neurosurgery. Stereotact Funct Neurosurg 58:108-113, 1992.
33. Roberts DW, Strohbehn JW, Friets EM, Kettenberger J, Hartov A. The stereotactic operating microscope: Accuracy refinement and clinical experience. Acta Neurochir Suppl 46:112-114, 1989.
34. Roberts DW, Strohbehn JW, Hatch JF, et al. A frameless stereotaxic integration of computerized tomographic imaging and the operating microscope. J Neurosurg 65:545-549, 1986.
35. Watanabe E, Watanabe T, Manaka S, et al. Three-dimensional digitizer (neuronavigator): New equipment for computed tomography-guided stereotaxic surgery. Surg Neurol 27:543-547, 1987.
36. Rhoten RP, Luciano M, Barnett GH. Computer-assisted neuroendoscopy (CANE). Neurosurgery 40: 635-638, 1996.
37. Galloway RL, Maciunas RJ, Latimer JW. The accuracies of four stereotactic frame systems: An independent assessment. Biomed Instrum Tech 25:457-460, 1991.
38. Wang MY, Maurer CR Jr, Fitzpatrick JM, et al. An automatic technique for finding and localizing externally attached markers in CT and MR volume images of the head. IEEE Trans Biomed Eng 43:627-637, 1996.
39. Barnett GH. Stereotactic techniques in the management of brain tumors. Contemp Neurosurg 19:1-9, 1997.

16

Image Cyberknife Radiosurgery

John R. Adler, Jr., M.D. • Achim Schweikard, Ph.D. • Martin J. Murphy, Ph.D.
Steven L. Hancock, M.D.

Stereotactic radiosurgery has become a widely accepted alternative to surgery and radiation therapy for some neurosurgical conditions. By combining the targeting principles of stereotaxy with a tightly collimated, focused high-energy radiation source, noninvasive destruction of small brain lesions is possible.[1] For selected brain tumors, this treatment represents an effective alternative to conventional open neurosurgery, radiation implantation, or standard fractionated radiation therapy. In addition, some tumors that are outside of the brain but adjacent to the base of the skull can also be treated by current stereotactic methods. For example, it has been demonstrated that radiosurgery is useful for some head and neck cancers.[2] Although the scope of disease that is amenable to radiosurgical treatment is expanding, further development of stereotactic radiosurgery has been hampered by the shortcomings of existing technology.

Stereotaxy frames perform two critical functions during radiosurgery—fixation and localization. Although required to maintain the target in a rigid relationship with the radiosurgical device, cranial fixation is both painful and confining for the patient. The discomfort is sufficiently severe that children undergoing radiosurgery generally must be given a general anesthetic. Radiation biologists have suggested that tumor control and tolerance of surrounding neural structures may be improved by the use of fractionated treatment; however, frames interfere with such treatment.[3] Even with rigid skeletal fixation, frame movement can occur over the several days or weeks required for fractionation. In addition, invasive frames capable of accurate refixation are impractical for radiosurgery. Although removable frames that use bony prominences and dental molds to achieve cranial fixation are under development, the overall accuracy of targeting during fractionated treatment is presently unclear.[4] Moreover, such devices are unlikely to prove useful for children or edentulous adults. Precisely focused irradiation of other sites in the body may also be beneficial; however, the principles of radiosurgical localization and fixation using frame-based stereotaxy are extremely difficult to apply to regions of the body beyond the cranium. These problems seem inherent to any stereotaxy system that relies on an external frame that is rigidly attached to the patient.

Radiosurgery achieves a steep radiation dose gradient by focusing narrow, highly collimated beams about a precise point. To accomplish this, the target is carefully positioned at the isocenter of the treatment machine. All commercially available radiosurgical instruments employ such fixed isocenters. The Gamma Knife uses a specific fixed array of cobalt-60 sources whose beams converge on a single point. Standard linear accelerator-based radiosurgical devices rotate up to 360 degrees around fixed rotational axes. Although these designs work well when treating spherical targets, it is not ideal for tumors and vascular malformations with irregular shapes. Standard radiosurgical methods treat such irregular volumes by constructing arrays of adjacent treatment spheres. Despite state-of-the-art radiosurgical planning software, the treatment of nonspherical shapes is time consuming and inevitably requires significant dose heterogeneity. This compromise also undermines the reliability of estimates of dose-response for both tumor control and treatment complications.

Besides limiting the expansion of radiosurgery into fractionated therapy, treatment beyond the cranium, and effective treatment of irregular volumes, existing radiosurgical approaches require highly specialized, labor-intensive technology that benefits a very limited group of patients. This has resulted in a relatively high cost per procedure. To circumvent all these limitations, a radically new technology that uses frameless localization, a lightweight radiation source, and a robotic delivery system has been developed by Accuray Inc. (Santa Clara, Calif.) (Fig. 16-1, *A*). The first of these instruments, called the Cyberknife, is installed at Stanford University (Fig. 16-1, *B*).

FRAMELESS STEREOTAXY

All the stereotactic instruments devised over the past 50 years must be rigidly anchored to the patient's skull. These devices provide a point of attachment for an external coordinate system and a mechanism for fixing the skull in a precise position for biopsy or treatment. The Cyberknife does not require rigid skull fixation. Instead, the location of the treatment volume can be accurately identified by using x-ray imaging to find and track the patient's skeletal features.[5] This approach represents a radical departure from conventional stereotaxy.

The Cyberknife features two diagnostic x-ray sources and two real-time imaging cameras. These cameras and sources are rigidly fixed at known positions relative to each other and a robotic manipulator that holds a small linear accelerator (LINAC), the high-energy x-ray source for treatment. The diagnostic x-ray sources and imaging cameras provide a stationary frame of reference for locating the patient's cranium (Fig. 16-2). As with all other forms of stereotaxy, this system is based on the assumption that the target within the brain maintains a fixed relationship with respect to the skeleton. Once skeletal landmarks have been located in the camera's coordinate system, the position of the predefined target lesion has also been determined. The location of skeletal landmarks is defined by a process of image correlation: real-time x-ray images from the treatment room are compared with images generated from a CT scan that is used as the basis for treatment planning.

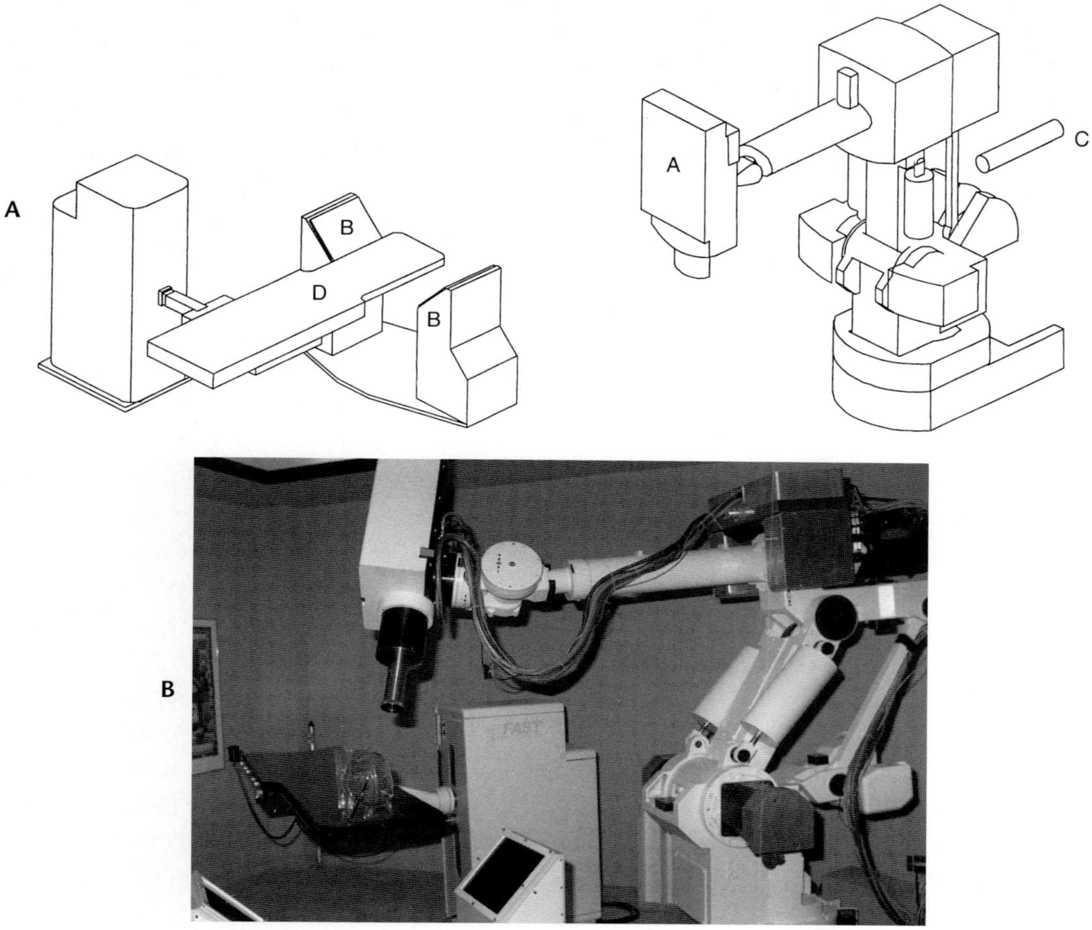

Figure 16-1. A, Components of the Cyberknife: *A*, Linear accelerator (LINAC); *B*, orthogonal x-ray cameras; *C*, one imaging x-ray source; *D*, treatment couch. **B,** The Cyberknife installed at Stanford University.

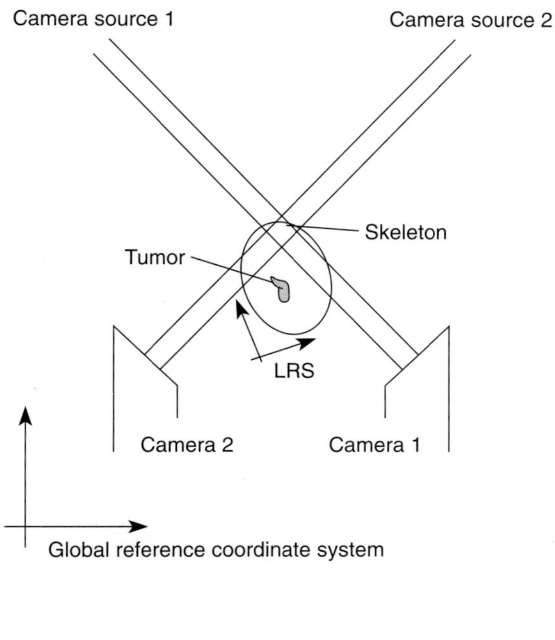

Figure 16-2. Two diagnostic x-ray sources and imaging cameras provide a stationary frame of reference for locating the patient's cranium, which is fixed to the local reference system *(LRS)*.

IMAGE-GUIDED TARGETING USING IMAGE CORRELATION

The targeting system of the Cyberknife uses digitally reconstructed radiographs (DRRs) that emulate the potential views of the patient obtained by the two x-ray cameras that image the patient in real time during radiosurgery. The DRRs are derived from the patient's treatment planning CT scan. This family of DRRs is generated by moving the patient's image in the CT coordinate system to a variety of precisely defined positions and orientations that span the expected range of patient positions and orientations during treatment. The precise geometry of the x-ray camera system is replicated in a camera model within the computer's software and is referenced to the CT system of coordinates. When the patient is positioned within the frame of reference defined by the treatment room's cameras, two DRRs calculated from the CT will match the pair of real x-ray images taken of the patient during treatment. Because of this approach, treatment planning coordinates can be directly translated from CT into the frame of reference of the treatment room cameras. This information is subsequently used to aim a robotic manipulator.

Without a frame, the patient cannot be expected to maintain the same precise position throughout both treatment and CT scanning. To compensate for this, real x-ray images are compared and correlated with the DRRs to define the patient's actual position during treatment. When x-ray images taken during treatment match one of these pairs of DRRs, the precise orientation of the patient and the target is defined. If the patient's position does not precisely match the DRR, the patient's position can be inferred by mathematical interpolation between the real images and the family of DRRs. When this measurement of position is completed, the treatment plan coordinates (e.g., the lesion isocenter) can be directly translated into the frame of reference of the camera system and, from there, to manipulator coordinates. The manipulator retargets the high-energy radiation beam to maintain its fix (i.e., position and orientation) on the actual position of the lesion.

The entire position measurement process, which includes live image acquisition and correlation, can be done in seconds. As a result, the robotic manipulator can locate and follow small movements made by the patient's head (or other skeletal feature) in real time.

The present image guidance system measures changes in the patient's translational position during treatment over a range of 2 cm in each of three directions. A more sophisticated version of the technique is under development that will track rotational orientation as well. Until these orientation measurements are possible, patient treatments employ a Laetinen noninvasive head restraint to eliminate significant rotations of the head by anchoring the head at the nasion and external auditory canals.

To measure the system's overall targeting and tracking precision, four clinical treatments have been simulated using a radiographic film phantom. This analysis demonstrated absolute root mean square (RMS) targeting errors of 0.5, 2.2, 3.1, and 3.9 mm and an RMS error of 0.6 mm in measuring relative motion. Fig. 16-3

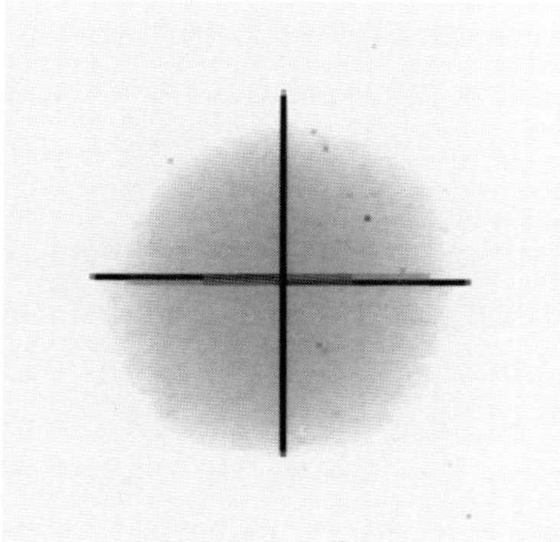

Figure 16-3. The dose distribution obtained with a radiographic film phantom during a simulation trial. The crosshairs mark the precise center of the intended target.

shows the actual dose distributions for the best of the simulation trials where the collimator size was 12.5 mm. A spherical dose was targeted at the precise center of the radiographic film (marked by the crosshairs). These tests of absolute targeting precision combine the inaccuracies inherent in the image guidance system, the robotic pointing of the LINAC, and isocenter definition during treatment planning. This overall system accuracy is comparable to and has the potential to outperform even conventional image-guided frame stereotaxy, which is limited both in the precision with which discrete fiducials can be located and by the mechanical flexure of stereotaxy frames.[6]

HIGH-ENERGY RADIATION SOURCE

The Cyberknife uses a novel lightweight 6 MeV LINAC. Because this device runs at a much higher "X-band" frequency than conventional medical "S-band" LINACs, it has been possible to significantly reduce the size and weight of critical components. Traditional medical LINACs weigh 3000 to 4000 pounds; the accelerator used in the Cyberknife weighs only 280 pounds. Despite the small size of this X-band LINAC, the performance of this radiation source is comparable to that of medical S-band machines. For radiation fields less than 7 cm with a source-axial distance of 100 cm, the radiation output is approximately 300 rads/min. Two independently scaled dosimetry systems are used to measure LINAC output. These devices have a precision of $\pm 1\%$ or 1 MU, whichever is greater. Unlike current radiosurgical systems, the Cyberknife can be turned on or off easily so that particularly radiation-sensitive structures such as the optic nerves will not be treated.

MANIPULATOR

The low weight of the LINAC and the accessibility to the patient's head afforded by image-guided localization permits the use of a robotic manipulator to orient the radiation beam. This manipulator allows automated positioning and pointing of the LINAC. The mechanical system is both flexible and precise, being capable of positioning the linear accelerator at any point over the treatment sphere at a distance of 60 to 100 cm with an absolute precision of 0.5 mm in position and ±0.0001 radians in orientation. These error measurements, which compare favorably with other stereotaxy instruments, have been repeatedly verified using a laser source.

The mechanical design of the Cyberknife makes it possible to easily reposition the isocenter. Consequently, the LINAC can be retargeted during treatment in response to small patient movements. When movement is detected by the real-time imaging system, a change in isocenter is calculated, and the new coordinates are sent to the manipulator. This feedback is used to adjust the location of the isocenter dynamically with respect to the robot's reference coordinate system. The manipulator can track the motion of a lesion without having to alter predetermined treatment paths. The robot travels at a speed of approximately 1.5 cm/sec, and head movement updates can be provided as frequently as every few seconds. Irradiation of the target is not continuous but is delivered from an arbitrary series of several hundred nodes (i.e., point and shoot). Although treatment time depends on the number and complexity of the paths, standard radiosurgical arcs take less than 5 or 6 minutes.

Present-day radiosurgical technology permits cross-firing over 2π steradian above the equator of the stereotaxy frame that encircles the head. Because of the localization and mechanical systems used in the Cyberknife, the potential range of direction available for radiosurgical targeting is increased to 3π. This increased capacity for cross-firing also makes possible improved dosimetry. Given the unique advantages of a robotic delivery system, a specialized treatment planning system has been developed.

NONISOCENTRIC TREATMENT PLANNING

Conventional LINAC-based radiosurgical systems are constrained to movement of the beam along circular arcs. As a consequence, the treated volume is ideally spherical.[7-9] This is problematic for nonspherical tumors. The mechanical gantry of the Cyberknife is unlike any standard LINAC-based radiosurgical instrument. Since the robot arm has six joints that can be moved simultaneously under computer control, it is possible to move the radiation beam along arbitrary spatial paths. In particular, the robot arm can simultaneously rotate and translate the high-energy radiation source.

A beam placement together with a pointing direction is termed a beam configuration. During treatment the beam is activated at a series of configurations. At each of these the duration of beam activation determines an intensity or weight. Forward treatment planning computes and visualizes a dose distribution based on a specific set of beam configurations and weights. Inverse treatment planning defines beam configurations and weights given the set of dose parameters needed to treat a specific condition. To accomplish this, the individual constructing a plan identifies a region of high dose (RHD), which is defined as the volume receiving 80% or more of the maximum radiation dose. An appropriate dose distribution for a given target should then satisfy the following constraints:

1. Critical and/or radiation-sensitive healthy structures near the tumor (e.g., nerves, vessels, and sensitive brain) receive a very low dose.
2. In most cases the dose inside the target is highly uniform (i.e., the dose in the tumor is both lower-bounded and upper-bounded).
3. The RHD should cover the entire target and match the target shape.
4. The drop-off around the RHD should be as sharp as possible (i.e., the generalized distance between the 80% isodose surface and isodose surfaces of lower values should be very small).

Several methods for evaluating radiosurgical and radiotherapeutical dose distributions are in clinical use. The most common paradigms being used are dose-volume histograms[7-10] and color representations of two-dimensional distributions overlying tomographic images. These techniques can be used to evaluate a distribution with respect to constraints 1, 2, and 4. However, the treatment planning system designed for the Cyberknife also uses three-dimensional isodose surfaces overlying reconstructions of anatomic regions, tissue-volume ratios,[7] and integrals over dose-volume histograms (the integral of the dose-volume histogram divided by the tumor volume) for evaluation.

With current LINAC-based radiosurgical systems, the patient couch is moved manually in addition to moving the accelerator. Although improved dose distributions could be achieved in many cases, to fully exploit combined gantry/couch movements would require a large set of beam directions and/or complex motions of the radiation source, and for practical reasons, these complex beam paths cannot be generated with conventional LINACs. Since the Cyberknife has six degrees of freedom, it offers full kinematic flexibility for placing and directing the radiation beam in three dimensions. To make full use of this added flexibility, treatment planning methods based on geometric algorithms have been developed. The following approach divided into three subtasks and emphasizing inverse planning is used.

1. Selection of beam configurations
2. Computation of beam weights
3. Motion planning (computation of a collision-free path connecting beam configurations)

Each subtask is regarded as an entirely geometric planning problem. The constraints for appropriate dose distributions are expressed by geometric requirements alone. Steps 1 and 2 are based on a geometric model of the physical characteristics of the photon beams produced by the accelerator. Since each of the three subtasks is considered separately in planning, the path connecting the beam configurations does not influence distribution. However, the inverse planning component must ensure that a path is executable and does not cause collisions or occlusion of the on-line vision of the x-ray imaging system.

Fully computerized optimization of distributions is problematic and is not used for the following reasons:

1. The constraints describing an adequate dose distribution are in conflict. For example, in many cases it is difficult to achieve accurate matching between the shape of the target and region of high dose and simultaneously achieve a sharp dose drop-off around the RHD.

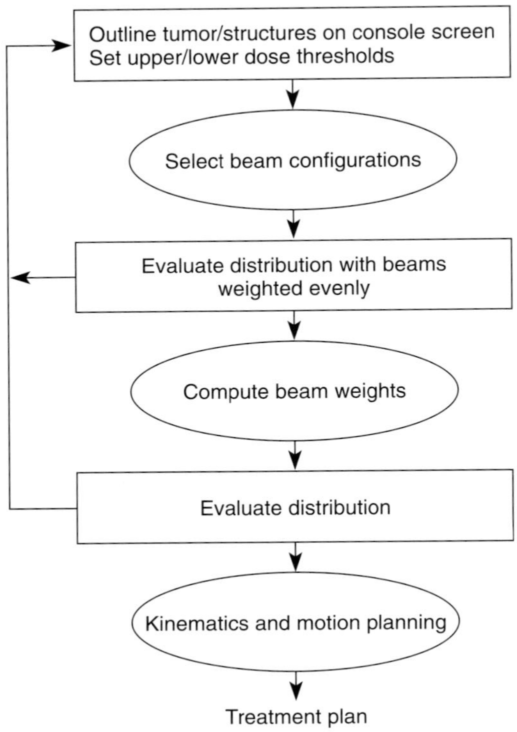

Figure 16-4. Paradigm for beam selection.

2. Although the described planning problem is nonlinear, optimization methods will only yield a local optimum, with no information about global optima.
3. The results of optimization depend on the settings of internal system parameters. Small changes in these values can yield widely diverging results. It is difficult to make the influence of such parameters and trade-offs transparent to the end user (i.e., surgeon).

For similar reasons we have not included poorly characterized radiobiologic considerations or complication probabilities into algorithmic planning.

Since complete methods are used for subtasks 2 and 3, the correctness of an output given a specific input can be clearly established based on algorithmic principles. Furthermore, computing time can be bounded in advance. For step 1, complete algorithmic solutions are problematic for combinatorial reasons. Therefore an extended set of standard paradigms for selecting beam configurations has been developed that takes advantage of the fact that the beam can be rotated and translated along arbitrary paths in space. These paradigms are direct extensions of current methods used in LINAC-based radiosurgery.

To plan a treatment, the user outlines the tumor and anatomic structures close to the tumor on the computer console. Fig. 16-4 illustrates paradigms for beam selection. The beam presently used in the Cyberknife is cylindric (i.e., the beam cross section is circular). For sphere-shaped targets, a spherical RHD is op-

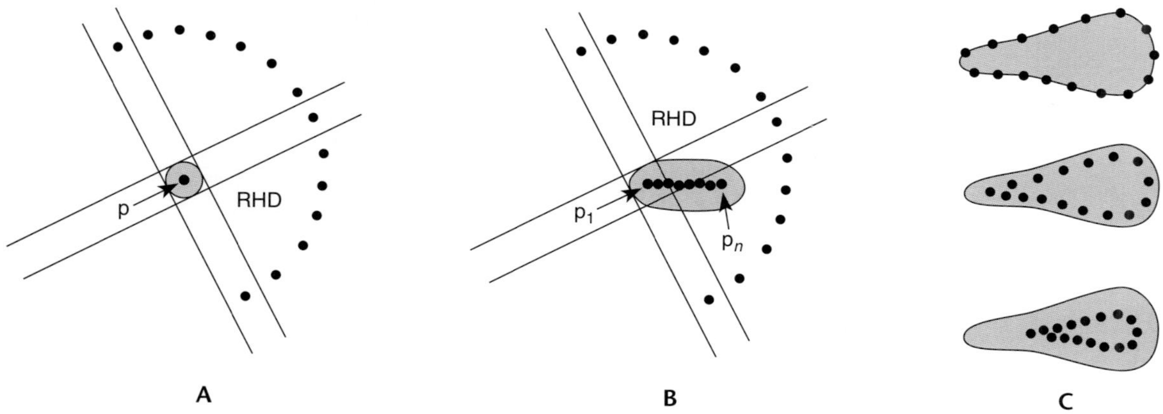

Figure 16-5. Achieving the RHD. **A,** Single isocenter is generated when all beam axes cross a single point. **B,** Series of equally spaced isocenter points results in cylindric RHD. **C,** RHDs for more complex shapes can be generated (bottom) by first placing a grid of isocenter points on the surface of the volume to be treated and then resolving each point into a series of beam configurations. Automatic beam weighting methods are used to homogenize this RHD.

timal. Such an RHD is generated by a series of beams in which the axes of each crosses a single point (p) (Fig. 16-5, A) called the isocenter. If all beams have equal weights, the RHD is spherical and this procedure is called a single-isocenter procedure.

A first generalization of this procedure is shown in Fig. 16-5, *B*. A series of points $p_1, \ldots, p_n$ is evenly spaced along a line segment. As in the single-isocenter procedure, a set of beam directions is computed for each point. We thus call the points $p_1, \ldots, p_n$ isocenter points. The resulting RHD is a generalized cylinder.

Spheres and generalized cylinders are adequate for many tumors. However, Fig. 16-5, C, demonstrates beam configurations for treating still more general shapes. In this case the system computes a representation of the tumor surface. A grid of isocenter points on the tumor surface is then determined. This grid can be retracted or expanded interactively. Each isocenter point is resolved into a series of beam configurations, as with the single-isocenter procedure. Automatic beam weighting is necessary to homogenize the RHD.

In the weighting phase the user can set upper and lower dose thresholds for the tumor and normal brain structures. Based on geometric algorithms, it can be decided whether the specified distribution can be achieved.[11,12] The beam configurations are linked to an executable path for the robot. System kinematics and planning techniques allow for the type of treatment administered by standard radiosurgical systems. Thus distribution characteristics achievable with earlier systems are also achievable with the Cyberknife.

Fig. 16-6 shows a sample case with a nonspherical tumor. Fig. 16-7 shows multiple slices taken from a phantom study for this case. Note the close spatial correspondence between inputted tumor shape and the actual dose distribution visible in the phantom.

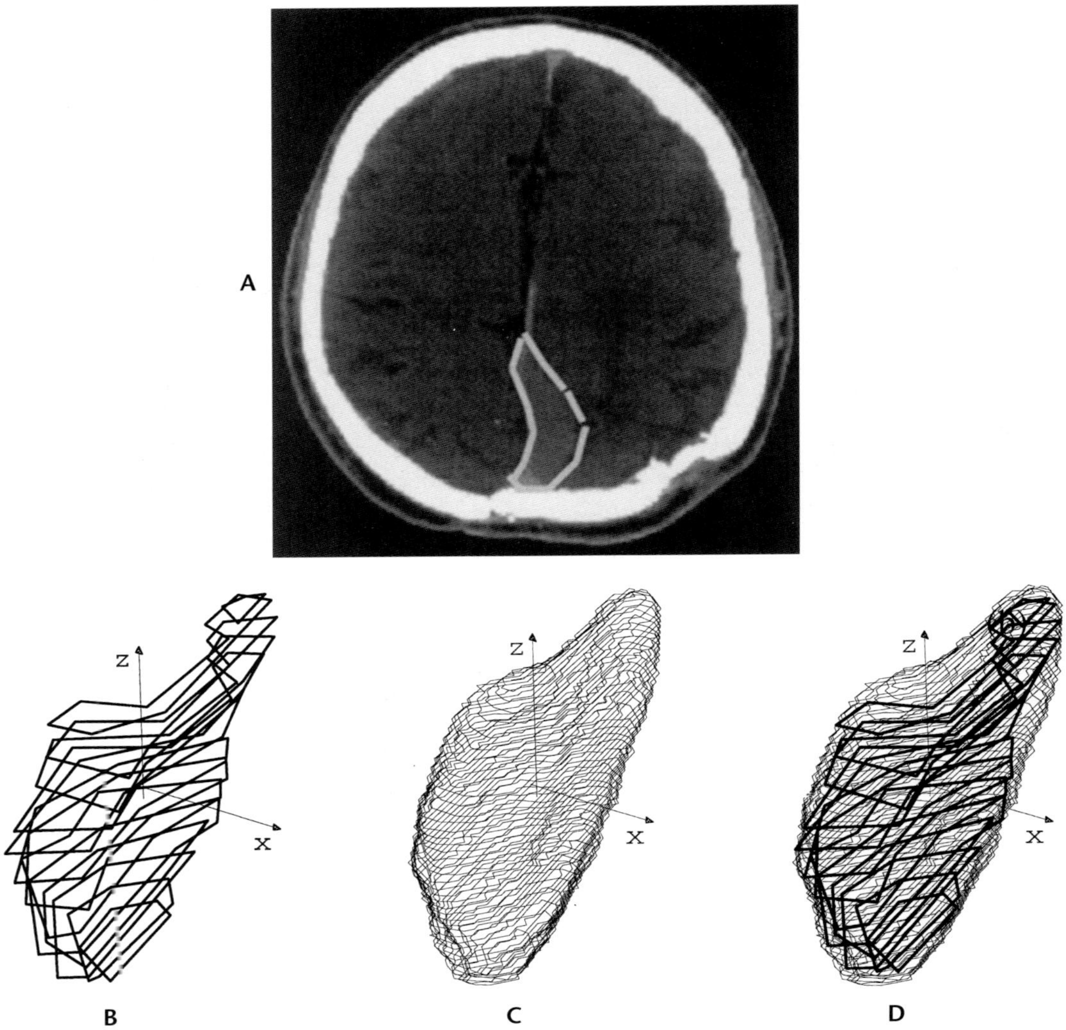

Figure 16-6. A, Sample case of nonspherical tumor. **B,** Geometric representation of tumor surface. **C,** RHD (80% isodose line) generated by treatment planning system. **D,** Superimposition of C on *B*.

CLINICAL EXPERIENCE

As of March 1, 1997, over 30 patients have been treated using the Cyberknife technology under an investigational device exemption supervised by the FDA. Brain metastasis, solitary or multiple, was the indication for treatment in the vast majority of patients, and nearly all had prior whole-brain radiation therapy. Three benign lesions were treated: one patient had a large fibrous tumor of the orbit and two patients had Von Hippel-Lindau and hemangioblastomas of the middle to lower cervical spinal cord. Because of the benign tumor's intimacy with critical structures of the central nervous system (optic nerve and spinal cord), each treatment was given in three fractions using a total dose of 21 Gy. Follow-up imaging

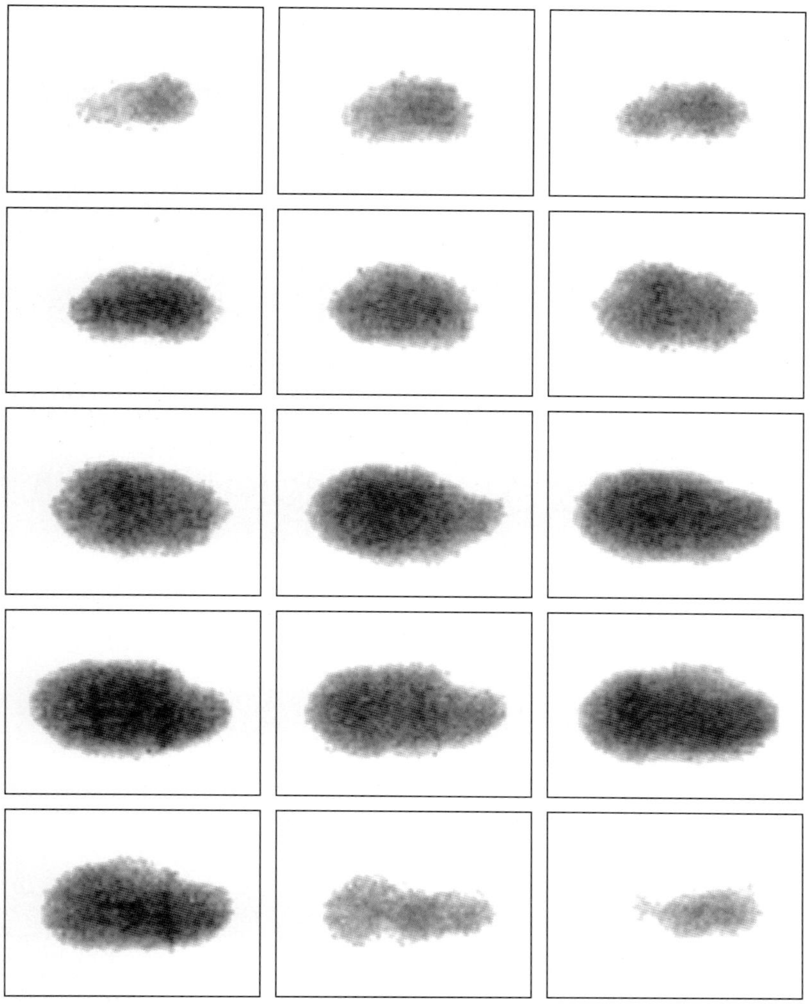

Figure 16-7. Series of slices from phantom study for treatment of tumor shown in Fig. 16-6, *A*.

to date confirmed that treatment with the Cyberknife results in a clinical response that closely mirrors that which can be achieved with other forms of radiosurgery.

SUMMARY

The Cyberknife is designed for state-of-the-art radiosurgery. The robotic manipulator with its six degrees of freedom of motion and its unique compact X-band LINAC provide a system that is capable of homogeneously irradiating tumors and vascular malformations of virtually any shape and delivering fractionated treatment. An image guidance system functions in real time to position and point the robotically mounted LINAC. Although the Cyberknife does not use skeletal fixation, the overall accuracy of localization compares favorably with radiosurgical systems that use invasive stereotaxy frames. To fully utilize the system's capabilities, a new method of treatment planning has been developed. Improved patient comfort, decreased treatment time, and the potential to treat extracranial targets are further benefits that this approach to radiosurgery offers. Clinical testing of this instrument is under way at Stanford University and five other institutions worldwide. Although the initial use of the Cyberknife will be restricted to neurosurgical procedures, new modifications that are being developed will permit treatment of lesions throughout the body.

References

1. Leksell L. Stereotaxis and Radiosurgery. An Operative System. Springfield, Ill.: Charles C Thomas, 1971.
2. Kaplin ID, Adler JR, Hicks WL, Fee WE, Goffinet DR. Radiosurgery for palliation of base of skull recurrences from head and neck cancers. Cancer 10:1-16, 1992.
3. Hall EJ, Brenner DJ. The radiobiology of radiosurgery: Rationale for different treatment regimes for AVM and malignancies. Int J Radiat Oncol Biol Phys 25:381-385, 1993.
4. Sofat A, Kratimemos G, Thomas DCT. Early experience with the Gill-Thomas locator for computed tomography directed biopsy of intracranial lesions. Neurosurgery 31:972-974, 1994.
5. Adler JR. Image-based frameless stereotaxic radiosurgery. In Maciunas RJ, ed. Interactive Image-Guided Neurosurgery. Park Ridge, Ill.: American Association of Neurological Surgeons, 1994, pp 81-89.
6. Maciunas RJ, Galloway RL, Latimer JW. The application accuracy of stereotactic frames. Neurosurgery 35:632-695, 1994.
7. Nedzi LA, Kooy HM, Alexander E III, Svensson GK, Loeffler JS. Dynamic field shaping for stereotactic radiosurgery: A modeling study intern. Int J Radiat Oncol Biol Phys 25:859-869, 1993.
8. Lutz W, Winston KR, Maleki N. A system for stereotactic radiosurgery with a linear accelerator. Int J Radiat Oncol Biol Phys 14:373-381, 1988.
9. Podgorsak EB, Olivier A, Pla M, Lefebvre PY, Hazel J. Dynamic stereotactic radiosurgery. Int J Radiat Oncol Biol Phys 14:114-126, 1988.
10. Winston KR, Lutz W. Linear accelerator as a neurosurgical tool for stereotactic radiosurgery. Neurosurgery 22:454-464, 1988.
11. Schweikard A, Bodduluri M, Tombropoulos RZ, Adler JR. Planning, calibration, and collision avoidance for image-guided radiosurgery. In Proceedings of the IEEE International Workshop on Intelligent Robots and Systems (IROS), 1994, pp 854-861.
12. Schweikard A, Tombropoulos RZ, Kavraki L, Adler JR, Latombe JCL. Treatment planning for a radiosurgical system with general kinematics. In Proceedings of the IEEE International Conference on Robotics and Automation, 1994, pp 1720-1727.

17

Definition of Functional Anatomy

Gene H. Barnett, M.D.

To ensure the best surgical management of primary brain lesions, assessment of the relationship of the abnormality or surgical approach to functionally eloquent cortex may be critical. Earlier in this century Penfield and Jasper[1] performed a series of elegant mapping studies of the human brain and established a predictable relationship between brain surface anatomy and function. This work was extended by other investigators using intraoperative or chronic indwelling electrodes in the surgical treatment of epilepsy.[2]

The plasticity of cortical function in children is well established but is believed to be relatively immutable in the adult. During the electrode era of brain mapping it was suggested that adult function may significantly depart from established anatomy, particularly in the presence of a slowly expanding lesion such as a low-grade tumor or vascular malformation.[2] However, much of this work was performed without the aid of imaging techniques that could confirm that the investigators had defined anatomic structures correctly. More recently, investigational noninvasive means of mapping brain function, such as PET,[3,4] functional MRI,[3-11] magnetoencephalography or magnetic source imaging,[12-15] and transcutaneous magnetic stimulation,[16,17] have demonstrated the validity of Penfield and Jasper's observations, provided noninvasive means of defining functional anatomy in individual patients, and shed new light on the issue of cortical functional plasticity in the adult.[14,18,19]

Today three-dimensional imaging techniques provide excellent visualization of the brain. These techniques range from complex (e.g., fusion with other imaging modalities)[20] to comparatively simple (e.g., preoperative image manipulations performed by today's surgical navigation systems [SNSs]).[21,22] If the relationship between cortical and functional anatomy in the adult is essentially fixed, then the anatomic information provided by SNSs may be sufficient to accurately infer function and obviate or indicate the need for more complicated or investigational means of functional mapping.

To better define the role of SNSs in determining cortical anatomy, we directly compared functional and anatomic localization information obtained through

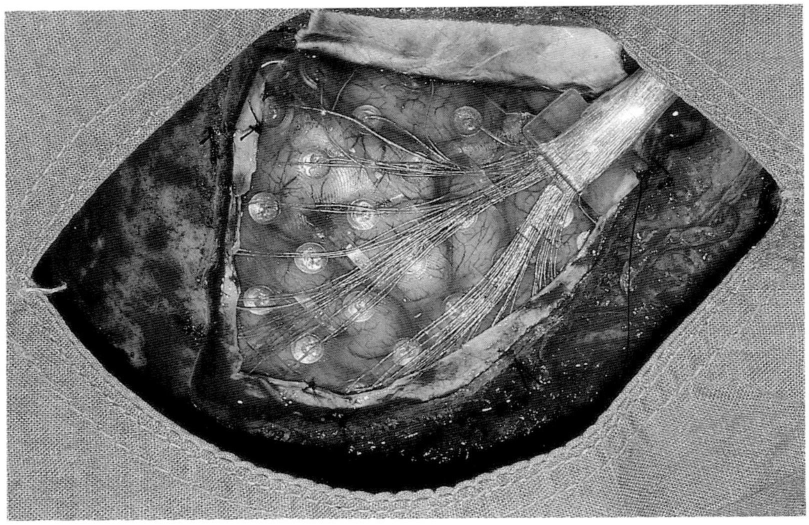

Figure 17-1. Chronic subdural electrode array used to map motor sensory areas. In this case the tumor was in the primary sensory area and contained functional tissue. The patient opted for resection, which resulted in a permanent cortical sensory deficit in the left upper extremity.

electrophysiologic monitoring, three-dimensional surface reconstructions (3DSRs), and "oblique" displays generated tangentially through the cortex using an SNS for a selected group of patients with lesions in or near rolandic or speech areas. In addition, we reviewed perioperative and sustained neurologic deficits in a series of 135 adult patients undergoing craniotomy for tumor in these areas.

Twenty patients with lesions judged to be near functionally eloquent cortex or in whom the surgical trajectory might be near such areas underwent volumetric MRI without and with the administration of intravenous contrast. The 3DSRs were performed on a Kuboda Pacific Titan 3000 graphics supercomputer using AVS software. A prototype ViewPoint SNS was used to render multiplanar image displays tangentially through cortical structures.[21,22]

The definition of functional anatomy (e.g., central structures), lesion location, and their relationship were assessed for each modality. In ten cases either prolonged neurophysiologic mapping using recording and stimulation techniques (Fig. 17-1)[14] or intraoperative mapping of evoked sensory or motor potentials were performed and correlated with the images.[23]

We also reviewed the perioperative and sustained postoperative deficits in 135 patients undergoing SNS-assisted craniotomy. Patients with lesions with extensive subcortical extensions or larger than 5 cm in diameter were excluded.

The surgical technique for tumor resection is described elsewhere. It was assumed that enhancing lesions encompassed nonfunctional tissue and that nonenhancing lesions may incorporate functional tissue. When possible, lesions were removed in an en bloc fashion to minimize the effects of brain shift.

Table 17-1. Imaging Data

Anatomic Definition	SNS Multiplanar Display	3DSR
Rolandic structures		
No previous surgery	Excellent	Good to excellent
No previous radiation therapy/ surgery	Good to very good	Poor
Local edema	Enhances visualization	Impairs visualization
Subcortical lesions	Very good to excellent	Poor

CLINICAL EXPERIENCE

Patient Population

A total of 135 patients underwent 139 craniotomies. Their average age was 47.3 years (range 18 to 82 years). High-grade primary glial neoplasms accounted for 40% of the lesions; low-grade tumors, 15%; metastases, 21%; meningiomas, 17%; and radiation necrosis or miscellaneous tumors, 4%. One patient died from venous infarction after surgery.

Imaging (Table 17-1)

Multiplanar imaging proved equal or superior to 3DSR in all cases. Tangential planes through the motor-sensory cortex clearly demonstrated rolandic features (see Fig. 17-4, *A*) irrespective of the presence of tumor, edema, or changes caused by previous surgery or irradiation. Real-time manipulation of these planes in the operating room required little additional time in the surgical planning mode. Since these were contrast studies and the depth of planes was variable, the relationship of subcortical lesions or trajectories to cortical anatomy was easily visualized.

Logistically, the acquisition of 3DSRs proved more complicated. Because dural enhancement in the volumetric contrast study obscured surface reconstruction, a second noncontrast volumetric acquisition was necessary. In patients who had undergone previous surgery and irradiation and those with significant brain edema, cortical features were often lost (see Fig. 17-4, *B*). Often the location of subcortical lesions was also difficult to deduce (Fig. 17-2).

Electrophysiology

In the 10 cases in which electrophysiologic mapping was performed, correlation between phase reversal and the inferred central sulcus was absolute for the multiplanar image displays derived from the SNS as well as the cases in which the 3DSRs allowed visualization of the motor area. Correlations with inferred speech areas were generally good, although not absolute.

A

B

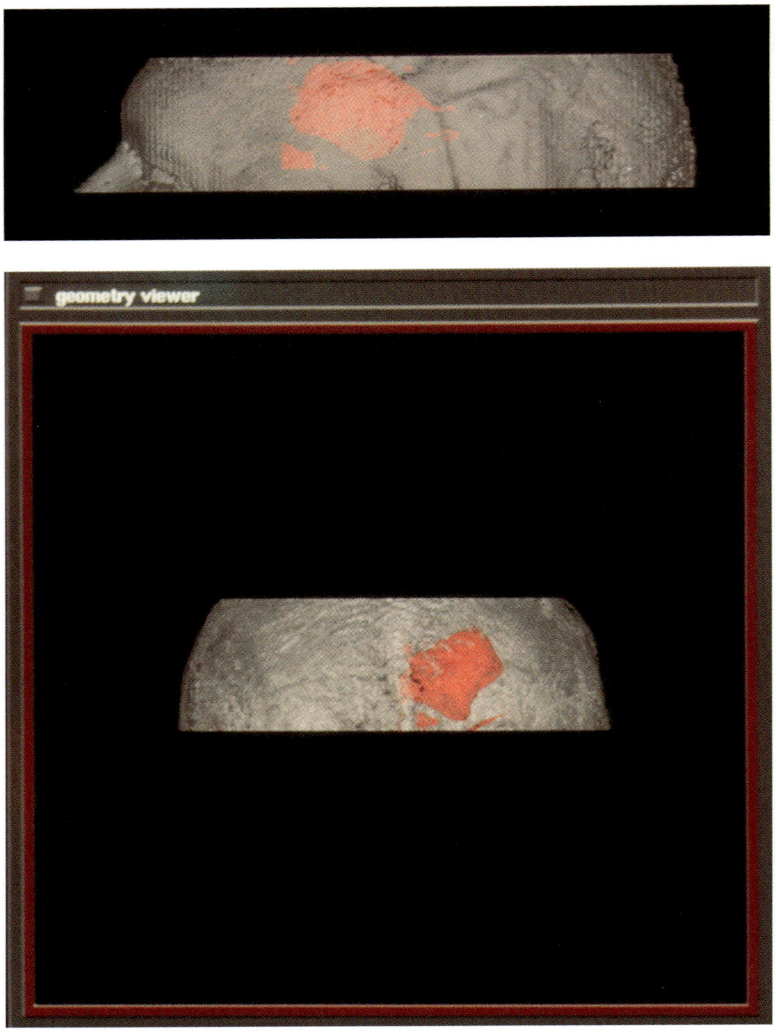

Figure 17-2. A, Lateral 3DSR with patient's scalp rendered translucent clearly visualizes orange tumor. **B,** However, no information on depth is given until display is rotated as shown here or if image is viewed stereoscopically.

Complications

In all except one patient complications were limited to those anticipated from SNS imaging of the anatomic area operated on. Nineteen percent of these patients with lesions in or near eloquent cortex experienced temporary worsening of symptoms with sustained deficits occurring in 6%. The permanent Broca's aphasia that occurred in one patient with a left frontal lobe glioblastoma was not anticipated.

Representative Cases

Case 1. Conventional imaging showed a right frontal tumor near the motor sensory complex in a 23-year-old woman who presented with a generalized sei-

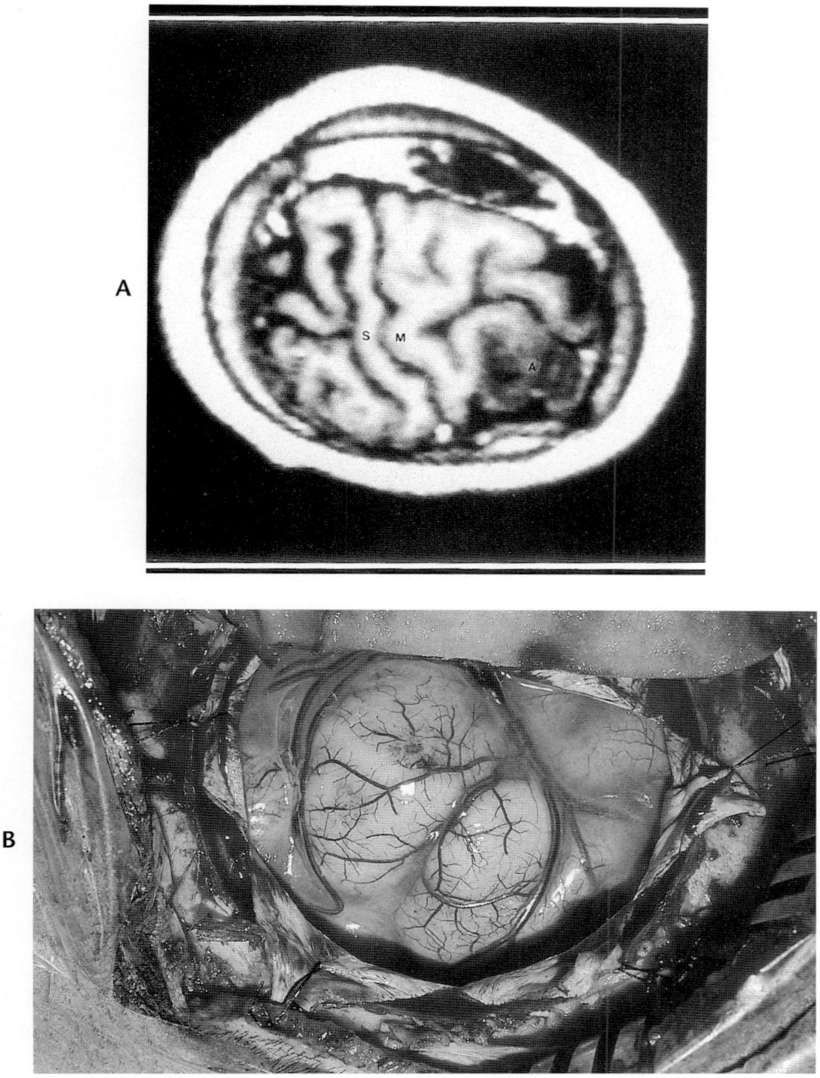

Figure 17-3. A, Tangential plane produced by SNS preoperatively to assess surgical risk of a patient with a right frontal lobe tumor. This image shows the lesion to be in the middle frontal gyrus. Rolandic features such as the pre- and postcentral gyri (inferred to be the motor and sensory areas) are clearly defined. **B,** Resection of this mixed glioma was confirmed by radiography to be complete and produced no deficits.

zure. A contrast-enhanced volumetric MR image was obtained and preoperatively manipulated using the SNS to produce a plane showing the relationship of the tumor to the rolandic complex. The tumor was found to be in the middle frontal gyrus anterior to the inferred motor strip (Fig. 17-3, *A*). Resection of this mixed glioma (Fig. 17-3, *B*) was shown to be complete on radiography and the patient experienced no deficit.

Case 2. A tangential multiplanar image display and 3DSR showed metastasis at the junction of inferior frontal gyrus and motor cortex in a patient who pre-

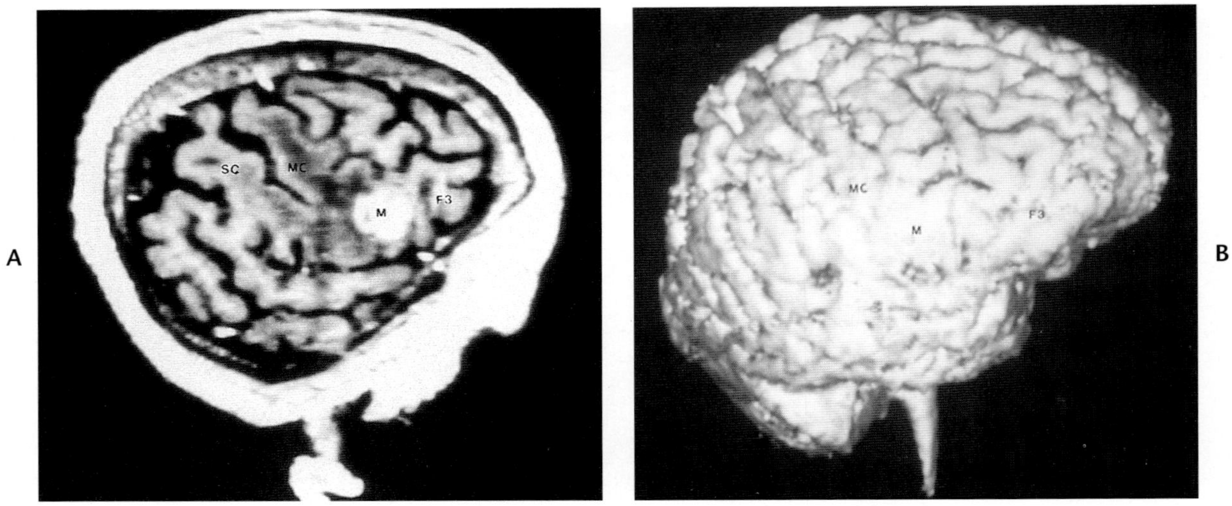

Figure 17-4. A, Tangential multiplanar image display of metastasis *(M)* at junction of inferior frontal gyrus *(F3)* and motor cortex *(MC)*. **B,** 3DSR of the same patient. The multiplanar image display more clearly shows the relationship of the lesion to the rolandic structures. Motor cortex can be recognized by its characteristic relationship to sensory cortex *(SC)*.

sented with left facial seizures (Fig. 17-4). The multiplanar image display generated by the SNS more clearly shows the location of the lesion with respect to functional anatomy and requires only a single enhanced MRI data acquisition. The motor cortex can be recognized by its characteristic relationship to the sensory cortex.

Case 3. This tangential multiplanar image display suggested that the posterior portion of this low-grade glioma extended into the inferior portion of the motor strip (Fig. 17-5, A). Intraoperative recordings using strip electrodes (Fig. 17-5, B) to stimulate and record somatosensory evoked potentials (Fig. 17-5, C) confirmed these anatomic inferences. Speech dominance had been defined earlier by intracarotid amobarbital testing.

Case 4. This 35-year-old man had undergone previous resection, radiation therapy, and brachytherapy for a superior right parietal glioblastoma. A 3DSR of the brain showed excellent representation of the surface anatomy on the left, unoperated side, but the anatomy (tumor, motor, and sensory strips) on the right was obscured by edema and gliosis (Fig. 17-6, A). A tangential multiplanar image display through this area, however, clearly showed the enhancing tumor and the parallel dark edematous white matter patterns of the pre- and postcentral gyri (Fig. 17-6, *B*).

Case 5. The single unexpected complication occurred in this 65-year-old woman in whom a left frontal glioblastoma had been thought to occupy the middle frontal gyrus. She awoke with severe Broca's aphasia that was permanent. The lesion actually involved a portion of inferior frontal gyrus (Fig. 17-7), but this case confirms that anatomic inference of speech localization alone may be hazardous.

A

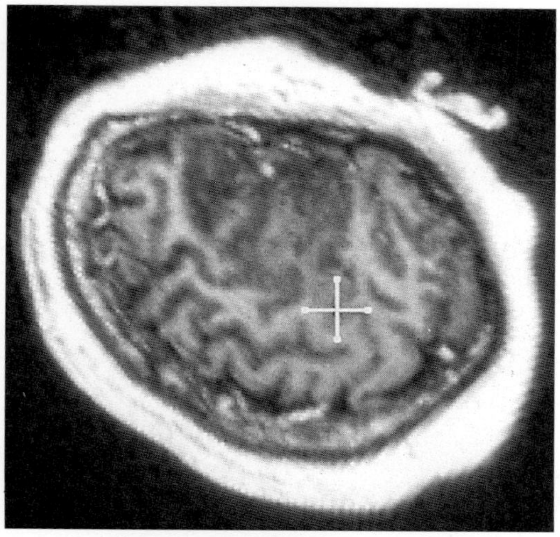

Figure 17-5. A, Tangential multiplanar image display suggested that the posterior portion of this low-grade glioma extended into the inferior portion of the motor strip. **B,** Intraoperative recordings using strip electrodes were used to stimulate the cortex and record somatosensory evoked potentials. Electrodes 1 and 2 are over the motor strip. **C,** Somatosensory evoked potentials confirmed the anatomic inferences derived from multiplanar image display.

B

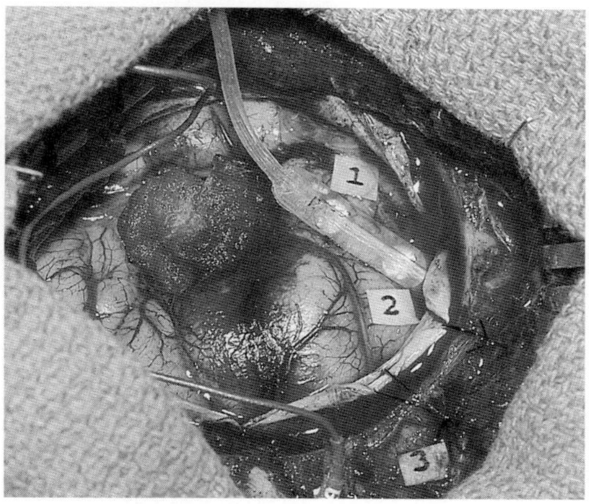

C

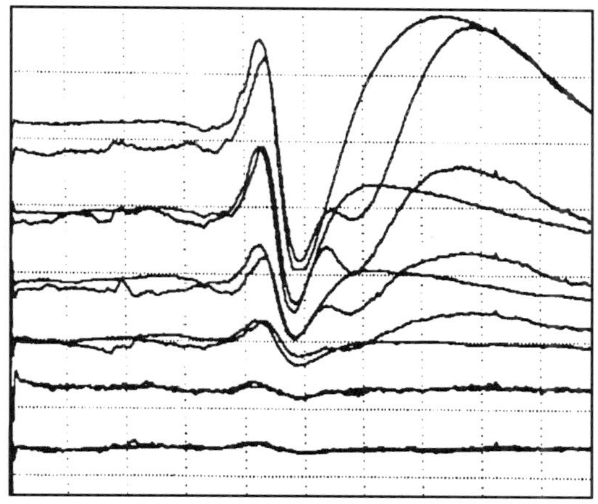

A

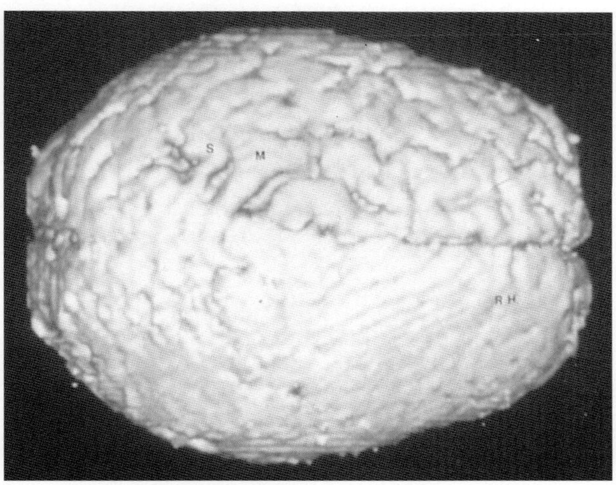

B

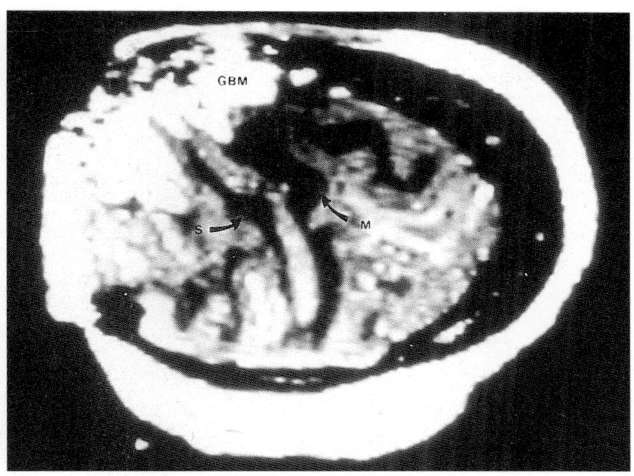

Figure 17-6. Large recurrent glioblastoma *(GBM)* involving right superior motor *(M)* and sensory *(S)* strips and superior parietal lobe. **A,** Although cortical surface of left hemisphere is well visualized on 3DSR, virtually all structures on the right hemisphere *(RH)* are obscured because of previous surgery, radiation therapy, and edema. **B,** Definition of tumor to functional anatomy is much better appreciated on the multiplanar image display. The rolandic structures are well defined by edematous (dark) white matter.

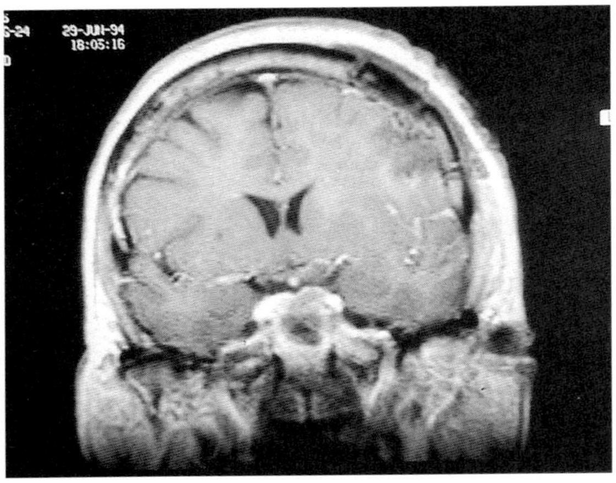

Figure 17-7. An unexpected expressive aphasia occurred in this patient after surgery. The lesion was interpreted preoperatively to lie exclusively within middle frontal gyrus, but it actually involved inferior speech areas as well.

DISCUSSION

Common planar CT or MRI often allows determination of surface anatomic features.[24] Transverse and sagittal studies may show the central sulcus and rolandic structures, and coronal displays can show the major divisions of the frontal, parietal, and temporal lobes. These limited imaging planes, however, have proved to be unreliable indicators of anatomic function when edema or masses intrude on them.[5,15] My experience suggests that in many cases multiplanar image displays can provide useful information about brain surface anatomy without being affected by lesions or edema and is equal or superior to 3DSR. However, unlike 3DSR, which in this case required more than one acquisition of data, multiplanar image displays require only a contrast-enhanced volume study that is routine in surgical navigation.[21,22] Today's complex image-processing techniques may be able to produce elegant autosegmentation of cortical and subcortical structures using complex algorithms, but many techniques still require multiple image acquisitions. Multiplanar image display by some SNSs requires no additional image processing[21,22] and can be used to infer the locations of primary motor, sensory, and to a limited degree speech areas before or during surgery.

Previous surgery appears to degrade conventional image interpretation due to gliosis and obliteration of sulcal cerebrospinal fluid spaces. Local brain edema was observed to produce similar distortions. Although 3DSR of the cortex was typically uninterpretable in these settings, the multiplanar image display was uniformly able to show the motor/sensory complex. In some cases subcortical edema actually enhanced the display of these surface features.

Electrophysiology confirmed the primary and sensory cortex anatomy as inferred by multiplanar image display in all cases as well as speech areas in selected cases. Although labor intensive, such motor stimulation and sensory recording techniques remain the gold standard by which newer noninvasive functional imaging studies are assessed.[2,10,23,25] Unfortunately, neither standard electrophysiology nor these imaging techniques provide much useful information on the relationship between the function of subcortical tracts and lesions.

Although most patients in this series had rapidly growing primary or metastatic lesions, several had low-grade glial neoplasms and meningiomas. None of these insidious lesions appeared to affect the location of functional anatomy. Although normal anatomy was at times *displaced* by mass effect, in no case was function relocated. The number of cases in this study is so small that results should be interpreted with caution. These findings are in contrast to some recent reports of cortical plasticity in adults; however, the cases reported usually resulted from significant peripheral deafferentation or childhood injuries to the central nervous system.[14,18,19] There is little compelling evidence that *clinically significant* cortical functional reorganization occurs when central lesions are acquired in adulthood.

Functional imaging promises to become more readily available as new investigational techniques evolve. Many, if not all, of these methods have been or could be merged with SNS technology to enhance definition of cortical brain function. PET has been shown to accurately map motor, speech, visual, and even higher cognitive function.[3,4] Lack of availability and poor spatial resolution have limited its use, however. Functional MRI appears to be an exciting technology capable of spatially mapping motor, visual, and receptive speech with good resolution.[3-5,8-11,25] However, it appears to measure flow and not function, it may not be sensitive in the presence of tumor,[9] and motor speech is not reliably assessed due to head movement. Nonetheless it may become the most widely available functional imaging method because it can usually be performed on high-field MRI devices. Transcranial magnetic stimulation may prove complementary to functional MRI.[16,17] Functional mapping using magnetoencephalography or magnetic source imaging is extremely elegant and overcomes most of the technical problems that limit functional MRI[12-15]; however, the high cost of the equipment is likely to prohibit its widespread adoption unless it proves clearly superior to these other techniques.

SUMMARY

This series suggests that the tangential multiplanar image display produced by some SNSs may allow accurate inference of functionally eloquent cortex. This relationship appears particularly strong for motor and sensory cortex, more so than for speech. In many cases this information may obviate the need for more rigorous testing of function using invasive or esoteric noninvasive methods. In other cases it may alert the surgeon to pursue functional MRI, transcranial stimulation, electrophysiologic mapping, or awake craniotomy.

None of the patients in this series were children. Any conclusions should not be extended to pediatric neurosurgical patients since brain function is known to be more plastic in this group.

References

1. Penfield W, Jasper H. Functional localization in the cerebral cortex. In Epilepsy and the Functional Anatomy of the Human Brain. Boston: Little, Brown, 1954, pp 41-155.
2. Luders H, Lesser RP, Dinner DS, Morris HH, Hahn JF, Friedman L, Skipper G, Wyllie E, Friedman D. Commentary: Chronic intracranial recording and stimulation with subdural electrodes. In Engel J Jr, ed. Surgical Treatment of the Epilepsies. New York: Raven Press, 1987, pp 297-321.
3. Ramsey NF, Kirkby BS, Van Gelderen P, Berman KF, Duyn JH, Frank JA, Mattay VS, Van Horn JD, Esposito G, Moonen CT, Weinberger DR. Functional mapping of human sensorimotor cortex with 3D BOLD fMRI correlates highly with H2(15)O PET rCBF. J Cereb Blood Flow Metab 16:755-764, 1996.

4. Scheifer U, Skalej M, Kolb R, Grodd W, Ahle M, Herzog H. Cerebral activity during visual stimulation: A positron emission tomography and functional magnetic resonance imaging study. Ger J Ophthalmol 5:109-117, 1996.
5. Binder JR, Rao SM, Hammeke TA, Yetkin FZ, Jesmanowicz A, Bandettini PA, Wong EC, Estkowski LD, Goldstein MD, Haughton VM, et al. Functional magnetic resonance imaging of human auditory cortex. Ann Neurol 35:662-672, 1994.
6. Bucholz RD. The central sulcus and surgical planning. AJNR 14:926-927, 1993.
7. Cao Y, Towle VL, Levin DN, Balter JM. Functional mapping of human motor cortical activation with conventional MR imaging at 1.5 T. J Magn Reson Imaging 3:869-875, 1993.
8. Fried I, Nenov V, Ojemann SG, Woods RP. Functional MR and PET imaging of rolandic and visual cortices for neurosurgical planning. J Neurosurg 83:854-861, 1995.
9. Mueller WM, Yetkin FZ, Hammeke TA, Morris GL III, Swanson SJ, Reichert K, Cox R, Haughton VM. Functional magnetic resonance imaging mapping of the motor cortex in patients with cerebral tumors. Neurosurgery 39:515-520, 1996.
10. Roberts TP, Zusman E, McDermott M, Barbaro N, Rowley HA. Correlation of functional magnetic source imaging with intraoperative cortical stimulation in neurosurgical patients. J Image Guid Surg 1:339-347, 1995.
11. Rueckert L, Appollonio I, Grafman J, Jezzard P, Johnson R Jr, Le Bihan D, Turner R. Magnetic resonance imaging functional activation of left frontal cortex during covert word production. J Neuroimaging 4:67-70, 1994.
12. Ganslandt O, Steinmeier R, Kober H, Vieth J, Kassubek J, Romstock J, Strauss C, Fahlbusch R. Magnetic source imaging combined with image-guided frameless stereotaxy: A new method in surgery around the motor strip. Neurosurgery 41:621-628, 1997.
13. Kamada K, Takeuchi F, Kuriki S, Oshiro O, Houkin K, Abe H. Functional neurosurgical stimulation with brain surface magnetic resonance images and magnetoencephalography. Neurosurgery 33:269-273, 1993.
14. Mogilner A, Grossman JA, Ribary U, Joliot M, Volkmann J, Rapaport D, Beasley RW, Llinas RR. Somatosensory cortical plasticity in adult humans revealed by magnetoencephalography. Proc Natl Acad Sci USA 90:3593-3597, 1993.
15. Sobel DF, Gallen CC, Schwartz BJ, Waltz TA, Copeland B, Yamada S, Hirschkoff EC, Bloom FE. Locating the central sulcus: Comparison of MR anatomic and magnetoencephalographic functional methods. AJNR 14:915-925, 1993.
16. Krings T, Buchbinder BR, Butler WE, Chiappa KH, Jiang HJ, Cosgrove GR, Rosen BR. Functional magnetic resonance imaging and transcranial magnetic stimulation: Complementary approaches in the evaluation of cortical motor function. Neurology 48:1406-1416, 1997.
17. Urban PP, Hopf HC, Fleischer S, Zorowka PG, Muller-Forell W. Impaired corticobulbar tract function in dysarthria due to hemispheric stroke. Functional testing using transcranial magnetic stimulation. Brain 120(Pt6):1077-1084, 1997.
18. Pons TP, Garraghty PE, Ommaya AK, Kaas JH, Taub E, Mishkin M. Massive cortical reorganization after sensory deafferentation in adult macaques. Science 252:1857-1860, 1991.
19. Ramachandran VS, Stewart M, Rogers-Ramachandran DC. Perceptual correlates of massive cortical reorganization. Neuroreport 3:583-586, 1992.
20. Alexander E III, Kooy HM, van Herk M, Schwartz M, Barnes PD, Tarbell N, Mulkern RV, Holupka EJ, Loeffler JS. Magnetic resonance image-directed stereotactic neurosurgery: Use of image fusion with computerized tomography to enhance spatial accuracy. J Neurosurg 82:271-276, 1995.
21. Barnett GH, Kormos DW, Steiner CP, Weisenberger J. Use of a frameless, armless stereotactic wand for brain tumor localization with two-dimensional and three-dimensional neuroimaging. Neurosurgery 33:674-678, 1993.
22. Barnett GH, Kormos DW, Steiner CP, Weisenberger J. Intraoperative localization using an armless, frameless stereotactic wand [Technical note]. J Neurosurg 78:510-514, 1993.
23. Wood CC, Spencer DD, Allison T, McCarthy G, Williamson PD, Goff WR. Localization of human sensorimotor cortex during surgery by cortical surface recording of somatosensory evoked potentials. J Neurosurg 68:99-111, 1988.
24. Iwasaki S, Nakagawa H, Fukusumi A, Kichikawa K, Kitamura K, Otsuji H, Uchida H, Ohishi H, Yaguchi K, Sumie H, et al. Identification of pre- and postcentral gyri on CT and MR images on the basis of the medullary pattern of cerebral white matter. Radiology 179:207-213, 1991.
25. Jack CR Jr, Thompson RM, Butts RK, Sharbrough FW, Kelly PJ, Hanson DP, Riederer SJ, Ehman RL, Hangiandreou NJ, Cascino GD. Sensory motor cortex: Correlation of presurgical mapping with functional MR imaging and invasive cortical mapping. Radiology 190:85-92, 1994.

18

Intraoperative Magnetic Resonance Imaging

Eben Alexander III, M.D. • Ron Kikinis, M.D.
Peter M. Black, M.D., Ph.D. • Ferenc A. Jolesz, M.D.

The neurosurgeon's knowledge of normal and pathologic anatomy is key to successful visual guidance. Because of the relative visual homogeneity of the brain, the neurosurgeon has far fewer anatomic landmarks to guide him than surgeons operating in other regions of the body. This challenge has inspired the development of stereotactic techniques to accurately guide the neurosurgeon.

Over the past five decades a variety of stereotaxy frames and imaging modalities have been developed to assist the neurosurgeon. Skull x-ray films, pneumoencephalography, and arteriography were some of the imaging modalities originally used for operative guidance. More recently, three-dimensional anatomic structural information has been derived from CT and MRI. The attached stereotaxy frame has been used to guide a probe (e.g., biopsy needle, lesioning electrode, and laser guide) to the target point. Stereotaxy frames use geometric paradigms to guide the neurosurgeon to the imaged target from prescribed entry points.

Recent technical developments have bypassed the frame by physically linking computerized three-dimensional image reconstructions to the patient in the operating room through the use of registration fiducials or surface anatomy (frameless stereotactic systems). Passive arms and wands (e.g., the ISG wand and The Operating Arm) provide spatial information in a robust fashion for definition of multiple sites. These points are then mapped onto the preoperative imaging space for display both preoperatively (for surgical planning) and intraoperatively (with multidimensional displays on a cathode ray tube monitor beside the operating table).

With both frame and frameless techniques, image acquisition occurs prior to the biopsy or resection, which in most cases is accomplished in the operating room some distance from the imaging device. Soft tissue positional shifts during actual lesion resection greatly degrade the fidelity of the image data relative to physical reality during the procedure. The problem is that such techniques rely on preoperatively acquired imaging data that can rapidly change once a procedure has begun. Thus the principal shortcoming of conventional frame and frameless systems is that the images are derived from preoperatively acquired image data. Significant anomalies such as failure to obtain diagnostic tissue may necessitate starting the entire procedure over, from patient transport to revised imaging.

The use of three-dimensional computerized models of MR images has enhanced neurosurgical planning for both frame and frameless neurosurgery. Three-dimensional MRI and CT reconstructions using frameless stereotactic systems enhance the surgeon's visualization during neurosurgical procedures.[1-10] With these imaging modalities, detailed three-dimensional computer models of the patient's head can permit a virtual reality (or more appropriately, enhanced reality) approach for preoperative planning and surgical procedures.

INTRAOPERATIVE SYSTEM

The Departments of Surgery (Neurosurgery) and Radiology of the Brigham and Women's Hospital (affiliated with Harvard Medical School) collaborated with scientists from General Electric Medical Imaging Systems to design and build a research surgical suite with a prototype open MRI scanner for interventional radiologic and surgical procedures (Fig. 18-1). The prototype GE Signa Advantage SP system was installed at the Brigham and Women's Hospital in January 1994. This was designed to assess the feasibility of real-time MRI during major open operative procedures.[11-13]

This system is a 0.5-tesla high-resolution whole body interventional imaging system. It was designed to allow space for a surgeon and assistant to perform major surgical procedures on the patient in the imaging field (Fig. 18-2). MR-induced radiofrequency (RF) signals from the body are enhanced through reconstruction techniques to provide multiplanar and, after image processing, three-

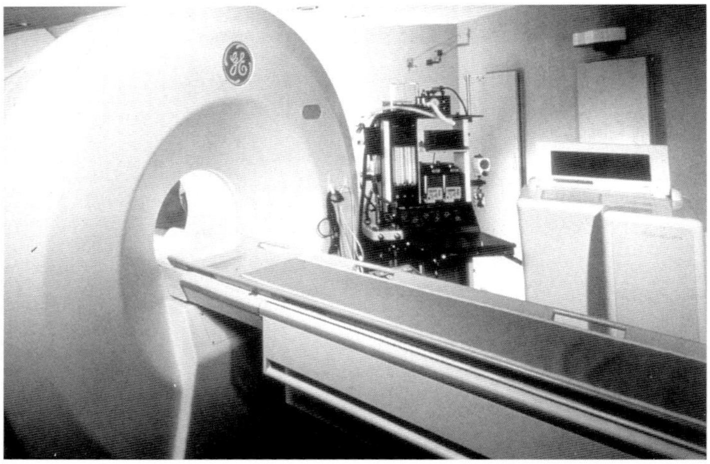

Figure 18-1. One of the two large tori is seen, with the patient couch entering the axis (standard for most cases). The fully MRI-compatible anesthesia machine and surgical instrument cabinet are seen on the right.

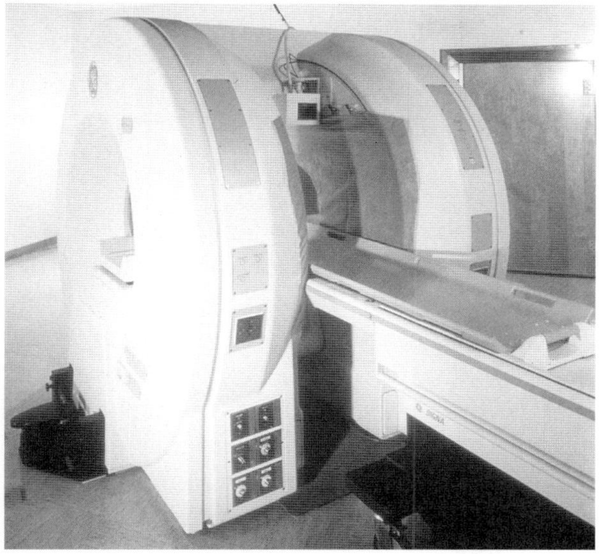

Figure 18-2. View through the tori shows the patient couch docked perpendicular to standard, giving room directly over the patient's head for the surgeon only. The couch occupies the assistant's position. This is useful for very large patients (coat size >50). The two large tori of the GE MRT system, standing on edge, are seen. The liquid crystal display screen is visible between them, above the operative field.

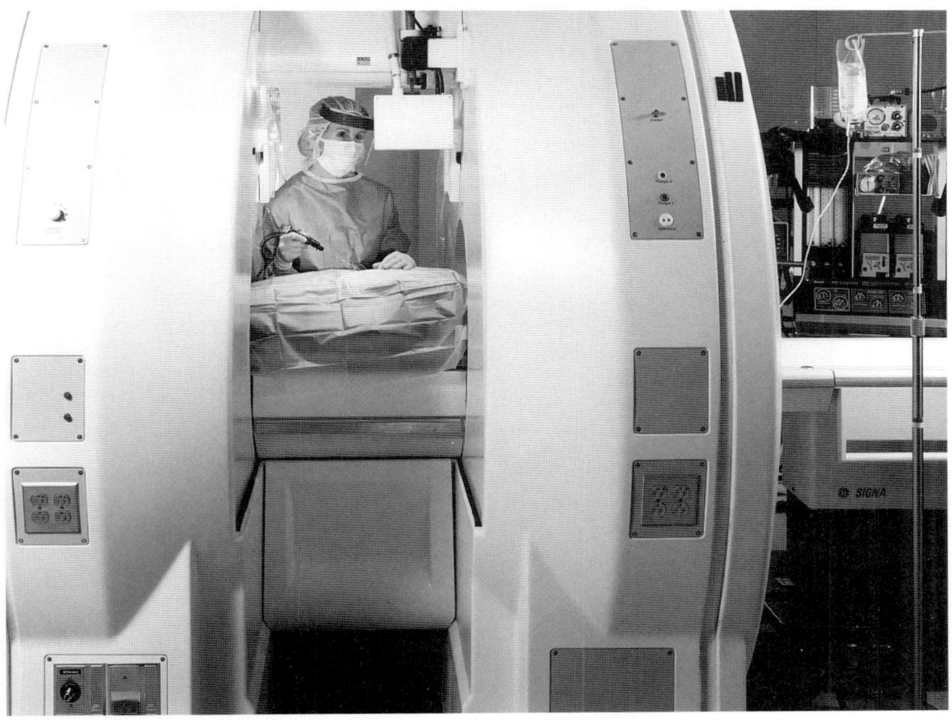

Figure 18-3. Patient being positioned down the axis of the two tori. The surgeon has access to the patient from the right, and an assistant has similar access to the patient from the opposite side. The surgeon holds Pixsys pointer (LED linked to overhead video cameras to precisely localize the pointer and biopsy vector). The respirator is visible to the right, behind the patient couch.

dimensional images of the patient's anatomic structures. This unique open-magnet configuration improves patient positioning options and allows easy access to the patient during operative procedures. The system was designed to permit good image quality with short scan times and access to the surgical field. It is currently the interventional MRI system with the best combination of high-field strength and surgical access.

The basic design of the imaging magnet was revised into two large parallel torus-shaped magnets placed side by side. This represents the arrangement that gives the surgeon and an assistant the best manual access while preserving image resolution. The patient couch may be positioned through the central openings of the two magnets (Fig. 18-3) or brought in between them (although the latter arrangement does not permit space for the assistant). Combined with specially designed flexible surface coils the system offers image resolution similar to the standard 0.5-tesla Signa system from GE. Redesign and manufacture of many of the instruments used for intracranial procedures has been a major component of the overall project.

SYSTEM DESIGN

The Signa Advantage SP system uses shielded gradient coils and power supplies with low-noise digital RF transceivers and frequency synthesizers: both surface flex coils (linear drive/transmit/receive) and a Quadrature drive transmit/receive head coil are available for imaging. The patient couch may be docked in either the axial position through the tori or in a transverse position between the two tori from the side.

The superconducting 0.5-tesla magnet is designed for whole body imaging. Passive shimming enables fine tuning as well as long-term stability of magnetic homogeneity throughout the 30 cm diameter spherical imaging volume (homogeneity 15 ppm throughout the volume). The bore diameter is 55 cm, with a gap between the two tori of 56 cm (some models have a 60 cm gap, but production costs were significantly higher).

The upper service module above the visualization space contains a laser alignment light, three-scan plane pointer charge-coupled device (CCD) video cameras, two table side image displays (liquid crystal) that provide real-time scanning information to the operating physician and assistant, and a patient observation camera and lighting. Standard cathode ray tube display monitors are incompatible with the magnetic field, although they are used in the technician control area.

A built-in intercom system within the magnet enclosure allows communication between the surgeon, the assistant, the patient (if awake), and the operator at the console outside the treatment room. The acoustic environment involves levels of approximately 85 decibels during active scanning, which necessitates intercom communications.

The patient transport table consists of a contoured cradle with a fixed table height. Guard rails double as IV injector boards and arm support and security rails. This couch supports patients weighing up to 300 pounds. The table is designed to be rigidly docked to the magnet subsystem in either the axial or side orientation but can hold a patient whether or not it is docked to the magnet. The connecting latch makes the table easily removable from the treatment area, which simplifies patient loading in routine and emergency situations.

The gradient subsystem of the Signa Advantage SP system offers a minimum slice thickness of 3.0 mm for two-dimensional and 0.7 mm for three-dimensional resolution. The minimum echo time is 2.5 msec with a millimeter field of view of 4 cm diameter.

The digital RF transceiver permits proton imaging at 21 MHz for 0.5-tesla field strength. The synthesizer eliminates RF-induced phase error image artifacts. A Quadrature drive transmit/receive head coil is available with an inner diameter of 28 cm. This has the advantage of an improved signal-to-noise ratio compared with similar linear coils that reduces imaging time. The RF power monitor has a preprogrammed rate of power deposition per kilogram of patient body weight that limits the power levels.

In addition to the head coil, transmit/flex coils are designed for proton imaging in this system. These coils are specifically designed to maximize the signal-to-noise ratio and enhance overall imaging capabilities through the use of small field of view thin slice imaging and to enhance the surgeon's access to the patient through a wide range of positioning and coil placement scenarios. These flex coils are designed to wrap around specific regions of anatomy following the natural curvature of the body surface. These coils are compatible with all Signa Advantage SP system pulse sequences and appropriate imaging options. The current image display processor allows for four on one image display with up to 256 gray scale levels on any one image.

DEFINITION OF IMAGE ORIENTATION

The stereotactic navigating (Pixsys) device is an essential component of the system. This optical tracking system was built directly into the intraoperative MRI system to allow a light-emitting diode (LED)–based navigational system to visualize the homogeneous volume of the magnetic field as a three-dimensional mapping space. The interactive scan plane locator uses a Pixsys system with triple CCD cameras to define multiplanar images of anatomic structures. The three CCD cameras are mounted in the overhead beam between the two superconducting magnet tori, allowing unobstructed visualization of the entire imaging space and operating area. LEDs on various instruments and localizer devices provide specific spatial information to the CCD cameras. With this Pixsys localization system, different instruments and structures (including the patient) within the imaging space provide spatial information to be correlated with the MRI anatomic data. The hand-held pointer with LEDs is designed to move freely through the imaging space to define anatomy and interactively define scan planes on a real-time basis. It may also be locked in position on a flexible surgical support arm.

Software analysis using an interactive Sun 4/670 workstation permits the location of these LEDs to be pinpointed within the three-dimensional operating space. When it is used in conjunction with image acquisition, the surgeon achieves near real-time localization. The system has provided precise navigation in which the tracking tip has been accurate within 1 mm.

Orientation of scans is controlled in real time by the operating physician or assistant. The slice thickness is changed interactively through the operator. Acquisition modes included two-dimensional standard multislice imaging up to 120 slice locations (256 × 256 pixel). In addition, three-dimensional volume imaging includes 12 through 124 slice locations in a gradient echo mode, depending on the pulse sequence.

IMAGE ACQUISITION

Images are obtained in axial, sagittal, coronal, oblique, or double oblique planes through a defined point in the imaging space using a wide variety of pulse sequences. The surgeon easily defines images in any desired plane relative to regions of interest and various approach vectors through interactive scan plane control with the hand-held Pixsys unit.

Image acquisition leads to reconstruction using two-dimensional and three-dimensional Fourier transformation techniques. The current software allows scan plane definition along the axis of the pointer in horizontal and vertical planes as well as in planes perpendicular to that axis. In addition, standard orthogonal sagittal, coronal, and axial images are defined through a specific point along the axis of the pointing device.

There are several noteworthy advantages of the current Signa Advantage SP system for intraoperative MR visualization. The pulse sequences available are listed as follows:

Two-dimensional recovery
Two-dimensional spin echo
Two-dimensional sequential gradient echo and three-dimensional volume acquisition
Two-dimensional multiplanar gradient recalled
Two-dimensional and three-dimensional spoiled gradient recalled
Three-dimensional steady-state, free precession
Two-dimensional time of flight
Three-dimensional time of flight including magnetization transfer
Three-dimensional multislab

Several enhancements are compatible with the various pulse sequences available: flow and respiratory compensation, electrocardiographic and peripheral pulse gating, explicit and graphic saturation, fat/water (spectral) saturation, image intensity correction, phase and frequency offset, etc.

In the two-dimensional mode a 3 to 20 mm slice thickness in 0.1 mm increments is available depending on the pulse sequence used. This includes an interleave option for multislice imaging. For the three-dimensional mode, 12 through 124 contiguous slice volume imaging with 0.7 to 5.0 mm slice thickness in 0.1 mm increments is available. The field of view ranges from 4 to 30 cm in 1 cm increments, which is continuous in all planes. The system offers the ability to scan off-

Advantages of the GE Signa SP System

1. A 0.5-tesla magnetic field, which is the highest of any "open" or interventional MRI system
2. Ample wide, vertical access to patient, allowing major surgical procedures
3. Interactive scan plane control to register images to surgical/interventional devices in the control of the surgeon (may replace conventional stereotactic blind approaches in several settings)
4. Front entry/side entry and vertical (sitting capabilities, used especially for dynamic spinal imaging) patient positioning possible
5. Integrated surgical services (lighting, anesthesia, and therapy devices such as Nd:YAG laser, high-speed cranial drill, and Selector ultrasonic aspirator)
6. All of the MR imaging capabilities of standard 0.5-tesla superconducting diagnostic MR system in an intraoperative setting

center and asymmetric field of views. Phase encoding is available from 128 to 512 matrix size in steps of 32, and the frequency coding is either 256 or 512.

Imaging time may be optimized to adjusting fractional (0.5, 0.75, or 1.5) or multiple number of excitations (multiple number of excitations of 1 to 150) when using imaging techniques with a defined contrast (repetitive time), resolution (matrix), and signal-to-noise ratio. The advanced display package offers interactive three-dimensional reformatting of planar images to create images in any defined plane at any angle. This package provides up to 256 stored images for paging mode, which also allows for a temporal and spatial loop with multiple display of up to four windows.

INSTRUMENTATION ISSUES

There are several technical limitations to working within a magnetic field. The principal limitation relates to avoiding the use of any ferromagnetic materials because of the risk that such objects would be strongly attracted by the powerful magnetic field, leading to free-flying metal missiles in the field. Nonferromagnetic materials such as aluminum, copper, bronze, titanium, and ceramics must be incorporated into the magnetic operating room instrument environment. Series 300 stainless steel instruments may be used for parts of a procedure, although significant imaging artifacts are seen. Many of these compatible materials create significant imaging distortions and artifacts that must be considered in assessing their suitability in a given surgical setting. Instrument design includes a full set of MRI-compatible materials, including a ceramic scalpel, appropriate drills and rongeurs, a modified brain biopsy needle (e.g., titanium, aluminum carbide, or carbon fiber), bipolar coagulation devices, ultrasonic aspirator, and suture needles. In addition, equipment used for anesthesia, coagulation, high-speed drilling, monitoring, etc. had to be redesigned for the MRI environment. The head-holder was modeled on the three-point fixation system used in standard neurosurgical operating rooms. This unit, with a base that is fixed to the movable MRI patient table, needed to be designed to fit within the core of the magnet, accurately hold the patient in the desired position, and allow for adjustments as required.

An MRI-compatible microscope was developed and has been used intraoperatively at the Brigham and Women's Hospital since June 1996. The microscope is configured to fit between the magnets and over the shoulder of the surgeon. It has a mobile stand and is pneumatically driven. This allows for fine control with a mouth clutch. A beam splitter for intraoperative video and two-dimensional or three-dimensional reconstruction image presentation is being developed. Imaging is easily performed with the microscope in position in the field.

An MRI-compatible nonirrigating bipolar coagulator was originally provided by Codman. Currently a Codman gravity irrigating system is being used. The MRI-compatible drill was designed in collaboration with Midas Rex, Inc. Ohmeda developed an MRI-compatible ventilator and associated anesthesia equipment. Patient monitoring devices were obtained from Bruker. Preliminary work is being done with surgical endoscopes (rigid endoscopes and camera and light source) and flexible endoscopes.

Sterile surgical draping materials were designed by Baxter, Inc. These surgical drapes and sterile instrument pockets (to prevent excessive passage of instruments in and out of the operative field) are affixed to the internal aspects of the magnet where the surgeon is positioned, allowing 360-degree sterile fields around the surgeon and the assistant. This provides a sterile operating environment equivalent to that found in conventional operating rooms and suitable for major operative procedures.

SOFTWARE CONFIGURATION

Present Software

Currently high-speed graphic and general-purpose computers, a Connection Machine CM-2, and an IBM PVS coarse parallel processor are used to segment and register MRI data sets using a Pixsys triple CCD imaging system to correlate MRI spatial information with the system's spatial environment. The Signa Advantage SP system has immediate implications for accessing anatomic points in real time for purposes of biopsy or functional lesioning. It also holds tremendous promise for complex neurosurgical resections, especially for infiltrative tumors or those with intimate attachments to critical neural and vascular structures, as well as for operative resection elsewhere in the body. It offers the promise of excellent anatomic structure definition throughout the operative field with real-time updates of critical surgical anatomy.

The current software configuration consists of MR images in planes either along the axis of the Pixsys pointer probe (default orientation is closest to horizontal) or perpendicular to that axis at a user-defined distance from the probe tip. Standard axial, sagittal, and coronal images may also be displayed through a point defined by the surgeon with the hand-held pointer. These images are displayed in a liquid crystal screen in the visual field of the operating surgeon and the assistant. The probe path and annotated extension may be visualized on the MR image. A Buckwalter arm is currently used to stabilize the probe once the path has been selected. A calibration sequence is used to verify the registration accuracy of the Pixsys localizer with the three-dimensional orientation of the MR images.

The Surgical Planning Laboratory at the Brigham and Women's Hospital and Harvard Medical School has developed a prototype system of video registration that allows alignment of three-dimensional physical space in the operating room with the three-dimensional reconstructed MR images.[1,2,6] A laser registration technique allows high-resolution surface mapping to align the patient's physical surface with that of the patient's reconstructed MR image.[3-5] We have also incorporated SPECT images through computerized image fusion to provide additional information for surgical guidance.[14] Additional preoperative information such as pertinent neuroanatomy from functional MRI or transcranial magnetic stimulation[15] offers high-resolution motor, visual, or speech localization in a given patient.

Future Software Development

The main thrust of current development involves a highly sophisticated system for image reconstruction with a virtual reality presentation, giving the surgeon all of the anatomic information needed to safely resect a given lesion without sensory overload. Complex preoperative data sets consisting of MRI, CT, SPECT, and PET as well as functional information from magnetic source imaging, vector evoked responses, and/or magnetic stimulation of motor pathways may all be combined into a functional-anatomic data set that is manipulated as surgery progresses using high-resolution MRI updating of the spatial-anatomic information generated preoperatively. Technical development of a display that offers magnified three-dimensional imaging that corresponds with the surgeon's field of view while operating is a major challenge.

Although the Signa Advantage SP system was designed to provide significant enhancement of open surgical resections, these simple point-related functions (biopsy, electrode placement for recording and functional lesions, etc.) will be improved using real-time visualization. Combination of this global multimodality real-time imaging system with the magnification and minimally invasive capabilities of flexible endoscopes will offer sophisticated guidance for small surgical robots that use ultrasonic aspiration and laser capabilities to resect tumors without the need for open craniotomy.

Thermal Lesioning

This system also has the ability to display tissue temperature as an image contrast parameter. This significant capability allows surgeons to monitor and control thermal ablation using laser, RF or focused ultrasound heating, or cryogenic cooling to create central nervous system lesions or perform tumor ablation.

Hynynen et al.[16] determined the feasibility of temperature-sensitive MRI for the detection of local temperature elevations at the focus of a low-power ultrasound beam in the rabbit brain. Acoustic power levels were sonicated at 3.5 to

17.5 watts. MR images were obtained 2 hours, 48 hours, 10 days, and 23 days after the sonications. Forty of 43 (93%) of the lowest power (3.5 watts) sonications were visible on temperature-sensitive MR images of brain in 28 rabbits and did not result in any short- or long-term histologic or MRI evidence of tissue damage. A contrast-to-noise ratio of approximately 6 and a temperature elevation of 7° to 8° C were observed. They concluded that temperature elevations induced by means of focused ultrasound exposures that do not cause damage in the in vivo rabbit brain can be detected on temperature-sensitive MRI. This imaging is not possible with other direct or indirect (x-ray, ultrasound, or CT) imaging techniques. The higher field strength of this system (0.5 tesla) makes it more suitable for more demanding tasks than other interventional MRI systems currently available.

NEUROSURGICAL EXPERIENCE

The system is optimal for frameless stereotactic biopsies using the optical digitizer, which allows interactive image plane acquisition and image updating on a scale approaching real time. The scanner is similar to a standard GE Signa scanner in that it runs the same software and includes a torus-shaped magnet. The principal difference lies in the scanner's field of view, which lies midway between two torus-shaped superconducting magnets separated by two steel beams. The two magnets combined produce a 0.5-tesla magnetic field that can produce images equal in quality to many commercially available medical scanners. The area between the two magnets can be draped sterilely and used as an operative field.

Intraoperative lesion localization for biopsy or resection, for example, is simple without the use of a frame. Catheterization of slitlike ventricles is likewise easily accomplished. Accomplishment of such surgical goals as complete tumor resection, correct ventricular catheter placement, total disc fragment removal, and the like can be confirmed by intraoperative imaging. Biopsy of subtle pathologic conditions visible only with MRI, often associated with subtle pathologic findings, is safer than with frame-based systems because the needle is visualized at the precise target location. One thus avoids the necessity of acquiring additional tissue samples (with the risk of additional sampling) for frozen section to confirm needle position, which is often problematic with frame-based systems. In addition, the promise of such techniques as intraoperative functional imaging of the brain, image-guided endoscopic laser resection, or focused ultrasound destruction of tumors emerge as possible future applications.

The value of this system becomes quite evident during difficult neurosurgical tumor resections, especially of infiltrative tumors bordering on critical neurologic structures. Critical blood vessels or the ventricular system can easily be avoided (with 1 mm accuracy) with real-time visualization. Difficult deep resections are readily performed because of the ease of image acquisition and the robust interactive definition of desired scan planes using the hand-held Pixsys pointer. A complete volumetric data set around a region of interest is obtained within 2 to 3 minutes without having to move the patient relative to the operative field. This offers a significant advantage over other interventional MRI systems, where image acquisition may take up to an hour on average and involve patient movement

Table 18-1. Neurosurgical Procedures Using the GE Signa Advantage SP System Cases at Brigham and Women's Hospital as of October 1997

Procedure	No. of Procedures
Biopsy	73
Shunt catheter/drainage/biopsy	22
Craniotomy	109
Laser tumor ablation	3
Transsphenoidal resection	5
Spinal	3
	215

out of the operative area with disruption of the sterile surgical field. Our clinical neurosurgical experience with the GE system is given in Table 18-1.

ENHANCED REALITY IN THE OPERATING ROOM

Virtual reality represents a rapidly growing field within computer science that encompasses the construction of simulated environments through computers. Since the major output of current computers has been visual or graphic, most early efforts in virtual reality have been directed at constructing visual worlds. Auditory simulation is also quite straightforward and easily incorporated into the virtual reality environment. Future developments will involve blending of other sensory modalities (e.g., tactile, olfactory, vestibular, or visceral) until one is able to completely immerse oneself in the virtual world.

How is the concept of virtual reality useful to the surgeon? By combining the wealth of signal information (e.g., MRI, CT, angiography, SPECT, PET, magnetic source imaging, magnetic stimulation cortical map data, and vector evoked responses) within one integrated three-dimensional computer model of the patient, one can greatly enhance the level of information about the surgical environment. A combination of imaging modalities offers a better understanding of the exact anatomy of a lesion and its surrounding vessels and neural pathways. One is thus able to perform more complete and safe resection or lesioning.

Virtual reality involves constructing a "real" model within the computer, and the challenge to current software engineers is to provide an effortless blend of visual presentations to the surgeon to provide the safest and most efficacious surgical intervention. Enhanced reality might be a more appropriate term for this surgical system since the computer model consists of a rich blend of information from many modalities to construct the most complete structure possible.[4,12,13]

SUMMARY

This novel technology will revolutionize several aspects of neurosurgery. Frameless stereotactic procedures can be performed under direct visualization. Intraoperative lesion localization for biopsy or resection will be readily accomplished without the use of a stereotaxy frame. In addition, the extent of tumor resection, lesioning electrode position, degree of spinal decompression, etc. can be confirmed intraoperatively in real time. The combination of the "microscopic" advantages of fiberoptic endoscopy with this "macroscopic" global visualization MRI system will offer significant enhancement of surgical orientation and analysis during operative procedures. Finally, the promise of such techniques as intraoperative functional brain imaging, image-guided laser resection (including the use of robotic agents), and focused ultrasound destruction of lesions emerge as exciting future applications.

Progress in minimally invasive techniques will follow the more widespread use of compact robotic surgical probes guided with advanced real-time imaging. Sophisticated virtual reality, supported by a robust intraoperative MRI device, offers the potential for a truly revolutionary surgical tool. Entire new vistas in neurosurgical intervention may open, mirroring the fundamental quantum leap that followed the introduction of the operating microscope a half century ago.

We are grateful to the many people whose work and dedication made the clinical implementation of this intraoperative system possible; in particular, Amir Zamani, M.D., Richard Schwartz, M.D., Liange Hsu, M.D., and Carl Winalski, M.D. (Department of Radiology), Marvin Fried, M.D., Paul Morrison (Section of ENT), George Topulos, M.D. (Department of Anaesthesia), Nobi Hata, M.D., Shin Nakajima, M.D. (Surgical Planning Laboratory), Robert Newman, Ray Kelley, and Susan Koran (GE application specialists), Angela Ruddy-Kanan, Cathy Holley, and Carol Richards (nursing staff), and Maureen Ainslee, Holley Isbister, and Cheryl Page (MRI technologists).

References

1. Wells WR III, Kikinis R, Altobelli D, Lorenson W, Ettinger G, Cline H, Gleason PL, Jolesz F. Video registration using fiducials for surgical enhanced reality. In Proceedings Fifteenth Annual Conference of the IEEE Engineering in Medical and Biological Society, 1993.
2. Gleason PL, Kikinis R, Altobelli D, Wells W, Alexander E III, Black PM, Jolesz F. Video registration virtual reality for nonlinkage stereotactic surgery. Stereotact Funct Neurosurg 63:139-143, 1994.
3. Grimson E, Lozano-Pérez T, Wells W, Ettinger G, White S, Kikinis R. An automated registration method for frameless stereotaxy, image guided surgery and enhanced reality visualization. IEEE Trans Med Imaging, 1996.
4. Jolesz FA, Shtern F. The operating room of the future. Invest Radiol 27:326-328, 1992.
5. Grimson WEL, Ettinger GJ, White SJ, Lozano-Pérez T, Wells WM, Kikinis R. An automatic registration method for frameless stereotaxy, image guided surgery, and enhanced reality visualization. IEEE Trans Med Imaging 15:129-140, 1996.
6. Cline HE, Lorenson WE, Kikinis R, Jolesz F. Three-dimensional segmentation of MR images of the head using probability and connectivity. J Comp Assist Tomogr 14:1037-1045, 1990.
7. Kikinis R, Shenton M, Jolesz FA, Gerig G, Martin J, Anderson M, Metcalf D, Guttmann C, McCarley RW, Lorenson W, Cline H. Routine quantitative analysis of brain and cerebrospinal fluid spaces with MR imaging. J MRI 2:619-629, 1992.
8. Ettinger GJ, Leventon ME, Grimson WEL, Kikinis R, Gugino V, Cote W, Sprung L, Aglio L, Shenton M, Potts G, Alexander E. Experimentation with a transcranial magnetic stimulation system for functional brain mapping. In Proceedings of CVRMed/MRCAS'97, Grenoble, France, March 1997, pp 477-486.
9. Kikinis R, Gleason PL, Moriarty TM, Moore MR, Alexander E, Stieg PE, Matsumae M, Lorenson WE, Cline HE, Black PM, Jolesz FA. Computer assisted interactive three-dimensional planning for neurosurgical procedures. Neurosurgery 38:640-651, 1996.
10. Black PM, Moriarty T, Alexander E III, Stieg P, Woodard EJ, Gleason PL, Martin CH, Kikinis R, Schwartz RB, Jolesz FA. Development and implementation of intraoperative magnetic resonance imaging and its neurological applications. Neurosurgery 41:831-842, 1997.

11. Schenck JF, Jolesz FA, Roemer PB, Cline HE, Lorenson WE, Kikinis R, Silverman SG, Hardy CJ, Barber WD, Laskaris ET, Dorri B, Newman RW, Holley CE, Collick BD, Dietz D, Mack DC, Ainslie ME, Jaskolski P, Figuera MR, von Lehn JC, Souza SP, Dumoulin CL, Darrow RD, St. Peters RL, Rohling KW, Watkins RD, Eisner DR, Blumenfeld SM, Vosburgh KG. Superconducting open configuration MRI system for image-guided therapy. Radiology 195:805-814, 1995.
12. Alexander E III, Moriarty TM, Kikinis R, Jolesz FA. Innovations in minimalism: Intraoperative MRI. Clin Neurosurg 43:338-352, 1996.
13. Moriarty TM, Kikinis R, Jolesz FA, Black PM, Alexander E III. Magnetic resonance imaging therapy: Intraoperative MR imaging. Neurosurg Clin N Am 7:323-331, 1996.
14. Schwartz RB, Holman BL, Garada BM, Carvalho PA, Folkerth R, Schwartz MS, Loeffler JS, Shrieve DC, Polak JF, Black PM, Alexander E III. Dual isotope single-photon emission computerized tomography used for prediction of histology and survival in patients after high-dose radiotherapy for malignant astrocytoma. Neurosurg Focus 1(3):1, 1996.
15. Ettinger GJ, Grimson WEL, Leventon ME, Kikinis R, Gugino V, Cote W, Karapelou M, Aglio L, Shenton M, Potts G, Alexander E. Noninvasive functional brain mapping using registered transcranial magnetic stimulation. In Proceedings of IEEE Workshop on Mathematical Methods in Biomedical Image Analysis, San Francisco, June 21-22, 1996.
16. Hynynen K, Vykhodtseva NI, Chung AH, Sorrentino V, Colucci V, Jolesz FA. Thermal effects of focused ultrasound on the brain: Determination with MR imaging. Radiology 204:247-253, 1997.

PART

IV

Socioeconomic Considerations

19

Social and Economic Impact of Surgical Navigation Systems

William E. Bingaman, M.D. • Gene H. Barnett, M.D.

Health care reform has led to an increasing demand for outcome analyses of new medical technologies. This process involves health, social, and economic outcome information gathered by a multidisciplinary team of scientists. The results will become increasingly important in determining health care resource allocation and acceptance of new technologies.[1-5]

Interactive surgical navigation systems (SNSs), also known as frameless stereotactic systems, have been developed as adjuncts to the surgical treatment of intracranial and spinal disease. Although the surgical efficacy has been established, their economic impact and effect on patient outcome remains undetermined.[6-12]

We performed a retrospective comparative review of SNS-assisted craniotomies and conventional craniotomies performed on patients with brain tumors at The Cleveland Clinic Foundation during 1992. The effect of this technology on operative time, hospital length of stay, and hospital cost—three variables related to patient outcome and cost—is presented.

BACKGROUND

Image-guided stereotactic craniotomy using frame or frameless techniques has several advantages over conventional methods of craniotomy that may favorably affect patient outcomes and cost. Accurate localization of intracranial lesions may allow for smaller craniotomies centered directly over the lesion that reduces the size of the wound and the amount of brain tissue exposed during surgery.[13-16] Similarly, accurate guidance to subcortical lesions reduces the amount of brain exploration needed, minimizing the chances of injury to surrounding brain. In addition, accurate delineation of lesion boundaries leads to faster, safer, and more complete lesion resection.[8,9,13-17] These factors may result in lower surgical morbidity and therefore reduced length of hospitalization and related costs.

Craniotomy using frame stereotaxy has several drawbacks compared with conventional techniques that has resulted in limited acceptance of this procedure. These include limited access to the patient's airway and surgical site; cumbersome logistics required for imaging, anesthesia, and surgery; patient discomfort caused by the frame; added cost in purchasing and maintaining a stereotaxy system; and limited orientation and localization information. The development of interactive SNSs not reliant on stereotaxy frames has overcome many of these limitations and increased flexibility in preoperative surgical planning.[9,12,16,18] Most important, the development of these devices has made real-time intraoperative orientation and localization possible.

Thus surgical navigation promises to become a more widely accepted and used technology in neurosurgery (and perhaps other surgical and radiologic arenas) than image-guided frame stereotaxy. Although use of this technology should improve patient outcome and reduce cost, its actual effect on these variables remains unknown. The impact on operative time remains controversial in the literature, no data exists on cost/benefit as compared with other treatment modalities, and no randomized studies on surgical outcomes have been performed.[8,9,11,12] We reviewed our early SNS experience at The Cleveland Clinic Foundation to formulate some initial answers to these questions.

STUDY DESIGN AND METHODOLOGY

The surgical benefits of SNSs are well substantiated in the literature.[9,11,12] To determine the economic impact on surgical therapy of brain tumors, we compared total hospital cost, operative time, and length of hospital stay for a group of patients treated by either conventional craniotomy or SNS-assisted craniotomy at The Cleveland Clinic Foundation from January 1992 through December 1992.

A retrospective chart review was performed for all patients treated for supratentorial brain tumors during 1992. We excluded those patients treated with frame-based stereotaxy, epilepsy procedures requiring more than one surgical procedure during the same admission for subdural mapping and resection, stereotactic biopsies without resection, and craniotomies for vascular malformations or other nonneoplastic disorders. All seven surgeons at this institution performed craniotomies during 1992, but the majority of SNS procedures were performed by one surgeon.

The SNS system used has been previously described.[6,9] In brief, the system has a sonic detector array mounted near the operative field and an ultrasonic emitter localization device. The localization device is sterilizable and fully compatible with intraoperative use. Preoperative MR imaging was typically performed. A craniotomy was considered "conventional" if frame or frameless computer-assisted techniques were not used.

Financial data were obtained from computer records of the accounting department. This included technical and operative charges during the hospital stay but excluded physician professional charges. Operative time was defined as total "cut to close" time, the time from incision to complete closure of the operative wound. This was obtained from anesthesia records. Hospital stay was defined as number of days from hospital admission to hospital discharge.

A total of 210 procedures were performed for supratentorial brain tumor during the study period. Eighty-five of these procedures were stereotactic biopsies and were excluded from analysis. Two charts were unavailable for review. One hundred twenty-three charts were reviewed, and 26 of these were excluded for reasons stated above (miscoded procedure, nonneoplastic disease, or more than one surgical procedure during the same admission). Ninety-seven procedures were included in the study. This included 48 craniotomies for primary central nervous system tumor, 27 craniotomies for meningioma, and 22 craniotomies for cerebral metastases.

TUMOR PATHOLOGY AND LOCATION

Patient information was stratified into two groups: craniotomies performed using SNS assistance and those performed using conventional techniques. These groups were then subdivided into cerebral glioma, meningioma, and cerebral metastasis categories.

Interactive surgical navigation was used in a total of 53 craniotomies. These included 26 craniotomies for cerebral glioma, 8 for meningioma, and 19 for cerebral metastasis. Forty-seven procedures were performed using conventional neurosurgical techniques. These included 22 craniotomies for primary cerebral glioma, 19 for meningioma, and 3 for cerebral metastasis.

Glioma

SNS-Assisted Surgery

In this group there were 11 cases of glioblastoma multiforme, 5 cases of anaplastic astrocytomas, 4 cases of low-grade astrocytomas, two cases each of gliosarcomas and oligodendrogliomas, and 1 case each of ganglioglioma and central neurocytoma (WHO classification).[19] The tumor involved the right parietal lobe in 8 cases, left frontal lobe in 6, right frontal lobe in 4, right temporal and left parietal lobes in 2 each, and right occipital, right occipital/temporal, bifrontal, and intraventricular locations in 1 each.

Two surgeons performed 24 cases and 2 cases, respectively. Eleven operations involved reopening a previous craniotomy site for reresection of tumor (reoperation glioma subgroup). Fifteen craniotomies were first-time resections (first operation glioma subgroup). Seven patients had received previous whole-brain radiation therapy; none had undergone stereotactic radiosurgery.

Conventional Surgery

There were 7 cases of glioblastoma multiforme, 6 cases of low-grade astrocytomas, 3 cases each of anaplastic astrocytomas and oligodendrogliomas, 2 cases of gangliogliomas, and 1 case of gliosarcoma. The tumor involved the right temporal lobe in 11 cases, left temporal lobe in 4, left frontal and right frontal lobes in 3 each, and intraventricular in 1.

Seven surgeons performed 2, 3, 4, 2, 7, 3, and 1 operation, respectively. Two craniotomies were performed as reoperations. Two patients had received previous whole-brain radiation therapy and none had undergone stereotactic radiosurgery.

Meningioma

SNS-Assisted Surgery

The tumor involved the right frontoparietal convexity, left frontal convexity, and left frontal parasagittal region in 2 cases each and the right frontal convexity and right vertex in 1 case each.

One surgeon performed all these craniotomies. One patient was having a reoperation. Seven of the meningiomas were considered of benign histology and one was a malignant brain invasion.[20]

Conventional Surgery

The tumor involved the tuberculum sellae in 4 cases, right frontal convexity and sphenoid wing in 3 cases each, left frontal convexity and left parietal convexity in 2 cases each, and right parietal convexity, right vertex, left frontal parasagittal region, olfactory groove region, and intraventricular region in 1 case each.

Seven surgeons performed 2, 2, 4, 1, 6, 2, and 2 operations, respectively. Three cases were reoperations. Eighteen meningiomas were of benign histology and one was malignant.

Metastases

SNS-Assisted Surgery

There were 12 cases of metastatic lung adenocarcinoma, 3 cases of ovarian carcinomas, 2 cases of carcinoma of the head and neck, and one case each of renal cell and breast carcinoma. The tumor involved the left frontal lobe in 5 cases, left occipital lobe and right frontal lobe in 4 each, right parietal lobe and right occipital lobe in 2 each, and right basal ganglia and left parietal lobe in 1 each.

Three surgeons performed 15, 3, and 1 operation, respectively. There were no cases of reoperative surgery. One patient has received previous whole-brain radiation therapy, and one patient had undergone stereotactic radiosurgery earlier.

Conventional Surgery

There were 2 cases of metastatic lung adenocarcinoma and 1 case of renal cell carcinoma. The tumor involved the right temporal lobe, right occipital lobe, and the left parietal lobe in 1 case each.

Three surgeons performed one operation each. There were no cases of reoperative surgery. One patient had previous whole-brain radiation therapy.

LENGTH OF STAY, HOSPITAL COST, AND OPERATIVE TIME

Table 19-1 shows the mean and median length of stay, hospital cost, and operative time for each group. The percent reduction in these variables for SNS-assisted glioma surgery as compared with conventional techniques is shown in

Table 19-1. Interactive Surgical Navigation vs. Conventional Craniotomy in the Treatment of Brain Tumors

	Glioma Surgery Subgroup		Meningioma Surgery Subgroup		Metastases Surgery Subgroup	
	SNS	Conventional	SNS	Conventional	SNS	Conventional
Length of stay (days)						
Mean	7.5	7.2	7.6	9.5	7.1	11.3
Median	7.0	7.0	5.0	7.0	4.0	9.0
Hospital cost						
Mean	$27,421	$24,569	$34,686	$36,046	$22,636	$30,915
Median	$24,462	$22,993	$19,473	$29,973	$19,259	$29,577
Operative time (min)						
Mean	237	254	167	378	159	229
Median	233	254	110	355	155	273

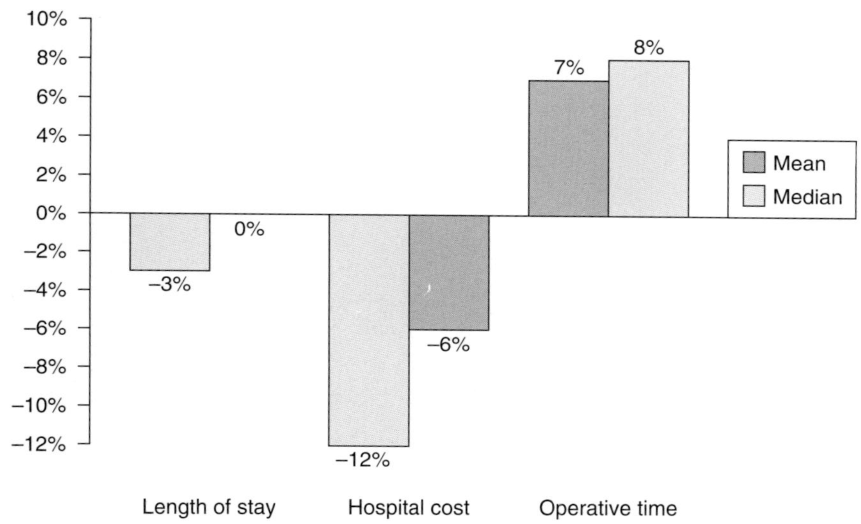

Figure 19-1. Reduction in length of stay, hospital cost, and operative time using interactive surgical navigation in glioma surgery.

Fig. 19-1. There was no effect on the length of stay, but there was a 6% increase in hospital cost and an 8% reduction in operative time (median values).

The glioma group was further broken down into reoperation and first operation categories. In the SNS glioma group there were 11 reoperations and 15 first operations. In the conventional glioma surgery group there were 2 reoperations and 20 first operations. Table 19-2 shows the values for length of stay, hospital cost, and operative time for both of these subgroups.

Fig. 19-2 gives the reductions in these variables for the SNS reoperation glioma subgroup. The length of stay was reduced 33%, the hospital cost 26%, and the operative time 13% (median values) with the use of an SNS. The same data for the first operation glioma subgroup is given in Fig. 19-3. Interestingly, opera-

Table 19-2. Interactive Surgical Navigation vs. Conventional Craniotomy in Glioma Subgroups

	RO With SNS	RO Without SNS	FO With SNS	FO Without SNS
Length of stay (days)				
Mean	5.7	7.5	9.0	7.2
Median	5.0	7.5	9.0	6.5
Hospital cost				
Mean	$23,526	$30,238	$30,759	$24,002
Median	$22,436	$30,238	$26,462	$22,871
Operative time (min)				
Mean	244	300	230	250
Median	260	300	213	244

RO = reoperation; FO = first operation.

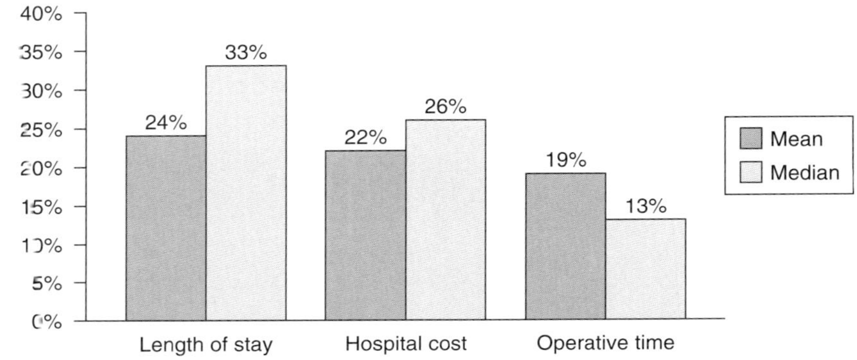

Figure 19-2. Reduction in length of stay, hospital cost, and operative time using interactive surgical navigation in reoperative glioma surgery.

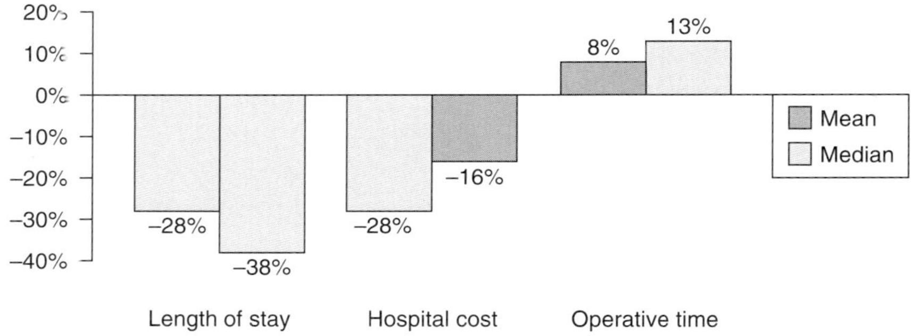

Figure 19-3. Reduction in length of stay, hospital cost, and operative time using interactive surgical navigation for first operation glioma subgroup.

tive time was reduced 13% with the use of an SNS, but hospital cost and length of stay were increased by 16% and 38%, respectively (median values).

In meningioma surgery the use of SNS was associated with a 29% reduction in the length of stay, a 35% reduction in hospital cost, and a 69% reduction in the operative time (median values) compared with conventional craniotomy techniques (Fig. 19-4).

Similarly, the percent reductions for SNS-assisted surgery in the metastasis group was reduced by 56% for length of stay, by 35% for hospital costs, and by 43% for operative time (median values) compared with conventional techniques (Fig. 19-5).

IMPORTANCE OF OUTCOME STUDIES

An essential issue in health care allocation is whether the benefits justify the costs incurred. Many experts believe that perhaps as much as one fourth to one third of all medical services are equivocal or inappropriate in terms of cost-bene-

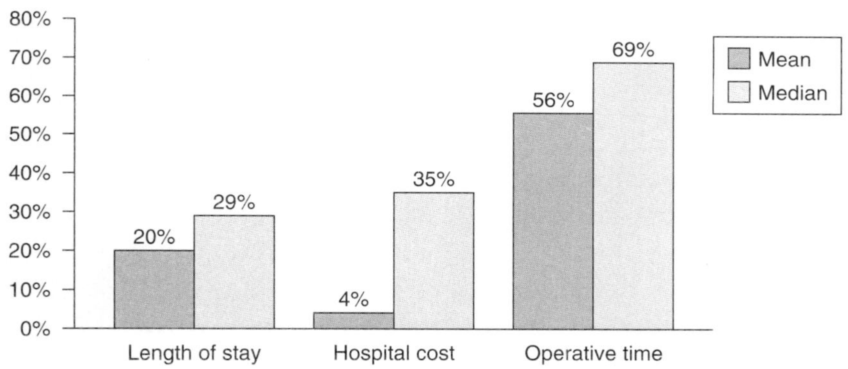

Figure 19-4. Reduction in length of stay, hospital cost, and operative time using interactive surgical navigation in meningioma surgery.

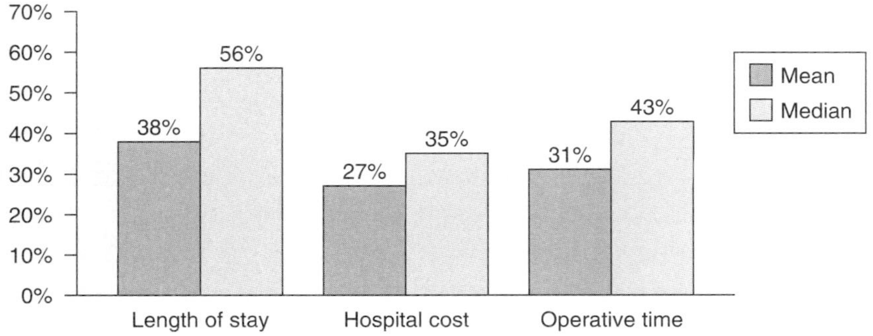

Figure 19-5. Reduction in length of stay, hospital cost, and operative time using interactive surgical navigation in metastasis surgery.

fit analysis.[5] A major reason for this is the lack of scientific data to support the effectiveness, costs, and cost-benefit ratios of different treatments for the same disease. To address this, Congress passed the Omnibus Budget Reconciliation Act in 1989 providing almost $600 million to support research on the outcomes, effectiveness, and appropriateness of medical care. The lack of specific outcome data, the increased funding to attain such data, and the recent attention concerning economic health care reform have accelerated the growth of a new kind of medical technology assessment. Outcome studies designed to assess marginal costs/benefits, opportunity costs, and other pertinent outcome data will likely become powerful weapons in the allocation of health care resources.[3]

The social and economic value of a medical procedure must be verified by valid data obtained through scientific investigation. Relevant data include the total cost of the illness, the incidence of that illness, and a host of data from comparisons of different treatment modalities. This includes outcome studies designed to measure health, satisfaction, and cost outcomes, resource-based cost evaluations of each treatment, variations in reimbursement between treatment modalities, and expenditures on research and development of individual therapies.[1]

The assessment of a new technology can be thought to occur in three stages. The first involves assessment of technologic characteristics. This might involve determining accuracy limits, resolution of imaging, etc. The second stage involves determining the efficacy of the proposed technology in treating a disease. The randomized, controlled clinical trial is the gold standard for this stage. The third stage involves determining the final points of interest—clinical, economic, and social outcomes. In the current age of limited health care resources this third stage of technology assessment becomes more important.[3]

The characteristics of the ideal SNS should include noninvasiveness, accuracy, exact reproducibility, simplicity of use, economy of time, versatility, and cost effectiveness.[21] Many centers are in the process of determining accuracy, reproducibility, and efficacy in treating intracranial and intraspinal pathology. This report represents a first step in examining the effect of SNS technology on social and economic outcomes. Not only will this type of information ultimately help to define the future of SNS devices in neurosurgery, it will also provide insight on the effectiveness of neurosurgical treatment of brain tumors.

OUTCOMES ANALYSIS

Operative Time

The use of interactive SNSs was associated with a consistently reduced operative time for all three types of brain tumor (Fig. 19-6), with the greatest reductions occurring in meningioma and metastasis surgery. Technology designed to reduce operative time is desirable for several reasons. A direct approach to the lesion permits a minimal scalp incision and bone flap, thereby reducing the time of opening and closure and obviating the need for lengthy intraparenchymal exploration. All of these factors should combine to reduce operative time.

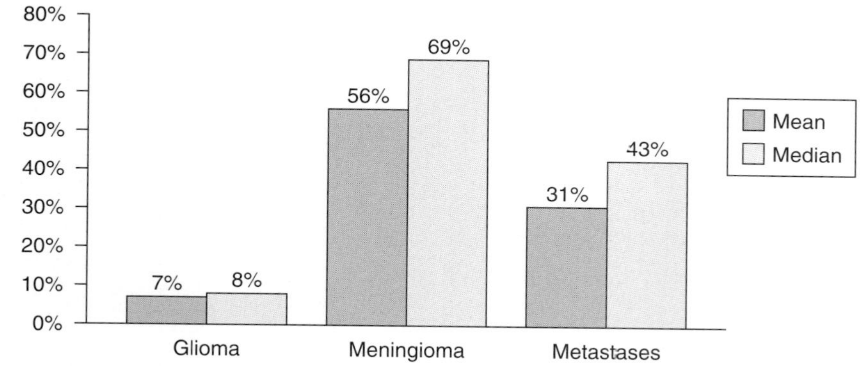

Figure 19-6. Reduction in operative time using interactive surgical navigation in glioma, meningioma, and metastasis surgery.

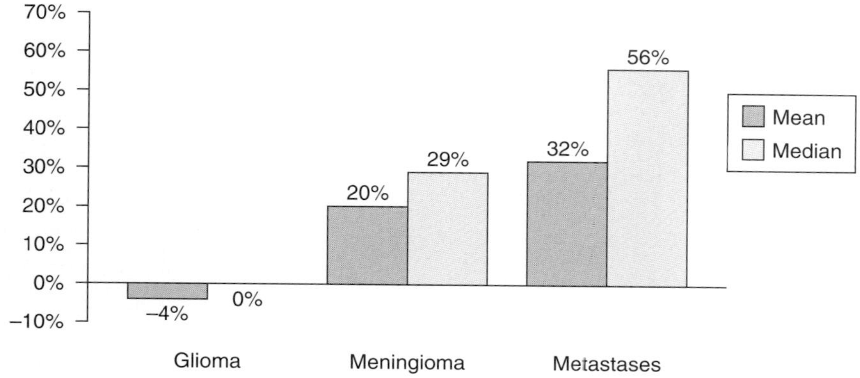

Figure 19-7. Reduction in hospital length of stay using interactive surgical navigation in glioma, meningioma, and metastasis surgery.

A reduction in the length of the operation also permits more efficient use of the surgeon's time and the hospital operating room facilities. Shorter operative time means more procedures can be performed by the surgeon. The economic impact of this aspect of SNS is difficult to determine accurately and was not assessed in this review. Reduced operative time is also an important variable influencing patient morbidity due to shortened exposure to anesthesia, reduced blood loss, and reduced risk of infection. Therefore technology that reduces operative time has important benefits extending beyond the simplistic measures of economic outcome used in this study.

Length of Stay

The use of SNSs was associated with reduced hospital length of stay in meningioma and metastasis surgery (Fig. 19-7). SNSs had no overall effect on the length of stay for the glioma group (Fig. 19-7) but reduced it for the reoperation glioma subgroup (see Fig. 19-2) and increased it for the first operation glioma subgroup (see Fig. 19-3).

The reduced hospital length of stay in the meningioma, metastasis, and reoperation glioma groups may result from reduced morbidity and increased efficiency of surgical therapy. Other factors likely play a role in length of stay determination and may especially influence the newly diagnosed glioma subgroup in which SNS was associated with an increased hospital length of stay. One such factor may be the individual surgeon's practice style. Thirteen of SNS-assisted surgeries performed in the first operation glioma subgroup were performed by one surgeon compared with only 2 of 20 in the first operation group using conventional techniques. In addition, the involvement of consultation services (medical neuro-oncology and radiation oncology) occurred frequently during the initial hospitalization for patients with newly diagnosed malignant primary brain tumors. This may have contributed to a prolonged hospital stay for additional treatment protocols to be synthesized.

Hospital Costs

Hospital costs associated with SNS-assisted meningioma and cerebral metastasis surgery were reduced, whereas those associated with SNS-assisted glioma surgery were increased (Fig. 19-8). Further analysis revealed that SNS was associated with cost reductions of 27% (see Fig. 19-2) in the reoperation glioma group and cost increases of 16% (see Fig. 19-3) in the first operation glioma group as compared with conventional craniotomy techniques.

The reduction in hospital cost associated with SNS-assisted treatment of meningiomas, metastases, and reoperation gliomas may reflect the clinical benefits of this technology that result in less morbidity, shorter use of costly operating room time, reduced hospital stays, and less expensive hospital charges.

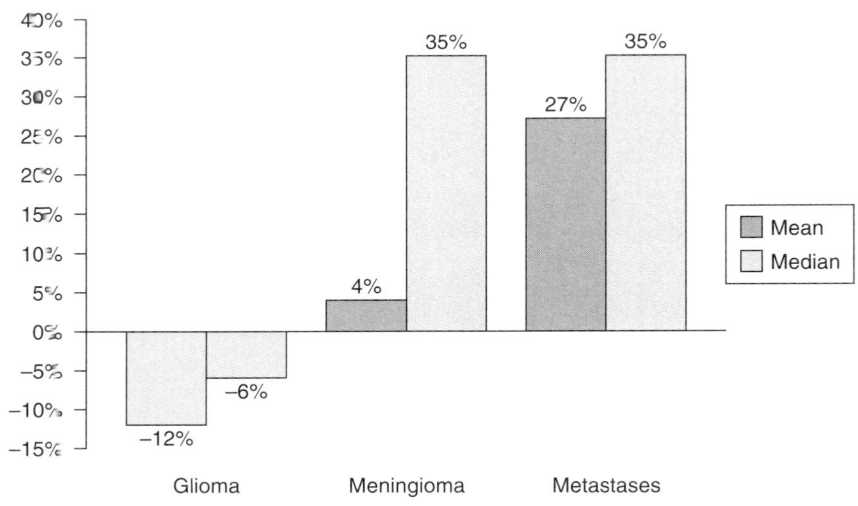

Figure 19-8. Reduction in hospital cost using interactive surgical navigation in glioma, meningioma, and metastasis surgery.

Cost increases associated with SNS-assisted treatment of newly diagnosed glioma patients may reflect the same individual practice bias as referred to in the length of stay discussion. For example, the principal SNS surgeon favored postoperative neuroimaging and screening for lower extremity venous thromboses (e.g., Doppler ultrasound or venograms); these studies were not routinely performed on other surgical services. Also, the additional imaging, procedural, and consultation charges incurred in the diagnosis and workup of newly diagnosed glioma patients serve to increase the technical hospitalization costs and may minimize any cost benefits from the use of SNSs. Further, the surgical risk of the two groups may not be directly comparable since the patients in the SNS group were commonly referred with inoperable lesions. An assessment based on surgical risk is in progress.

Potential Methodologic Problems

Although the results of this retrospective review are interesting, the reader must interpret the information presented with caution. Many factors inherent in the determination of hospital and surgical costs cannot be adequately controlled for in a retrospective analysis. Selection bias is one of the largest potential sources of error. This becomes apparent when one considers the individual numbers and characteristics of the tumors in each group (Tables 19-3 to 19-5). The meningiomas treated using SNSs consisted mainly of superficial convexity or parasagittal meningiomas. In contrast, the meningiomas treated by conventional surgery included nine anterior cranial fossa lesions. This disparity may account for part or all of the differences observed between the conventional and SNS meningioma groups. Although the glioma groups were comparable in number and pathology, the group treated by conventional techniques included fewer cases of reoperations. In addition, the conventional group included 15 tumors localized to the temporal lobe (out of 22 total). One might speculate that these tumors were more easily treated by standard temporal lobectomy, obviating the need for more sophisticated surgical technology. The cerebral metastases groups vary most in the number of tumors treated in each group.

Although all surgeons at this institution performed craniotomies in 1992, the majority of SNS procedures were performed by one surgeon. This may affect the data in several ways. First, individual practice methods vary from surgeon to surgeon. As suggested earlier, since the SNS cases in all groups were performed primarily by one surgeon, his practice methods may not reflect those of other surgeons; treatment approach and risk may also differ. Finally, overrepresentation of one surgeon in any group may cause inequality in operative time based on individual surgical skills.

Individual tumor characteristics such as size, presence of hemorrhage or hydrocephalus, specific location, presence of edema or intracranial tissue shifts, and tumor consistency are important factors determining patient outcome; however, the specific contribution is unknown. Further analysis will be required to assess the individual contributions of these variables to patient outcome and the use of SNSs.

Table 19-3. Glioma Patient Data

Sex/Age	Tumor Type	Tumor Location	Tumor Size	Surgeon	Reop	Prior Radiation	Postop Complications	Medical Risk Factors	Steroid Use	Operative Time (min)	Length of Stay (days)	Hospital Cost
Surgical Navigation												
M/42	GBM	L. frontal	5.0 cm	S.H.	No	No	None	None	No	385	9	$28,580
M/76	GBM	R. parietal	3.5 cm	S.H.	No	No	None	HTN, BPH	No	184	19	$33,489
M/66	GBM	R. frontal	NA	G.B.	Yes	Yes	None	DVT	Yes	180	5	$16,778
M/37	Oligo	Bifrontal	NA	G.B.	Yes	Yes	None	None	Yes	263	5	$23,700
F/34	LGA	L. frontal	NA	G.B.	Yes	No	None	None	No	262	5	$23,098
F/29	AA	R. occ./par.	NA	G.B.	Yes	Yes	None	DVT, seizures, s/p Ommaya with gram-pos. infection	Yes	258	2	$18,414
M/34	AA	L. parietal	NA	G.B.	Yes	No	Seizure, reop for wound leak	None	Yes	274	8	$37,679
M/37	GBM	R. parietal	2.5 cm	G.B.	Yes	Yes	None	Smoker	Yes	138	6	$17,269
M/44	AA	R. frontal	NA	G.B.	Yes	Yes	None	HTN	Yes	278	7	$24,399
M/32	Oligo	R. parietal	1 cm	G.B.	Yes	No	None	None	No	312	4	$21,774
M/42	AA	R. parietal	NA	G.B.	Yes	Yes	DVT	None	Yes	153	14	$34,356
F/27	LGA	R. frontal	Diffuse	G.B.	Yes	No	Bilateral calf DVT	None	No	382	6	$28,618
F/43	GBM	R. frontal	NA	G.B.	Yes	Yes	None	None	Yes	223	2	$16,729
M/69	Gliosarcoma	L. parietal	NA	G.B.	No	No	None	Smoker	Yes	205	4	$19,494
M/62	GBM	R. parietal	4 cm	G.B.	No	No	Hyponatremia	Smoker, PUD	No	159	7	$24,793
M/32	LGA	R. temporal	2.5 cm	G.B.	No	No	Gram-neg. meningitis	None	No	230	10	$27,491
M/46	AA	R. parietal	NA	G.B.	No	No	Atrial arrhythmia	Hypercholester-olemia	No	326	14	$57,896
F/44	GBM	L. frontal	3.5 cm	G.B.	No	No	None	None	No	190	3	$13,427
M/53	GBM	L. frontal	4 cm	G.B.	No	No	Depression, hyperglycemia	Asthma, ETOH abuse	No	196	10	$24,525
M/31	Neurocytoma	Intraventricular	NA	G.B.	No	No	Prolonged CSF drainage	None	No	300	16	$50,986
F/41	Mixed glioma	L. frontal	NA	G.B.	No	No	None	MVP, smoker	Yes	245	7	$26,809

M/68	GBM	R. parietal	3 cm	G.B.	No	No	Myocardial ischemia	Colon cancer	Yes	167	5	$20,471
F/45	GBM	R. frontoparietal	NA	G.B.	No	No	Prolonged placement	None	Yes	296	9	$56,487
F/43	GBM	L. frontal	4 cm	G.B.	No	No	UTI	None	No	235	7	$23,000
F/64	Gliosarcoma	R. parietal	5 cm	G.B.	No	No	None	Smoker	Yes	150	7	$26,114
F/26	Ganglioglioma	R. temporal	2 cm	G.B.	No	No	None	None	No	158	3	$16,563
Conventional Craniotomy												
M/60	AA	L. temporal	NA	S.H.	No	No	None	Prostate cancer, HTN	No	238	6	$25,085
F/11	LGA	R. temporal	2 cm	A.F.	No	No	None	None	No	320	5	$20,326
F/70	GBM	R. frontal	3 cm	Y.C.	No	No	None	None	No	210	11	$33,313
F/8	Ganglioglioma	R. temporal	2 cm	Y.C.	No	No	None	None	No	245	4	$16,142
F/37	LGA	R. temporal	1.5 cm	J.H.	No	No	None	Chronic UTI	No	145	7	$17,392
M/14	Oligo	L. frontal	NA	Y.C.	Yes	No	Hyperglycemia	IDDM, pancreatitis	No	295	8	$27,338
F/55	GBM	L. temporal	2.5 cm	J.H.	No	Yes	Persistent aphasia	None	Yes	232	7	$22,883
F/13	LGA	L. frontal	2 cm	Y.C.	No	No	None	None	No	262	6	$18,296
M/56	GBM	R. frontal	NA	I.A.	No	No	None	PUD	No	300	5	$22,858
M/3	LGA	R. temporal	2 cm	A.F.	No	No	Persistent fever (unknown origin)	None	No	342	12	$30,208
M/32	Oligo	R. frontal	Diffuse	Y.C.	No	No	None	None	No	375	6	$24,913
F/32	AA	R. temporal	8 cm	J.H.	No	No	None	None	No	168	8	$22,370
M/60	Gliosarcoma	R. temporal	NA	I.K.	No	No	Seizures	None	No	243	12	$34,435
M/33	LGA	Intraventricular	5 cm	I.A.	No	No	R. hemiparesis	HTN	No	305	7	$33,138
M/52	GBM	R. temporal	NA	S.H.	Yes	Yes	None	None	Yes	164	6	$16,462
M/51	GBM	R. temporal	NA	S.H.	No	No	None	None	No	278	9	$30,346
F/74	GBM	R. temporal	Diffuse	G.B.	No	No	CSF leak from wound	Breast cancer, hypothyroid	No	241	5	$22,765
M/16 mo.	Oligo	L. frontal	NA	J.H.	No	No	None	None	No	282	7	$21,336
F/63	AA	L. temporal	NA	Y.C.	No	No	None	Smoker	No	180	10	$23,103
M/61	GBM	L. temporal	NA	G.B.	No	No	None	None	No	207	7	$28,514
F/15	LGA	R. temporal	3 cm	A.F.	No	No	None	None	No	265	6	$28,782
M/19	Ganglioglioma	R. temporal	1 cm	Y.C.	No	Yes	None	None	No	300	5	$20,518

AA = anaplastic astrocytoma; BPH = benign prostatic hypertrophy; CAD = coronary artery disease; CHF = congestive heart failure; COPD = chronic obstructive pulmonary disease; DVT = deep vein thrombosis; HTN = hypertension; IDDM = insulin-dependent diabetes mellitus; LGA = low-grade astrocytoma; MVP = mitral valve prolapse; Oligo = oligodendroglioma; PUD = peptic ulcer disease; UTI = urinary tract infection.

Table 19-4. Meningioma Patient Data

Sex/Age	Tumor Location	Tumor Size	Surgeon	Reop	Prior Radiation	Postop Complications	Medical Risk Factors	Steroid Use	Operative Time (min)	Length of Stay (days)	Hospital Cost
SNS-Assisted Surgery											
M/60	R. frontal convexity	NA	G.B.	No	No	Renal failure, respiratory arrest, death	IDDM, HTN, smoker	No	101	26	$138,187
F/48	L. parasagittal	3 cm	G.B.	No	No	None	None	No	114	3	$14,214
M/78	R. frontoparietal convexity	NA	G.B.	No	No	None	Smoker	No	170	6	$20,861
F/46	L. parasagittal	2.5 cm	G.B.	No	No	None	None	No	385	3	$24,515
F/75	R. parieto-occipital convexity	NA	G.B.	Yes	No	None	None	No	275	10	$30,524
F/67	L. frontal convexity	1.5 cm	G.B.	No	No	A-V block, temporary aphasia	Angina, HTN	Yes	102	4	$17,656
M/40	R. frontoparietal convexity	NA	G.B.	No	No	None	None	No	83	6	$18,084
F/53	L. frontal convexity	1.5 cm	G.B.	No	No	None	Syncope, hypothyroid	No	105	3	$13,447
Conventional Surgery											
F/74	R. vertex	NA	I.K.	No	No	None	None	No	526	5	$32,032
F/74	L. frontal convexity	6 cm	Y.C.	No	No	Epidural hematoma requiring evacuation	HTN, hypercholesterolemia, CAD, aortic sclerosis	No	360	7	$34,174
F/49	Tuberculum sellae	1 cm	S.H.	Yes	No	Prolonged confusion	Smoker, chronic UTI, PUD	Yes	359	7	$29,973
F/15	Intraventricular	NA	A.F.	No	No	Disconnection syndrome	None	No	498	27	$68,724
F/41	R. parietal convexity	8 cm	S.H.	No	Yes	Epidural hematoma requiring evacuation	Non-Hodgkin's lymphoma	Yes	468	9	$42,272

M/68	L. frontal convexity	5 cm	G.B.	No	No	None	HTN, PUD, smoker	No	193	5	$25,461
F/35	Tuberculum sellae	NA	S.H.	Yes	No	None	MVP, PUD	Yes	643	5	$32,768
F/74	L. frontal parasagittal	NA	I.K.	Yes	No	Persistent CSF leak requiring skin grafting	HTN	No	290	23	$81,194
F/70	L. sphenoid wing	NA	G.B.	No	No	None	None	No	255	6	$23,679
F/59	R. sphenoid wing	NA	A.F.	No	No	Laryngeal edema, L. hemiplegia	IDDM, heart murmur	No	692	15	$56,896
F/48	L. parieto-occipital convexity	NA	S.H.	No	No	None	Aortic insufficiency	No	207	7	$18,747
F/61	Tuberculum sellae	3 cm	I.K.	No	No	None	IDDM, dementia, HTN	No	485	15	$42,712
M/67	R. frontal convexity	3 cm	S.H.	No	No	None	None	No	330	7	$23,753
F/64	R. olfactory groove	3 cm	Y.C.	No	No	None	Hypothyroid, pituitary tumor, HTN	No	480	7	$26,546
F/77	R. frontal convexity	NA	I.K.	No	No	None	None	No	232	4	$16,022
F/53	L. parietal convexity	2 cm	J.H.	No	No	None	None	No	150	3	$14,407
F/53	R. frontal convexity	NA	I.A.	No	No	UTI	PUD, hyperglycemia	No	350	9	$26,695
F/70	L. sphenoid wing	3 cm	S.H.	No	No	Stridor requiring tracheostomy, aspiration pneumonia	IDDM, malnutrition, steroid dependence, HTN, psychosis	Yes	355	11	$76,272
F/56	Tuberculum sellae	1.5 cm	I.A.	No	No	UTI, R. common peroneal palsy	IDDM	No	317	8	$12,556

CAD = coronary artery disease; HTN = hypertension; IDDM = insulin-dependent diabetes mellitus; MVP = mitral valve prolapse; PUD = peptic ulcer disease; UTI = urinary tract infection.

Table 19-5. Metastases Patient Data

Sex/Age	Tumor Type	Tumor Location	Tumor Size	Surgeon	Reop	Prior Radiation	Postop Complications	Medical Risk Factors	Steroid Use	Operative Time (min)	Length of Stay (days)	Hospital Cost
SNS-Assisted Surgery												
M/67	Lung adenocarcinoma	L. occipital	NA	G.B.	No	No	None	Lung cancer	Yes	155	4	$17,400
F/47	Ovarian carcinoma	L. frontal	3 cm	S.H.	No	No	None	HTN, ovarian cancer	No	192	4	$18,814
M/59	Lung adenocarcinoma	L. parietal	2.5 cm	G.B.	No	Yes	None	Lung cancer, atrial fibrillation, CHF, smoker	No	167	4	$19,259
F/75	Lung adenocarcinoma	L. occipital lobe	2 cm	G.B.	No	No	None	Lung cancer	No	165	10	$27,674
M/45	Large cell lung carcinoma	R. frontal	NA	G.B.	No	No	None	Smoker	Yes	124	2	$14,077
M/60	Renal cell carcinoma	R. parietal	2.5 cm	G.B.	No	No	None	Renal cell carcinoma, liver failure, HTN	No	155	3	$15,475
F/34	Breast carcinoma	R. caudate	3 cm	G.B.	No	No	None	Metastatic breast cancer, HTN	No	240	10	$26,901
M/58	Large cell lung carcinoma	L. frontal	NA	G.B.	No	No	R. hemiparesis, prolonged placement	Myasthenia gravis	Yes	160	21	$40,149
F/55	Lung adenocarcinoma	L. occipital lobe	5 cm	G.B.	No	No	None	Lung cancer	No	140	3	$15,233
M/70	Laryngeal carcinoma	L. occipital lobe	2 cm	I.K.	No	No	None	CAD, carotid stenosis, smoker, ethanol abuse	No	116	4	$16,608
M/52	Lung adenocarcinoma	L. frontal lobe	2 cm	G.B.	No	No	None	PUD, ethanol abuse, smoker, gallstones, hepatitis	No	122	9	$29,268

M/57	Lung adenocarcinoma	R. frontal	2 cm	S.H.	No	No	None	Ethanol abuse, hematuria	No	85	8	$17,858
M/65	Laryngeal carcinoma	R. occipital	5 cm	G.B.	No	No	None	HTN, COPD, smoker, laryngeal carcinoma	No	72	3	$15,036
M/63	Prostate carcinoma	R. occipital	5 cm	G.B.	No	No	DVT	ASCHD	No	270	3	$20,106
M/51	Lung adenocarcinoma	R. frontal	1 cm	S.H.	No	No	None	Lung cancer	No	295	7	$31,722
F/59	Ovarian carcinoma	L. frontal	1 cm	G.B.	No	No	None	Ovarian cancer, atrial arrhythmia	No	115	4	$19,203
F/76	Lung adenocarcinoma	L. frontal	NA	G.B.	No	No	None	COPD, smoker, CHF, UTI	No	97	16	$39,307
M/64	Lung adenocarcinoma	R. frontal	3 cm	G.B.	No	No	None	Lung carcinoma	No	105	14	$22,811
F/45	Ovarian carcinoma	R. parietal	2 cm	G.B.	No	No	None	Ovarian cancer	No	240	6	$23,187
Conventional Surgery												
M/52	Lung adenocarcinoma	L. parieto-occipital	3.5 cm	S.H.	No	No	None	Lung cancer	No	120	9	$22,819
M/60	Renal cell carcinoma	R. occipital	2 cm	Y.C.	No	No	None	Smoker, COPD, renal cell cancer	No	273	9	$29,577
M/65	Lung adenocarcinoma	R. temporal	7 cm	I.K.	No	Yes	Sepsis, atrial fibrillation, death	DVT, head and neck cancer	No	294	16	$40,348

CAD = coronary artery disease; CHF = congestive heart failure; COPD = chronic obstructive pulmonary disease; DVT = deep vein thrombosis; HTN = hypertension; PUD = peptic ulcer disease; UTI = urinary tract infection.

SUMMARY

SNS-assisted surgical therapy of brain tumors and other neurosurgical disorders is increasing. To determine its effect on patient outcome, we compared hospital cost, hospital length of stay, and total operative time for craniotomies in patients with brain tumors using SNS and conventional techniques.

SNS-assisted craniotomy was associated with decreases in hospital cost, operative time, and hospital length of stay in patients with meningioma, cerebral metastasis, and recurrent glioma. Interactive surgical navigation was associated with a reduced operative time for newly diagnosed glioma patients but increased hospital costs for those patients. Its use had no effect on hospital length of stay for glioma patients.

Although our review has demonstrated no detrimental effects of SNSs on hospital cost, length of stay, or operative time, many variables were not controlled for and the results should be interpreted cautiously. Further multicenter clinical investigation is necessary to more accurately predict the effect of this technology on patient outcome.

The importance of outcome studies relates to allocation of health care resources. Advances in surgical technology such as surgical navigation are important in achieving efficient and safe neurologic therapies. Further investigation on the effect on patient outcome is desirable to validate their use and secure additional funding for future development.

References

1. Bean JR. Stereotactic radiosurgery: At the threshold or the crossroads? Neurosurgery 33:1114-1115, 1993.
2. Drummond M, Labelle SG. Health economics: An introduction for clinicians. Ann Intern Med 107:88-92, 1987.
3. Fuchs VR, Garber AM. The new technology assessment. N Engl J Med 323:673-677, 1990.
4. Selai CE, Rosser RM. Good quality quality? Some methodological issues. J R Soc Med 86:440-443, 1993.
5. Volpp K. Costs, benefits, and the changing ethos of medicine. JAMA 269:1708, 1993.
6. Barnett GH, Kormos DW, Steiner CP, Weisenberger J. Intraoperative localization using an armless, frameless stereotactic wand. J Neurosurg 78:510-514, 1993.
7. Kato A, Yoshimine T, Hayakawa T. A frameless, armless navigational system for computer-assisted neurosurgery. J Neurosurg 74:845-849, 1991.
8. Leggett WB, Greenberg MM, Gannon WE. The viewing wand: A new system for three-dimensional computed tomography-correlated intraoperative localization. Curr Surg 48:674-678, 1991.
9. Barnett GH, Kormos DW, Steiner CP. Use of a frameless, armless, stereotactic wand for brain tumor localization with two-dimensional and three-dimensional neuroimaging. Neurosurgery 33:674-678, 1993.
10. Maciunas RJ, Galloway RL, Fitzpatrick JM. A universal system for interactive image-directed neurosurgery. Stereotact Funct Neurosurg 58:108-113, 1992.
11. Drake JM, Prudencio J, Holowka S. Frameless stereotaxy in children. Pediatr Neurosurg 20:152-159, 1994.
12. Guthrie BL, Adler JR. Computer-assisted preoperative planning, interactive surgery, and frameless stereotaxy. Clin Neurosurg 38:112-131, 1992.
13. Zamorano L, Dujovny M, Chavantes C. Image-guided stereotactic centered craniotomy and laser resection of solid intracranial lesions. Stereotact Funct Neurosurg 55:398-403, 1990.
14. Gomez H, Barnett GH, Estes ML. Stereotactic and computer-assisted neurosurgery at the Cleveland Clinic: Review of 501 consecutive cases. Cleve Clin J Med 60:399-410, 1993.
15. Moore MR, McL Black P, Ellenbogen R. Stereotactic craniotomy: Methods and results using the Brown-Roberts-Wells stereotactic frame. Neurosurgery 25:572-578, 1989.
16. Kelly PJ. Stereotactic craniotomy. Neurosurg Clin N Am 1:781-799, 1990.
17. Pillay PK, Hassenbusch SJ, Sawaya R. Minimally invasive brain surgery. Ann Acad Med 22(Suppl):459-463, 1993.

18. Roberts DW, Strohbehn JW, Hatch JF. A frameless stereotaxic integration of computerized tomographic imaging and the operating microscope. J Neurosurg 65:545-549, 1986.
19. Zulch KJ. Histological Typing of Tumors of the Central Nervous System. Geneva: World Health Organization, 1979.
20. Wilkins RH, Rengachary SS. Neurosurgery. New York: McGraw-Hill, 1985.
21. Hariz MI, Fodstad H. Stereotactic localization of small subcortical brain tumors for open surgery. Surg Neurol 28:345-350, 1987.

20

One-Year Outcome Data After Resection of Malignant Glioma

Gene H. Barnett, M.D. • James G. Walsh, R.N., B.S.N.
Charles P. Steiner, B.S. • Joseph P. Weisenberger, R.T.

The extent of surgical resection is considered by many to be an important long-term prognostic indicator of survival in patients with primary malignant astrocytoma (glioblastoma, anaplastic astrocytoma, and anaplastic oligodendroglioma).[1-10] Stereotactic techniques have been advocated to reduce the extent of tumor resection in patients with primary malignant brain tumors and thus the postoperative wound and neurologic morbidity.[3,11-18] Although the early postoperative merits of craniotomy using surgical navigation systems (SNSs) are well described for these lesions,[4,18-23] there is little information on the extended outcome in these patients. We present 1-year outcome data on a series of patients undergoing resection of malignant astrocytomas.

STUDY POPULATION

Demographic data on all patients undergoing resective craniotomy for brain tumor using SNS guidance were prospectively entered into a computer database. Routine clinical and radiologic surveillance examinations were performed on all patients at 2- to 3-month intervals thereafter.

These data were retrospectively reviewed for purposes of this analysis. Patient age, sex, diagnosis, and postoperative wound or sustained neurologic morbidity were extracted as well as functional status at 1-year follow-up using the Karnofsky Performance Scale (KPS).[24] For purposes of this study, those patients with a KPS score of 90 to 100 were classified as "excellent," 70 to 80 as "good," 50 to 60 as "fair," and less than 50 as "poor." When information was not recoverable from the database or patient records, the patient, family, or family physician was interviewed by phone.

Surgical complications were defined as postoperative wound disorders requiring reoperation or protracted hospitalization or treatment or sustained neurologic deficits resulting in a decrease in the KPS score by 20 points or more.

For newly operated lesions, minimal access craniotomies, typically 1½ to 2 inches in diameter, are planned using an SNS. For previous craniotomies using conventional scalp and bone flaps, it is usually necessary to reopen the entire flap, although on occasion a minimal access approach can be performed using only a portion of the previous incision. A detailed description of operative technique was presented in Chapter 5.

Over a 21-month period 33 patients with malignant glioma underwent 35 resective craniotomies using SNS assistance (Table 20-1). Twenty-three patients had glioblastomas, 8 had anaplastic astrocytomas, and 2 had anaplastic oligodendrogliomas. Ten of the 24 glioblastoma operations and 4 of the 11 anaplastic

Table 20-1. Patient Data

Age	Diagnosis	Reop?	Complications	One-Year Outcome
38	AO	Yes		Excellent
41	AA	Yes		Excellent
44	AA	Yes		Poor
30	AA	Yes		Deceased
34	AA			Excellent
43	AA			Excellent
29	AA			Excellent
46	AA			Good
34	AO			Fair
34	AA			Excellent
29	AA			Deceased
34	GBM	Yes	Wound	Good
35	GBM	Yes		Fair
40	GBM	Yes		Deceased
44	GBM	Yes	Abulia	Deceased
46	GBM	Yes	Hemiparesis	Fair
49	GBM	Yes		Deceased
75	GBM	Yes		Deceased
75	GBM	Yes	Wound	Good
34	GBM	Yes	Wound	Deceased
44	GBM	Yes		Deceased
42	GBM			Deceased
42	GBM			Excellent
53	GBM			Excellent
62	GBM			Fair
66	GBM			Poor
68	GBM			Deceased
75	GBM			Lost to follow-up
39	GBM			Deceased
57	GBM			Good
48	GBM			Excellent
74	GBM			Poor
74	GBM			Lost to follow-up
78	GBM			Deceased
62	GBM			Poor

AA = anaplastic astrocytoma; AO = anaplastic oligodendroglioma; GBM = glioblastoma.

glioma operations were reoperative procedures. Resection was complete (>95%) in all patients when this was the preoperative goal (Fig. 20-1). Patients with anaplastic lesions were younger than those with glioblastomas (mean 37 [range 29 to 46] vs. 55 [range 34 to 78] years). Two patients with glioblastoma were lost to follow-up.

Overall, 9 (82%) of the anaplastic glioma and 12 (55%) of the glioblastoma patients were alive 1 year after surgery. For previously unoperated anaplastic glioma patients, 1-year survival was 86% (6/7), whereas 67% (8/12) of glioblastoma patients had 1-year survival rates. One-year survival after reoperation was 75% for the anaplastic glioma group and 40% for the glioblastoma group. Functional outcomes for the groups are shown in Figs. 20-2 to 20-7. Three reoperations in glioblastoma patients resulted in wound infections and two patients had sustained neurologic deficits. There were no operative deaths.

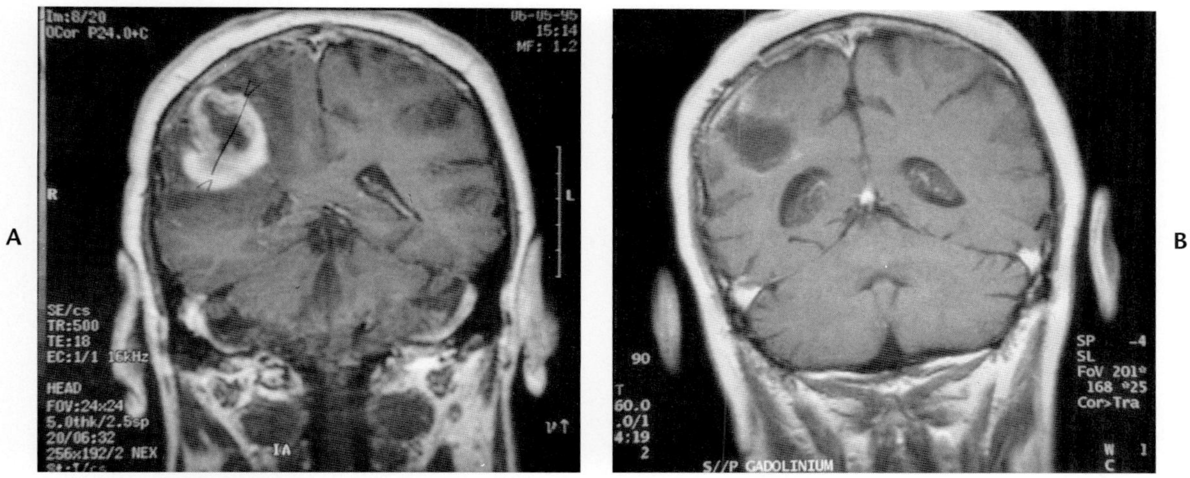

Figure 20-1. Glioblastoma before **(A)** and after **(B)** SNS-assisted resection shows nearly complete resection usually can be achieved if that is the surgical goal.

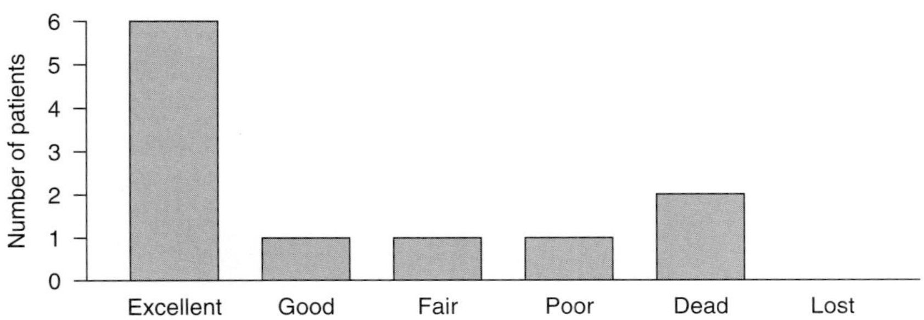

Figure 20-2. Outcome of all patients with anaplastic gliomas at 1 year.

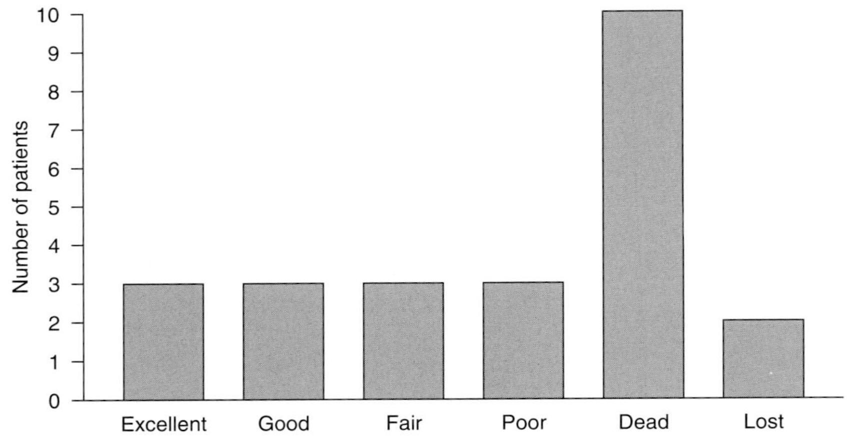

Figure 20-3. Outcome of all patients with glioblastoma at 1 year.

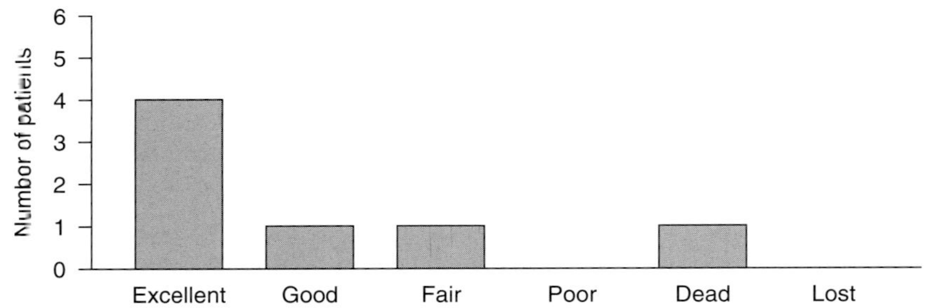

Figure 20-4. Outcome of patients with anaplastic glioma at 1 year who underwent first operation.

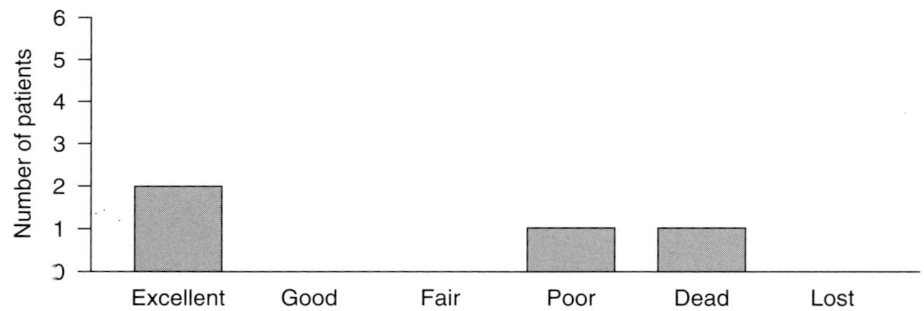

Figure 20-5. Outcome of patients with anaplastic glioma at 1 year who underwent reoperation.

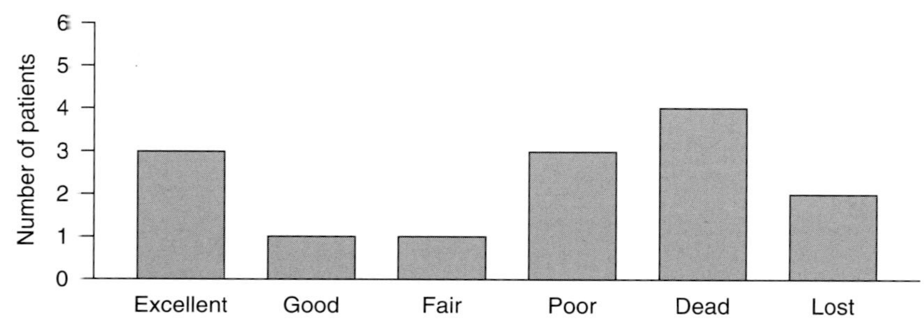

Figure 20-6. Outcome of patients with glioblastoma at 1 year who underwent first operation.

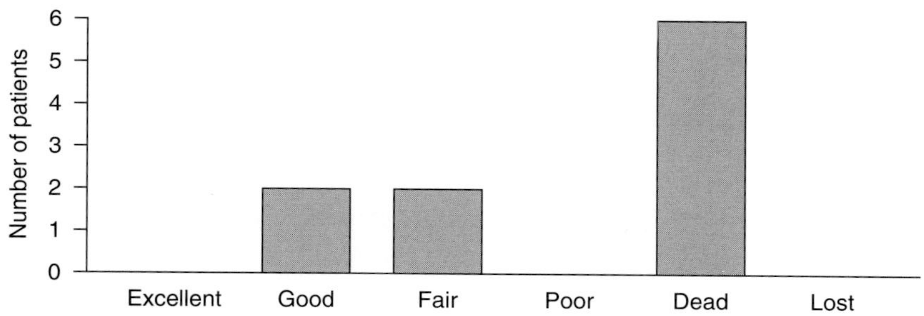

Figure 20-7. Outcome of patients with glioblastoma at 1 year who underwent reoperation.

OUTCOME ANALYSIS

The long-term prognosis for malignant glioma is poor; mean life expectancies are 11 and 18 months for glioblastoma and anaplastic glioma patients, respectively.* Therefore the goal of management of malignant glioma is to extend high-quality survival since these lesions are almost uniformly fatal. Numerous reports suggest that extent of surgical resection can be an important factor in extending survival of these patients.† It is likely that the fraction of tumor removed (e.g., 70% resection) is more significant than the volume of residual tumor. The Brain Tumor Cooperative Group showed that residual tumor (as determined by area on immediate postoperative CT scans) was a highly significant prognostic factor ($p<0.0001$).[10] Since surgical navigation can provide clearer definition of the tumor-brain interface and functional anatomy, surgical resection of these tumors can be maximized.[8-23,26,27] Our group previously confirmed that the extent of resection, as judged by postoperative MRI, was essentially complete when deemed feasible preoperatively.[18]

These results support the finding that extensive surgical resection of these lesions is associated with better than expected survival at 1 year. Nearly 90% and 70% of the anaplastic glioma and glioblastoma groups undergoing first operations were alive at 1 year, with 83% and 50% of those survivors having an excellent or good functional status, respectively. These results compare favorably to the 1-year survival of patients with glioblastomas and anaplastic gliomas reported in the literature. Hoshino[25] cited a 55% 1-year survival for glioblastomas and anaplastic gliomas from the Japanese brain tumor registry. Winger et al.[9] reported a 28% 1-year survival for glioblastoma patients overall and 67% for the malignant glioma patients (both anaplastic astrocytomas and glioblastomas combined) undergoing gross total resection. Similarly, Ammirati et al.[1] found a 69% 1-year survival for those having gross total resections of malignant gliomas. The report from Kelly's group on the outcome from volumetric resection of glioblastomas and anaplastic astrocytomas demonstrated 1-year survivals for nearly 40% and 90% of patients, respectively.[3]

---

*See references 1-3, 5-10, 15, 23, 25.

†See references 1-3, 5, 8-10, 23.

Reoperation for malignant glioma is usually associated with a poorer prognosis and increased risk of complications in comparison to first operations. Our data are consistent with these observations. Half of patients undergoing reoperation for anaplastic gliomas were alive at 1 year and had an excellent functional status. Sixty percent of patients undergoing reoperation for glioblastoma, however, were dead at 1 year, with only two alive with a good (70 to 80) KPS score.

SNS techniques appear to be a low-risk, effective means of helping to extend quality survival in both anaplastic glioma and glioblastoma patients undergoing first operations. Despite the small number of patients, a similar conclusion may be drawn for patients with anaplastic glioma in the reoperative group, because the two survivors had an excellent functional status 1 year after surgery. These data, however, call into question the role of aggressive reoperation for glioblastoma: 60% of patients were dead, only 20% had a good functional status, and wound and neurologic morbidity were 30% and 20%, respectively.

SUMMARY

These results should be interpreted with caution in view of the small number of patients and the fact that they represent only one surgeon's experience using SNS to assist craniotomy. Further potentially confounding factors include the use of perioperative chemotherapies and the use of brachytherapy in two patients with glioblastoma undergoing first operations. Nonetheless, SNS appears to be promising for the surgical management of these lesions. Further study is recommended.

We wish to thank Picker International (Highland Heights, Ohio) for hardware and software support of the frameless stereotactic program.

References

1. Ammirati M, Vick N, Liao YL, Ciric I, Mikhael M. Effect of the extent of surgical resection on survival and quality of life in patients with supratentorial glioblastomas and anaplastic astrocytomas. Neurosurgery 21:201-206, 1987.
2. Andreou J, George AE, Wise A, de Leon M, Kricheff II, Ransohoff J, Foo SH. CT prognostic criteria of survival after malignant glioma surgery. AJNR 4:488-490, 1983.
3. Devaux BC, O'Fallon JR, Kelly PJ. Resection, biopsy, and survival in malignant glial neoplasms. J Neurosurg 78:767-775, 1993.
4. Friets EM, Strohbehn JW, Hatch JF, Roberts DW. A frameless stereotaxic operating microscope for neurosurgery. IEEE Trans Biomed Eng 36:608-617, 1989.
5. Jelsma R, Bucy PC. The treatment of glioblastoma multiforme of the brain. J Neurosurg 27:388-400, 1967.
6. Levin VA, Hoffman WF, Heilbron DC, Norman D. Prognostic significance of the pretreatment CT scan on time to progression for patients with malignant gliomas. J Neurosurg 52:642-647, 1980.
7. Mahaley MS, Mettlin C, Natarajan N, Laws ER, Peace BB. National survey of patterns of care for brain-tumor patients. J Neurosurg 71:826-836, 1989.
8. Warnick RE. The role of cytoreductive surgery in the treatment of intracranial gliomas. Semin Radiat Oncol 1:10-15, 1991.
9. Winger MJ, Macdonald DR, Cairncross JG. Supratentorial anaplastic gliomas in adults. J Neurosurg 71:487-493, 1989.

10. Wood JR, Green SB, Shapiro WR. The prognostic importance of tumor size in malignant gliomas: A computed tomographic scan study by the Brain Tumor Cooperative Group. J Clin Oncol 6:338-343, 1988.
11. Barnett GH, Kormos DW, Steiner CP, Piraino D, Weisenberger J, Hajjar F, Wood C, McNally J. Frameless stereotaxy using a sonic digitizing wand: Development and adaptation to the Picker ViStar medical imaging system. In Maciunas RJ, ed. Interactive Image-Guided Neurosurgery. Park Ridge, Ill.: American Association of Neurological Surgeons, 1993.
12. Gomez H, Barnett GH, Palmer J. Contemporary stereotactic neurosurgery at the Cleveland Clinic. Review of 501 consecutive cases. Cleve Clin J Med 60:399-410, 1993.
13. Hassenbusch SJ, Anderson JS, Pillay PK. Brain tumor resection aided with markers placed using stereotaxis guided by magnetic resonance imaging and computed tomography. Neurosurgery 28:801-806, 1991.
14. Kelly PJ. Volumetric stereotactic surgical resection of intra-axial brain mass lesions. Mayo Clin Proc 63:1186-1198, 1988.
15. Kelly PJ, Hunt C. The limited value of cytoreductive surgery in elderly patients with malignant gliomas. Neurosurgery 34:62-67, 1994.
16. Kelly PJ, Kall BA, Goerss S, Earnest F IV. Computer-assisted stereotaxic laser resection of intra-axial brain neoplasms. J Neurosurg 64:427-439, 1986.
17. Moore MR, Black PM, Ellenbogen R, Gall CM, Eldredge E. Stereotactic craniotomy: Methods and results using the Brown-Roberts-Wells stereotactic frame. Neurosurgery 25:572-577, 1989.
18. Murphy MA, Barnett GH, Kormos DW, Weisenberger J. Astrocytoma resection using an interactive frameless stereotactic wand. An early experience. J Clin Neurosci 1:33-37, 1994.
19. Barnett GH, Kormos DW, Steiner CP, Weisenberger J. Intraoperative localization using an armless, frameless stereotactic wand. J Neurosurg 78:510-514, 1993.
20. Barnett GH, Kormos DW, Steiner CP, Weisenberger J. Use of a frameless, armless wand for brain tumor localization with two-dimensional and three-dimensional neuroimaging. Neurosurgery 33:674-678, 1993.
21. Guthrie BL, Adler JR. Frameless stereotaxy: Computer interactive neurosurgery. Perspect Neurol Surg 2(1):1-19, 1991.
22. Roberts DW, Strohbehn JW, Hatch JF, Murray W, Kettenberger H. A frameless stereotaxic integration of computerized tomographic imaging and the operating microscope. J Neurosurg 65:545-549, 1986.
23. Watanabe E, Watanabe T, Manaka S, Mayanagi Y, Takakura K. Three-dimensional digitizer (neuronavigator): New equipment of CT-guided stereotaxic surgery. Surg Neurol 27:543-547, 1987.
24. Karnofsky DA, Abelmann WH, Craver LS, Burchenal JH. The use of the nitrogen mustards in the palliative treatment of carcinoma: With particular reference to bronchogenic carcinoma. Cancer 1:634-656, 1948.
25. Hoshino T. A commentary on the biology and growth kinetics of low-grade and high-grade gliomas. J Neurosurg 61:895-900, 1984.
26. Barnett GH, McKenzie RL, Ramos L, Palmer J. Nonvolumetric stereotaxy-assisted craniotomy. Results in 50 consecutive cases. Stereotact Funct Neurosurg 61:80-95, 1993.
27. Roberts DW, Strohbehn JW, Friets EM, Kettenberger J, Hartov A. The stereotactic operating microscope: Accuracy refinement and clinical experience. Acta Neurochir Suppl 46:112-114, 1989.

Index

R

S

T